Making Medical
Spending Decisions

MAKING MEDICAL SPENDING DECISIONS

The Law, Ethics, and Economics of Rationing Mechanisms

MARK A. HALL

Professor of Law and Public Health
Wake Forest University
Bowman Gray School of Medicine

New York   Oxford
OXFORD UNIVERSITY PRESS
1997

Oxford University Press

Oxford   New York
Athens   Auckland   Bangkok   Bogota
Bombay   Buenos Aires   Calcutta   Cape Town
Dar es Salaam   Delhi   Florence   Hong Kong   Istanbul
Karachi   Kuala Lumpur   Madras   Madrid
Melbourne   Mexico City   Nairobi   Paris
Singapore   Taipei   Tokyo   Toronto

and associated companies in
Berlin   Ibadan

Copyright © 1997 by Oxford University Press

Published by Oxford University Press, Inc.,
198 Madison Avenue, New York, New York 10016

Library of Congress Cataloging-in-Publication Data
Hall, Mark A.
Making medical spending decisions :
the law, ethics, and economics of rationing mechanisms /
Mark A. Hall.
p.   cm.   Includes bibliographical references and index.
ISBN 0-19-509219-8
1. Health care rationing—United States.
I. Title.
RA410.53.H35   1997   362.1'0973—dc20   96-24738

1 2 3 4 5 6 7 8 9

Printed in the United States of America
on acid-free paper

For Mrs. Millspaugh,
Mr. Nelson,
Mrs. Arthur,
Dr. Brooks,
Dr. Dunne,
Prof. Currie,
and Prof. Murphy—
teachers, all of whom
epitomize the best of
their noble calling.

Preface

I entered academia in 1985 shortly after the revolution in Medicare payment known as "prospective payment." My job change caused me to join a health maintenance organization (HMO), and the ensuing birth of my daughter brought my first sustained adult contact with the medical establishment. I realized then that the fundamental issue in health care public policy for the rest of the century would be how cost-containment measures affect medical decisions. My attention at first was taken up with the particulars of various discrete legal and ethical problems such as how insurance contracts are interpreted by the courts, whether doctors should be motivated to consider costs, and what financially motivated decisions should be disclosed to patients. I spent several years exploring each of these as free-standing legal and social problems.

Gradually, I began to sense in both my thinking and that of others a broader conceptual framework for understanding these resource allocation issues in terms of comparative institutional analysis. This framework assumes, first, that human affairs are too complex for acceptable first-order decisions to be comprehensively prescribed. Abstract and analytical principles alone cannot determine what resources should be devoted to each patient and each treatment. Science is far too inexact and individual circumstances and values are far too multifarious. Therefore, the most we can hope for is to allocate decisional authority to the correct person or institution. We must also realize, however, that no one decision maker or institutional structure is optimal; each is plagued with various problems but each also has important advantages over the others. Because no one approach is ideal, we must strive for the least-imperfect mix of institutions and incentives. This can never be achieved until we have a clear impression of what each institutional structure has to offer, warts and all.

Here, I undertake this daunting task by examining three alternative medical spending decision makers: (1) patients paying for their treatment out of their own pocket; (2) doctors making cost/benefit trade-offs at the bedside; and (3) a variety of third parties, primarily insurers and government agencies, but also ideal democratic institutions such as citizen groups, imposing spending limits from outside the treatment relationship. Chapter 1 lays out the motivating premises for this approach to the issues, and it also contains a chapter-by-chapter plan for the book. A summary of conclusions can be found at the start of Chapter 7. Here, suffice it to say that my analysis relies heavily on a market mechanism in which consumers choose who will decide how medical dollars are spent through the types of insurance they select—a market mechanism that, at present, is seriously flawed. The most important message of this book is that we need to vastly improve the ability of ordinary people to understand and choose how their health insurance affects medical spending decisions.

Acknowledgments

While this book was being conceived and written over the course of the past five years, the following individuals have given generously of their time and attention to critique various draft portions and preliminary articles. I give my heartfelt thanks to Mary Anne Bobinski, Mark Boynton, Daniel Callahan, Larry Churchill, Michael Curtis, Charles Dougherty, Ruth Faden, Susan Goold, Diana Greene, Clark Havighurst, Alan Hillman, Martin Hollis, Alan Meisel, Paul Menzel, Haavi Morreim, Jeffrie Murphy, Steve Ortquist, Allison Overbay, Edmund Pellegrino, Craig Richardson, Marc Rodwin, Michael Shapiro, Sandra Tanenbaum, Robert Veatch, and Ron Wright. The book is much better for my having tried to convince them of my views, even though I did not always succeed.

Parts of this book are based on work that has appeared previously as "Rationing Health Care at the Bedside," 69 *NYU Law Rev.* 693 (1995); "Liberal and Communitarian Ethics of Insurance Selection," in *Health Care Crisis? The Search for Answers* (Misbin et al., eds.; Univ. Publishing Group, 1995); "The Problems with Rule-based Rationing," 19 *J. Med. & Philo.* 315–332 (1994); "Informed Consent to Rationing Decisions, 71 *Milbank Q.* 645–68 (1993); "The Ethics of Physician Bedside Rationing," 8 *Public Affairs Q.* 33–49 (1994); and "Health Insurers' Assessment of Medical Technology," 140 *U. Penn. Law Rev.* 1637–1712 (1992) (with G.F. Anderson). I appreciate the permission of each of these publishers to reprint portions of these works.

Preparation of this book was assisted in part by a grant from the Robert Wood Johnson Foundation in 1991 and by the hospitality of the Vermont Law School during the summer of 1992.

Contents

Making Medical Spending Decisions

1

Introduction: Who Decides?

THE INEVITABILITY OF MEDICAL SPENDING DECISIONS

When we are ill, we desperately want our doctors to do everything within their power to heal us, regardless of the costs. Medical technology has advanced so far, however, that literal adherence to this credo for every human frailty would consume much more than our country's entire economic output,[1] and, in the process, cause economic collapse.[2] Our potential medical demands are limitless. Bringing our massive medical prowess to bear on every physical and mental deficiency would mean treating each person's occasional insomnia, periodic lethargy, seasonal allergies, and minor aches and pains as if they were life-threatening illnesses. It would mean hours of psychological counseling each week, and personal fitness coaches and dietary trainers for everyone (not just for movie stars and other Californians). Ambulances staffed 24 hours a day would have to be as common as fire hydrants, parked throughout each town to respond instantaneously to any medical emergency. This is obviously hyperbole, but it illustrates what it would mean to take seriously the sentiment that nothing is more valuable than one's health and thus cost should be no object when it comes to medical care.[3]

No one in fact intends these sentiments to be taken so literally, but stopping short of this absurd state of affairs necessarily requires some sacrifice of marginal medical benefit in favor of other social needs. Any workable system for financing and delivering health care must face the fundamental problem of how best to

3

allocate limited medical resources among competing beneficial uses. Someone, somewhere must decide which items of potential medical benefit are not worth the cost.

Making these medical spending decisions is discussed in various terms, the most alarming of which is health care "rationing." Using such an emotionally charged term in this life-and-death context can polarize discussion and hamper rational analysis. This polarization was vivid during the national debate over President Clinton's sweeping proposals for health care reform. President Clinton adamantly asserted that his reforms would not cause rationing, a claim that was sharply disputed by his critics.[4] Despite their bitter clash, both sides of the political debate were in tacit agreement that it is desirable and feasible to avoid any health care rationing.

This stubborn refusal to acknowledge the need to ration is also shared by some respected policy analysts from academic and medical circles. They dispute my axiomatic starting premise that rationing in some form is inevitable. Instead, they argue that all our health care needs could be affordably met if we eliminated the large portion of "unnecessary" care that bloats the present health care budget.[5] This position is conceptually confused and empirically wrong. Conceptual confusion springs from the misunderstanding or misuse of the term "medically necessary." Using "need" to set limits on spending contradicts a fundamental trait of human psychology—that our needs are shaped by our wants, which are themselves shaped by available resources. What is possible is desired, and our wants become our needs. Therefore, over the long run, need is more *de*scriptive of how we actually spend money than it is *pre*scriptive of how money should be spent.[6]

As interpreted in practice, "medically necessary" lacks sufficient independent meaning to set a solid limit on how we spend health care resources. Few current expenditures are so devoid of any plausible medical benefit that they could be eliminated solely on the basis of being entirely unnecessary. This is best illustrated by the failure of "certificate of need" (CON) laws to control investment in health care facilities.[7] CON laws try to limit the capacity of the health care delivery system using objective measures of medical need. These laws require hospitals and other facilities to demonstrate a "need" in the community in order to receive permission to build or purchase new facilities and services. When put to the test, CON regulators have been forced to yield to the reality that need can be defined only by actual demands from doctors and patients, and under traditional systems of reimbursement, medical demands are almost limitless.[8] Consequently, CON laws have had almost no effect on total medical expenditures.

Consider, for example—after the development of X-ray machines costing $100,000 each, followed by computerized automated tomography (CAT) scanners that cost $1 million, and magnetic resonance imagers (MRI) at a cost of $3 million—whether there is now a widespread need for positive emission tomography (PET) scanners which approach $10 million: "They are remarkable medical detectives that reveal all sorts of information about chemical activity, show what parts of the brain you use when you move an arm or leg or think, and diagnose certain kinds of heart and brain disease and cancer."[9] Clearly, every hospital should have at least one.[10] Although not all medical spending entails such high-tech advances, most of it is for something that is plausibly superior to a cheaper alternative. Very little can be confidently eliminated as wholly unnecessary.

Suppose this were not the case, though. Suppose we could trim a thick layer of fat off the bulging physique of medical enterprise. We still would not control medical inflation over the long run without some form of rationing. Eliminating unnecessary care does not provide lasting relief because it is only a one-time savings that is quickly engulfed by the inevitable progress of medical advances. William Schwartz documents that the health care system historically has grown 7 percent per year even after discounting for general inflation. Immediate elimination of fully one-quarter of present health care spending would provide only a three-year respite, at which point spending levels would be back to where they were before and headed upward at the same steep pitch.[11]

It is sometimes thought that medical advances will eventually reduce medical spending by making people fundamentally healthier, but this assumption is equally flawed. Medical needs are inherently limitless because aging and illness are a permanent feature of the human condition. Much beneficial medical care results in people living to an older age where they are more frail and succumb to more chronic and expensive diseases. This does not mean we should suppress these innovations, only that the drive to conquer all forms of illness is ultimately doomed to failure. The course of history over this century demonstrates that, as medicine advances, so do both medical needs and medical spending.

For these various reasons, most policy analysts recognize that rationing in some form is desirable and inevitable. Every spending decision is necessarily a rationing decision simply because resources devoted to one person or one use are not available for someone or something else. If wants are limitless and resources are finite, it is impossible to maintain that rationing is avoidable in all its forms.

We have always rationed health care resources on a massive scale, but according to irrational and unjust principles.[12] Presently, we ration health care by denying it to those unfortunate individuals who lack insurance either because their employer does not provide it or because their level of poverty has not yet fallen to the desperate level required for Medicaid eligibility.[13] At the same time, we heavily subsidize health insurance for the upper and middle classes through a regressive tax policy that excludes from an employee's income the value of insurance premiums contributed by employers. Moreover, for those who are fully insured, we devote vast resources to save lives and restore health once an illness or accident occurs, but we spend only microscopic amounts in comparison on basic safety, health education, and health prevention measures.[14] Medical care is also rationed when insurance benefits are limited for mental health, dental, and nursing home services.

The haphazard and unprincipled basis on which rationing presently occurs effectively rebuts another argument raised by critics of rationing, namely, that rationing should occur only under numerous, morally demanding conditions that presently do not exist.[15] These critics impose unattainably utopian prerequisites for rationing, such as developing ethically unassailable and scientifically valid rationing criteria, insisting on their strict egalitarian application throughout all strata of society, and first eliminating all wasteful spending, both within medicine and elsewhere in society. These demands ignore the fact that any systematically thought-out rationing scheme, however flawed, is far superior to the thoughtless and inhumane way in which many uninsured people are now treated. A more considered form of resource allocation is the first step, not the last, toward social equity and broad-based reform.[16] Only with some better approach to rationing will minimally acceptable access to health care become affordable for everyone.

Despite these many powerful arguments, it is still controversial to speak in terms of rationing health care. In order to avoid drawing the fire of those who oppose any use of this term, I will instead lean toward the more neutral terminology of *resource allocation* or *spending decisions*. I will not entirely refrain from the "R" word, however. Its emotional baggage can help to dramatize the pervasive necessity of making medical spending decisions. Despite their differing emotional content, both rationing and allocation can fairly be used in the generic sense that refers to either implicit or explicit denial of marginally beneficial medical treatment out of consideration for its cost.[17] It is not necessary, as some have proposed, to define restricted senses of these terms that attempt to avoid the controversy that surrounds them.[18] Some of these specialized definitions are merely rhetorical techniques that hope to allow implicit rationing to occur by describing it with less inciting terms. I prefer to look that controversy square in the eye in order to gauge its full measure and to fashion the most compelling response.

ASKING THE RIGHT QUESTIONS

Let us begin with a cursory map of rationing: How, where, and by whom does it occur? Fundamentally, medical spending decisions are made at three different levels. At the macro or global level, society must decide, whether purposefully or by default, how much of its resources to devote to the medical enterprise. At present, the United States devotes about 14 percent of its total economic output to medicine; this is a figure that has been climbing steadily for decades.[19] Although there is no way to know for certain what the correct level of total spending is, there is broad consensus that the United States spends far more than it should for what it receives.

What we get for what we spend invokes the second, intermediate level of re-source allocation. Total medical spending must be allocated among preventive versus curative versus palliative treatment, and between acute versus chronic ail-ments. Total spending also must be allocated among mental versus physical, cardio-vascular versus endocrinology, and countless other subdivisions within medical practice. Here, too, there is undeniable evidence of misallocation. Most policy analysts believe we spend far too little of our medical budget on preventive care, and many believe that those who suffer from chronic ailments are neglected in favor of either futile or wasteful attempts at curing acute illness.

The third level of resource allocation consists of the micro treatment decisions made at the bedside level. Which patient receives which scarce organ for a life-saving transplant is the most dramatic example, but microlevel rationing also in-cludes more mundane questions such as when to use generic versus expensive antibiotics, whether an MRI scan is advisable, and whether a patient without insurance must be treated. Here, too, misallocation is easy to spot. Many individual items of care are massively overprescribed for those with insurance. "Almost half the coronary bypasses, the majority of Caesarean sections, and a significant pro-portion of many other procedures . . . are unnecessary or of questionable value."[20] Meanwhile, over 40 million Americans lack insurance at any point in time, so their access to basic care is severely hampered. Even more disturbing, there is strong evidence that patients with equivalent insurance and similar health conditions receive different treatment according to their race and socioeconomic status.[21]

These three levels of rationing are not hermetically divided. They blend into and influence each other in a disorderly, interconnected pattern that is not at all easy to demarcate or disentangle.[22] Accordingly, this summary does not provide much insight into how spending decisions are actually made. Understanding the nitty-gritty of how health care is rationed requires us to look at the institutions and processes in society that control the critical decisions at each of these levels and ask what their attractive features and ugly flaws are. These questions remain important regardless of the overall structure of a health care financing and deliv-ery system. Whether it is regulatory or competitive, public or private, we are plagued by two basic issues: (1) Who should decide what care is not worth the cost, and (2) what criteria of benefit should be used to make this determination?

The second of these problems is the one that has received more attention to date. Numerous volumes have been written on questions such as whether the short sup-ply of transplantable organs should be distributed based simply on random draw or according to who has been waiting the longest, or instead should be based on elaborate concepts of medical need or medical benefit.[23] This literature also gives extensive thought to routine medical technologies. It explores whether medical resources generally should be rationed according to age[24] or instead according to some more quantitative formula for effectiveness or value.[25] Others before me have debated at length whether medical benefit should be defined by the number of lives saved, the length of life, the quality of life, or some more intermediate goal such as diagnostic certainty, and whether judgments about people's social worth can be prevented from tainting these concepts.[26]

These are tremendously fascinating and important questions that deserve continuing inquiry, but they avoid what I see as a more fundamental question: Who should be the rationing decision maker?[27] This is the main question to which this book is devoted. Who makes medical spending decisions is of fundamental importance for four reasons. First, some decision-making processes obviate the need for an explicit consensus on substantive criteria. For instance, the competitive market mechanism leaves the substantive criteria to individual choice as in other sectors of the economy where rationing is largely hidden. In such a system, no consensus is necessary because we each decide what counts as sufficient medical benefit to justify the cost. Second, even if we adopt more collective forms of rationing, it is highly unlikely that we will agree on a single, substantive criterion, or a lexical ordering of several rationing criteria.[28] Therefore, the criteria question inevitably will be influenced by whatever decision-making framework we choose, whether political, medical professional, or market oriented. Third, even if agreement on general criteria is reached, their precise definition and application depend on the broad range of discretion exercised by whomever implements the criteria.

Finally, many, perhaps most, medical spending decisions are not made explicitly; instead, they are implicit in the institutional setting or the clinical style of individual practitioners. Substantive criteria can, by their nature, control only explicit decision making; implicit decisions are more amenable instead to the structural incentives that influence the people and institutions that exercise decision-making authority. Therefore, we cannot predict, understand, and evaluate these decisions without closely examining alternative decision-making mechanisms. As law professor Neil Komesar observes, "although important and controversial decisions about who decides are buried in every law and public policy issue, they often go unexamined, are treated superficially, or, at best, are analyzed in terms of the characteristics of one alternative."[29] My aim is to remedy this deficiency in our understanding of the social problem of how health care resources are allocated.

THE PLAN OF THIS BOOK

The structure of this book is formed from the earlier work of medical sociologist David Mechanic. He first articulated that health care spending decisions can be made through three fundamentally different mechanisms.[30] Cost-sensitive treatment decisions can be made by patients, by physicians, or by third parties—primarily private and governmental insurers but also various regulatory or review organizations. Elsewhere in our economy, cost/benefit trade-offs are usually made through the purchasing decisions of individual consumers. For example, nutrition resources are allocated at both the macro and micro levels through the aggregation of countless individual decisions of how much food to buy, of what quality, and from what source. This simple market mechanism is not generally available or desirable for health care because of the unpredictability of illness and the complexities of medical judgment. As discussed in Chapter 2, we purchase insurance rather than pay out of pocket because we want to protect ourselves from the uncertain costs of health care and the anxiety of making spending decisions under the strain of serious illness. Moreover, even without insurance, patients make few of their medical decisions themselves because the complexity of treatment compels us to delegate extensive authority to our doctors.

These two structural elements—insurance and physician agency—make consumer rationing unavailable for many health care purchasing decisions. Some role for consumer-based resource allocation may be preserved to the extent that insurance requires patients to pay deductibles and·co-insurance. Consumer rationing may also occur to the extent that informed-consent law places the ultimate authority in the hands of patients. But because consumers will always rely on insurance to insulate them from some health care costs, and because patients will always rely to a significant degree on their physicians' recommendations, medical spending decisions are necessarily made through the agency of insurance and the agency of physicians.

Insurers, either private or governmental, can make medical spending decisions through cost-sensitive rules about what treatment they will pay for. Until recently, this has seldom happened, but in 1994 Oregon became the first state to attempt explicit rule-based rationing for all of medicine. Oregon ranked over 600 condition–treatment pairings (e.g., surgery for appendicitis) according to their medical effectiveness for purposes of allocating limited Medicaid funding. Elsewhere in this country, efforts are underway to develop a host of much more detailed and nuanced clinical practice guidelines, which could also serve as rule-based tools for third-party resource allocation. In addition to insurers' payment rules, spending decisions can be imposed by other parties who are similarly outside the doctor–patient relationship. Courts, citizen groups or other ideal democratic processes, and physician administrators who review the work of treating doctors are each able to set limits or give directions on how medical resources are spent. All of these alternatives are discussed in Chapter 3.

The third fundamental alternative for allocating medical spending authority is for physicians to incorporate cost considerations into their clinical judgment. Authorizing physicians to make cost/benefit trade-off decisions at the bedside differs from centralized, rule-based rationing because it individualizes spending decisions to the circumstances of each patient, and it operates through professional incentives rather than bureaucratic authority. Bedside rationing, however, fundamentally compromises physicians' role-based ethic, which as discussed in Chapter 4 traditionally requires doctors to provide all care that offers any benefit, regardless of its cost. Physician bedside rationing is rendered even more controversial by the use of financial incentives to motivate doctors' performance. Whether and under what conditions this increasingly widespread practice is permissible is the topic of Chapter 5.

Whichever mechanism we choose for medical resource allocation, we also confront the problem of how the law and ethics of informed consent should apply to the resulting treatment decisions. Regardless of whether spending decisions are made by centralized bureaucratic rules or by individualized professional discretion, a critical ingredient in their legitimacy is whether patients are informed of and consent to the mechanism and the resulting denials of potentially beneficial treatment. This important topic is explored in Chapter 6.

A final set of analytical distinctions, which also form a troika, are necessary to understand how the remainder of this book is organized. Political theorist Fred Schauer explains that social decisions can be made at any one of three tiers.[31] The first determines what substantive action should be taken in the real world. For our purposes, this first-order inquiry is whom to treat and how much to spend. These are the substantive rationing criteria that I purposefully avoid for reasons explained above. The second level determines who should decide these first-level questions. This is the primary topic of this book. But there is also a third level of inquiry, which I reach in the concluding chapter: How do we decide who should decide? At this third level, the reader will quickly discover that I place great weight on the process of selecting health insurance. The gist of my position is that subscribers are bound by the choices made when they knowingly and freely select an insurance plan with a particular mix of resource allocation systems, whether under a public program or in a private market.

Placing heavy theoretical weight on informed insurance selection conflicts with the reality that many people have no choice whatsoever over the type of health insurance they receive, and even those with options have severely constrained choice because the full array of options they might desire are not available at prices they can afford. These serious imperfections require me to consider in Chapter 7 the extent to which my theoretical justifications depend on completely unconstrained choice among insurance plans.

As can be seen from this summary, most of this book engages in what Edward Rubin terms a "microanalysis of social institutions,"[32] one that seeks to assess the relative strengths, weaknesses, and characteristics of alternative mechanisms for allocating health care resources, drawing from both political economics and social theory. This book does not seek to determine which actual treatment decisions doctors, patients, and regulators should make. My resolution of the second-level issue is therefore somewhat vague and abstract: Medical spending decisions should be made through a mix of market, democratic, and professional mechanisms, as they each are best fit for particular dimensions of the problem. In developing this answer, I will strive (despite my academic tendencies) to be as concrete and pragmatic as I can. I take heed of Mary Ann Bailey's wise criticism that "rationing tends to be seen in terms of moral absolutes rather than as a practical problem in social choice—a search for a workable compromise . . . [over] what combination of institutions and processes can produce a health care rationing system [this country] can live with."[33]

Accordingly, I will not be wedded to a particular analytical framework or ideological perspective. I will undertake a pragmatic analytical critique, one that seeks to clarify for each rationing mechanism its basic rationale, its inherent limits, the evidence supporting both views, the potential for harm or manipulation, and the accommodations needed to make it work. Undoubtedly, I will not be entirely objective. My subjective views will almost certainly show through, influenced by my own life experiences as a middle-aged white married professional male in good health whose close relatives have never been seriously ill and who is a satisfied enrollee of an HMO. I cannot avoid these biases; I can only attempt to identify them as such in order better to encourage the reader's critical appraisal rather than blind acceptance. Only by open dialogue and candid assessment will we be able to generate the social consensus necessary to move purposefully ahead rather than to continue stumbling along as we have.

Notes

1. The U.S. gross domestic product per capita is about $23,000. To see how easy it would be to spend this amount each year on maximal health care, consider that it costs about this same amount on average simply to incarcerate a prisoner (not counting the costs of building new prison space). See also Lamm 1992, at 1512 ("[A] French study asked how much it would cost to give all the health care that is 'beneficial' to each citizen. The answer was five-and-one-half times the French gross national product.").

2. Although this is obvious hyperbole, it is in fact the direction in which health care spending trends are headed. See Waldo et al. 1991, at 231, 235 (projecting that U.S. health spending could reach as high as 43.7% of GNP by 2030).

3. See generally Veatch 1990, at 462; Elhauge 1994, at 1459. For another, more humorous illustration in the form of a parable about a society that values eating over all else, see Lave and Lave 1970.

4. Gaylin 1993, at 57, 64 (criticizing Clinton plan for failing to account for possibility of rationing); McCaughey 1994, at 21, 22 (criticizing Clinton plan for causing massive rationing); Lamm 1994 (criticizing Clinton plan for failing to acknowledge that rationing might be necessary).

5. See, e.g., Relman 1990a; Pellegrino and Thomasma 1988, at 185 (suggesting that rationing is not permissible except in times of disaster, epidemics, and the like or until all funding sources are exhausted and all waste and unnecessary care is eliminated).

6. See Callahan 1990, at 45; Eddy 1991b, at 782–88; Williams 1974, at 60; Elhauge 1994, at 1467.

7. See Ashby 1984; Steinwald and Sloan 1981, at 274; Salkever and Bice 1979.

8. Bovbjerg 1978.

9. Califano 1986, at 103.

10. Based purely on the concept of medical need, interpreted as meaning any medical benefit whatsoever, it would also be difficult to refuse permission for a "proton beam accelerator":

> It is a vision of the future that medical scientists have had for more than 40 years: Inside a space-age hospital room, a team of doctors activate an atomic accelerator. . . . In a few seconds, the proton beam kills cells in a cancerous tumor, leaving nearby healthy cells untouched. Now, this vision is no longer so far away. Last month, scientists at the Fermi National Accelerator Laboratory here unveiled the first proton beam accelerator built for hospital use. When the machine is ready for operation next year at Loma Linda University Medical Center near Los Angeles, many believe it will prove itself a major breakthrough in the war on cancer.
>
> Others, however, think the proton accelerator is a white elephant. They complain that its untested medical benefits and enormous price make it the ultimate example of medical technology run amok. Some doctors say proton therapy will prove useless in the treatment of most cancers. It is unquestionably the most expensive piece of medical equipment ever built. The cost—$40 million, including the special building needed to house the machine—dwarfs the cost of the next most expensive medical device. . . . At this state, Loma Linda officials say they can't even begin to guess what patients will be charged for treatment on the machine.
>
> Nevertheless, the device does have wide support. Proton therapy for cancer is believed to have a number of advantages over chemotherapy, conventional radiation and surgery. . . . Loma Linda is sure there will be enough patient demand for its machine. [At] Harvard, . . . [p]atients typically have a two-month wait for its machine, says Herman Suit, the chairman of Harvard Medical School's department of radiation medicine. "There's no excess capacity," he says (James 1988, at A1).

11. Schwartz 1987, at 221. See also Aaron and Schwartz 1990, at 418–19.

12. See Fuchs 1984; Schwartz 1989, at 21; Rosenblatt 1981.

13. In 1992, the poverty line for a family of four was $14,335. Medicaid eligibility often is set at less than half the poverty level and, in some states, may be set at less than one-quarter the federal poverty level. See Capilouto et al. 1992, at 453.

14. See, e.g., Califano, Jr. 1992, at 1535 ("[L]ess than three-tenths of one percent of our national health bill pays for health promotion and disease prevention.").

15. For assertions of this position, see, e.g., Etzioni 1991, at 88; Mehlman 1985; Angell 1985, at 1207 (arguing that a country that wastes $1 million a minute for Super Bowl commercials, $300 billion on defense, and $25 billion on tobacco should be prepared to spend "whatever is necessary for effective medical care"); Lowey 1980, at 697 (stating that "our society clearly has money to spend on luxuries and baubles").

16. See generally Callahan 1988, at 261.

17. See Mechanic 1979, at 19–21, 95–96.

18. See generally Evans 1983 (distinguishing rationing from allocation); Reagan 1988 (explaining that the word rationing is reserved for explicit, administrative decisions and does not include ordinary price allocation); see also Hadorn and Brook 1991 (advocating that rationing be used to describe only unfair and discriminatory denial of services based on inability to pay); Havighurst 1992 (arguing that rationing occurs only if the government precludes private purchase of health care).

19. Other industrialized countries spend only about 7–10 percent of their total economic output on health care. Schieber et al. 1994.

20. Califano 1992, at 1533.

21. Ford and Cooper 1995.

22. In theory, it is possible to conceive of a neat and tidy approach that sets a fixed global budget at the legislative level which is then allocated through regulatory authority to various intermediate levels within the health care system, leaving individual doctors and institutions to decide how best to treat particular patients within these allocations. This top-down, supply-side, regulatory approach is roughly how the British National Health Service works. In contrast, it is also possible to work from the bottom up through a demand-side system that starts with individual patients and doctors making discrete treatment decisions. These individualized decisions form into patterns of resource consumption within medicine that ultimately determine the total amount we spend. This free-choice system is roughly how the United States system was conceived until the mid-1980s. A third approach might target the intermediate level of resource allocation by setting budgets for categories of treatment, for groups of patients, and for sectors of the health care industry. These intermediate budgets, pushing downward, would determine the amounts available for individual treatment; aggregating upward, they would determine total spending. This is roughly how resource allocation occurs under managed care insurance; health maintenace organizations (HMOs) operate under fixed amounts per person, and the Medicare prospective payment system sets budgets according to diagnosis. Our fragmented financing and delivery system contains significant elements of each of these approaches.

23. The leading general discussions are found in AMA 1995a; Blank 1988, at 82–83, Fig. 3.1; Churchill 1987; Kilner 1990; Winslow 1982. An early general discussion is contained in Note 1969. The most recent treatment is the cogent and comprehensive analysis by Elhauge 1994. For a thorough discussion of rationing criteria used commonly throughout society, see generally Elster 1992.

24. See generally, e.g., Callahan 1987; Daniels 1988.

25. See generally Elixhauser 1993.

26. See, e.g., Harris 1985; Williams 1992.

27. See also Klein 1993b (advocating focus on the decisionmaking question); Goold 1996 (same).

28. For a thorough exposition of why this is so, see Elhauge 1994.

29. Komesar 1995, at 4.

30. Mechanic 1980. For further elaboration, see Mechanic 1986, at 147–48; Mechanic 1979, at 19–21, 95–96.

31. Schauer 1992.

32. Bailey 1994, at 41.

33. Rubin 1996.

2

Patient Spending Decisions

In most sectors of the economy, it would seem ludicrous to even consider whether the primary authority for making spending decisions should reside with someone other than consumers. Take, for instance, the production of automobiles. It would be inconceivably socialistic for the government to decide how many cars of each size, shape, and color to produce and who is to receive them, and we would view it as an equally repulsive form of corporate fascism to give the auto industry itself binding authority to make these decisions. Our society determines how many cars of what kind and quality go to which people through the aggregate forces of supply and demand, as expressed through millions of individual purchasing and nonpurchasing decisions. Government regulates the accuracy of information we receive through ads and sales pitches and it sets safety standards for quality defects that are impossible to detect by simple inspection. But these decisions are only at the periphery of the industry. The great bulk of decisions made by the auto industry are directly responsive to consumer desires.

Likewise, it is difficult to conceive of any other good or service where it is even plausible to frame the central inquiry of this book in the way I have. In almost every other area of commercial life, it is assumed without further inquiry that consumers decide how much to spend on what goods and services of which quality. We might debate precisely what role government officials or expert technicians should have in the shadows of the market, but the core resource allocation decisions are presumptively consumer-driven throughout almost all of the economy. Therefore, it is appropriate to start the analysis of health care allocation decisions by explaining why this same response does not end the inquiry here.

15

This chapter will explain and critique at some length the thinking of those who advocate a free-market approach to making medical spending decisions, an approach that places the dominant authority with individual patients at the time they seek treatment. It begins with a description of the remarkably strong case in favor of reforms that would radically alter the existing health care marketplace. This chapter then proceeds to explain in detail why markets are only a partial solution and why there are inevitable limits on the scope of individual patient authority. Because of these inherent limits, consumers themselves insist that substantial authority over how to spend medical resources be vested with government or with the providers of medical services—the very systems of decision making that are so inconceivable elsewhere in the economy.

Before undertaking this analysis, it is important to clarify a critical source of possible misunderstanding. In equating market-based reforms with patient decision making, I do not mean to say that the only way a market can function is to leave cost-sensitive treatment decisions with patients. Instead, a market system in health care will inevitably result in patients delegating authority to make these decisions to physicians or to third parties, primarily through consumers' informed choice in purchasing substantial amounts of health care insurance. It will soon be clear that I favor a market system for the selection of insurance despite my qualms about a consumer market for the selection of discrete items of treatment. My critique of market-based reforms in this chapter is aimed only at those who encourage patients to go without comprehensive insurance. Versions of market reforms that rely on comprehensive insurance are addressed throughout the remainder of the book, especially in Chapter 7.

THE CASE IN FAVOR OF MARKET REFORMS

The Moral Case

Proponents of market reform in health care make their case with a moral fervor that has almost a religious tone. They sanctify the merits of individual freedom and demonize the intrusions of centralized bureaucracies, whether of government or private insurance origins. Here are some leading examples:

If a free market is in operation, two important ethical concerns are advanced. The first, and most important, is the cause of truth. . . . The market makes transparent the true economic costs of health care services . . . , [u]nlike systems of centralized government planning, where masses of data must be collected, analyzed and applied in a vast enterprise of bureaucratic decision-making. . . . The second important ethical concern advanced by a free market is justice. Those who make enormous contributions of time and labor in the system will be able to reap the just desserts of their efforts, their due. In speaking of this "moral element in free enterprise," Friedrich A. Hayek observes, "It is the essence of a free society that we should be materially rewarded not for doing what others order us to do, but for giving some others what they want." An ancient principle of justice is reaffirmed when labor is rewarded in such a manner.[1]

Medicine controlled by the state ultimately serves only the state. After Romania's communist regime fell in 1989, Americans saw photographs of Romanian hospitals. On the one hand, a modern hospital with the latest technology and luxury conveniences was reserved for Communist party officials and key bureaucrats. On the other hand, hospitals for ordinary people were operated out of World War II army barracks. . . . Th[is] tragedy represent[s] the ultimate, logical consequence of a goal that is almost universally accepted by health policy analysts: the complete elimination of markets, prices, competition, and choice from the health care sector.[2]

Another rhetorical tactic is to put the issue in terms of a power struggle between the individual consumers who make up the proletariat and the hierarchy of government agencies or large insurance companies that would control them. Thus, the most thoughtful and convincing book advocating that patients make their own health care spending decisions is conspicuously entitled *Patient Power*, a theme that is repeated throughout its 650 pages. The authors maintain that severely limiting the scope of insurance would:

- Transfer power from large institutions and impersonal bureaucracies to individuals.
- Remove health care (as much as possible) from the political arena, in which well-organized special interests can cause great harm to the rest of us.
- Change the role of physicians, who would no longer serve as the principal agents of third-party payers, but would serve as the principal agents of patients, and help them to make informed choices.
- Change the role of employers, who would not be buyers of health care and would not make decisions for employees concerning their health insurance, but would be agents for individual employees and help them to make informed choices and to monitor the performance of competing insurers.[3]

This strain of libertarian moral and political theory strikes a strong chord with many people because of its deep foundations in American history and social life. America was founded on the spirit of rugged individualism that underlies the Bill of Rights and the Declaration of Independence. We are among the least socialistic of the western industrialized nations, with one of the lowest tax burdens. When health care reformers speak of a "uniquely American" solution to the health care crisis, they mean one that minimizes the role of government and centralized planning in favor of economic incentives and individual market transactions.

Market advocates quickly dispense with those who object that health care has a special importance that distinguishes it from ordinary consumer goods. These advocates observe that so, too, do many other necessities of life such as food, shelter, and education, which to a greater or lesser extent are nevertheless subject to market systems. As law professor Richard Epstein has put the point, the unique importance of health care demands that, in choosing between government and markets, we exercise extreme care in making the correct choice; it does not pre-determine an answer in favor of government.[4] Indeed, since elsewhere we almost always choose to minimize the role of government, this view of the issue puts the burden on advocates of government to explain what is wrong with a free market for health care.

This burden is made even heavier by a few simple observations on the obvious flaws of centralized decision making in medicine (points developed in much greater detail in Chapter 3). The government operates within constitutional and political constraints that require it to act evenhandedly, showing no undue favoritism or discrimination among its citizens. This biases government decision making to-ward simple, across-the-board solutions to complex problems, even when those problems require highly individualized responses. For instance, if the government is faced with the question of whether an MRI scan is appropriate for a particular medical condition, it is likely to give a yes-or-no answer, even though the best answer may well vary from one person to the next depending on how important it is for that individual to cure the condition. A professional dancer, basketball player, or amateur tennis player with a sprained knee may feel that it is much more com-pelling to spend $1000 for an MRI scan as a precaution to investigate the serious-ness of the injury than would an ordinary patient who might be willing to wait and see if the knee healed on its own. The market allows us to make these distinc-tions ourselves, but it would strike us as unjust for the government to impose these distinctions on us.

This MRI example typifies only one of a vast multitude of conditions and treat-ments; similar cases occur across the entire range of medical practice. "What is 'best' in a particular case will depend on the values and needs of the patient, the skills of the doctor, and the other resources available. The quality of the outcome depends a great deal on how the patient feels about it. What is an annoyance for one patient may mean the inability to keep a job for another with the same condi-tion."[5] The same observation can be made for automobiles, except the diversity of taste in size, color, shape and power of cars is much less important to us than a similar or greater diversity in tastes for procedures that directly affect our bodies and minds. If the government were to make these decisions for us all, it would reach much less nuanced, fine-tuned results than if we were each to decide for ourselves.

Accordingly, a market system employing individual patient choice is likely to produce a greater level of both objective and subjective health benefits than one that relies on centralized, "government-issue" answers. We have good reason to believe that people will actually feel better and do better if they can choose for themselves what treatment to receive than if everyone has to be treated exactly the same. Recall that John Stuart Mill, who developed the philosophical founda-tion for libertarian thought, was a utilitarian; his primary justification for individual liberty was that it leads to demonstrably better results, not that it is morally superior regardless of the results. Enhanced well-being creates a pragmatic as well as a moral foundation for private markets, a foundation that is stronger the more important the stakes are in individualizing decisions.

The especially strong desire to individualize health care decisions is reflected in the legal doctrine of informed consent. The law imposes on physicians much stronger duties to discuss treatment options in detail with their patients than it imposes on almost any other arena of economic activity.[6] The reasons spring from the unique importance of medical treatment and the special relationship patients have with their physicians. According to the landmark court decision,

the patient, being unlearned in medical sciences, has an abject dependence upon and trust in his physician for the information upon which he relies during the decisional process, thus raising an obligation in the physician that transcends arms-length transactions. . . . [I]t is the prerogative of the patient, not the physician, to determine for himself the direction in which he believes his interests lie.[7]

Although this law is motivated by the desire to avoid patient injury from invasive medical procedures, the same justifications also support patient control over how best to spend money, since decisions to save money by avoiding treatment have just as strong a potential to cause injury as do decisions to receive risky treatment.[8]

These very strong values of pluralism and individual autonomy are generally seen as consistent with market-based reforms. On the other hand, market reforms are inconsistent with what many observers have noted is an equally strong egalitarian strain in American attitudes about medicine. As discussed below, most of us believe that everyone has a basic human entitlement to medical care. This element of social justice is difficult to achieve with a purely market-based system. Our egalitarian instinct appears to require some measure of centralized government authority. It is possible, however, to reconcile the two objectives of individual pluralism and social egalitarianism so as to preserve a central role for the market and keep the government at bay. Egalitarian values are at least partially met if the government subsidizes those who are too poor to afford a minimally decent level of care, enabling them, too, to participate in the market on their own terms. Beyond this minimal subsistence level, whatever it might be,[9] most people do not feel there is a compelling case for perfect equality in health care,[10] any more than they do for education, housing, food, or other social obligations that are infused with special importance. Market reformers thus maintain that this mix of social values is best achieved if most health care spending decisions are consumer-driven.

The Economic Case

Those who are not convinced by this moral case might still be persuaded by the economic case in favor of patients paying for their own costs of medical treatment. Although it may be perfectly moral for an individual to remain oblivious to costs, doing so burdens others because we all pay for each others' health care choices through private or public insurance programs. This insight is captured in the conservative political witticism, "If you think Medicare is expensive, just wait until it's free." Full insurance coverage ultimately costs society more for the very reason that it appears cheaper to us as individuals. We demand, or are willing to accept, much more expensive treatment if we do not have to pay out of pocket. Because we do not pay individually for the resulting increases in insurance premiums, we can enjoy the benefits of expensive treatment by taking a free ride on society or on the insured group. This is why market reformers focus their attack on the excessive scope of insurance. Their solution to massive inefficiency in health care spending is to encourage consumers to make individual spending decisions on their own by paying for care out of pocket.

The economic case for increased patient cost sharing is not this simple, however. The psychic benefit that comes from being insured is just as important in economic theory as are the tangible goods and services that could be purchased by reducing the scope of insurance. Economists buy insurance just like all the rest of us because they, too, are willing to pay a price in advance rather than pay out of pocket when the need arises. The extra cost of paying in advance is worth not having to worry about expenses later on. It would be socially destructive to force consumers to forego health insurance when they are willing to pay the price for this security.

What economists object to, then, is not the simple availability of comprehensive health insurance. They object to the social policy of subsidizing insurance in a manner that hides its true costs from consumers. If consumers were made aware of the full economic effects of health insurance, economists theorize they would not be willing to purchase nearly as much and, as a consequence, they would willingly make many more of their own medical spending decisions. Reducing health insurance to a level actually desired by consumers given its costs will therefore result in a better allocation of societal resources and will lower total spending on medical care.

Economists convincingly point to the tax laws as the main culprit for excessive levels of health insurance.[11] Federal and state tax codes exclude from the calculation of personal income any amounts that employers contribute toward specified fringe benefits, including health insurance.[12] This tax shelter is the primary reason most private health insurance is provided through the workplace. Employees much prefer to receive an additional increment of compensation in the form of tax-free health insurance (or another fringe benefit such as a pension contribution) rather than as increased wages that might be used to buy the same or another benefit. When the employer buys health insurance, it does so with untaxed money, whereas when the employee buys health insurance, he does so only after taxes are taken out. This is true for both federal and state income and payroll taxes.

Assuming a marginal income tax rate of 50 percent (which is true for many middle-income workers combining federal, state, and local taxes), a dollar spent by the employer will purchase twice as much health insurance as a dollar recieved by the employee.[13] Therefore, even if the employee does not want more insurance as much as he wants more money, at this tax rate he prefers the additional insurance up to the point that it buys twice as much coverage as he would be willing to buy on his own. This goes a long way toward explaining why, in recent years, average wage increases have fallen nearly flat adjusted for inflation while fringe benefits constitute the fastest-growing component of labor costs.

To dramatize even further the effect of this tax subsidy, consider the differences in the kind of insurance that could be purchased with the same amount of money if it were spent by an employer rather than an individual. If the basic insurance coverage were the same and the difference were reflected entirely in the deductible amount, average consumers who bought their insurance with the same wages they use for other goods and services could, in current market conditions, replace a policy that has a $250 deductible with a policy that has a deductible of $2500 or more.[14] Stated in the reverse, even though it is extremely wasteful for most families to pay the extra premium needed to lower the deductible from $2500 to $250, most families are willing to allow their employer to do so instead of raising wages because the insurance deductibles that employees pay are taxed whereas employer-paid premiums are not.

Not only is this tax subsidy effect highly inefficient, it is inequitable. Tax deductions hold a disproportionate advantage for higher-income workers because they are subject to higher tax rates. If one views the government's decision not to tax health insurance premiums as an implicit payment for part of those premiums, then the government provides only half as much support to a low-income tax payer in a 15 percent tax bracket as it does to a middle-income tax payer in a 30 percent bracket who has the same insurance. Of the $600 per family that the federal government on average forgoes collecting each year on account of this tax exclusion, $1560 goes to families in the top fifth income group whereas only $270 goes to families in the bottom fifth.[15]

The primary economic consequence of widespread, comprehensive insurance is vastly increased spending on medical services. Evaluations of the appropriateness of many different types of treatment suggest that more than 25 percent of all health care spending is either entirely unnecessary or is of only questionable or marginal benefit.[16] This huge inefficiency results not just from the fact that fully insured patients are unconcerned about the costs of treatment, but also from the fact that medical services are especially unsusceptible to objective scrutiny by third parties, a point that is developed more in Chapter 3. Elsewhere in the economy, comprehensive insurance does not cause massive waste because other constraints substitute for market discipline when consumers purchase services through insurance. These other constraints are lacking in the health care market.

Take, for instance, the costs of repairing an automobile after an accident. Even when these costs are fully insured and therefore the car owner has no stake in shopping for the best deal, it is easy for the insurer to protect against abuse simply by enforcing the market prices that are charged for similar repair services when they are not insured. The portion of repair shop revenues paid by consumers out of pocket provides an objective benchmark for what prices are reasonable under automobile insurance. The fact that virtually all health care services are paid for by private or public insurance, however, means that this benchmark is almost entirely lacking for medical services.[17] Accordingly, insurers have been unable to rein in total medical spending simply by reference to the behavior of other doctors. The standard techniques—limiting charges to those that are "usual, customary, and reasonable," or evaluating treatment decisions through "peer review" by other doctors—are only able to detect highly aberrant behavior. They do nothing to address the bulk of medical practice, that is, the very behavior caused by the inflationary incentives of insurance.

Two short anecdotes serve to illustrate this point. One is a confession that a practicing surgeon in Manhattan made in a letter to *The New York Times*:

When I finished my [medical] training some years ago, the surgeon who directed my department was routinely allowed $800 from Medicare for a commonly performed surgical procedure. This was considered top dollar for such a procedure but was entirely commensurate with his skill and reputation. Acting upon the advice of my predecessors, . . . I began to bill $1,000 in order to "up" my profile for the same procedure—and, to my surprise, I began receiving higher fees than my former chief despite my nearly novice status. Neither I nor the American Medical Association complained about these arrangements.[18]

The other is a report of doctors speaking about the standard-setting process under Medicare peer review:

They'd get a group of doctors together and ask something like, "How long are you guys keeping patients in the hospital for gallbladders?" . . . If one doctor said 6 days, and another said 8, and a third said 12, they'd put down 12 as the standard. There was no attempt to be parsimonious, only to catch the very small percentage who were pulling truly outrageous things.[19]

The other source of inefficiency in the scope of insurance comes from state law requirements that mandate inclusion of certain categories of treatment. Often as the result of lobbying by special interest groups representing medical professionals, state legislatures have imposed a host of requirements on private insurers that force them to cover blocks of service that not all consumers would otherwise desire. Examples include items as frivolous as hairpieces and sperm bank deposits and items as peripheral as naturopathy and acupuncture, but also items of serious and widespread concern such as drug and alcohol treatment, organ transplants, and care for newborn infants. Calculations suggest that these coverage mandates increase the cost of insurance by 20–30 percent, thereby deterring a large number of people from buying any coverage at the same time that those with coverage use services even more excessively.[20]

Another consequence of state-mandated benefits laws is that employers substitute self-funded insurance for purchased insurance. This results from a federal law known as the Employee Retirement Security Act of 1974 (ERISA) which prevents states from regulating self-insured employers. Since larger employers constitute the healthiest and most stable portion of the insurance market, their increasing decision not to purchase health insurance has caused the not-so-gradual disintegration of the insurance market for medium and small employers. Those employers who are unable to self-insure are the only ones required to pay the high costs of these mandates. For this and other reasons, these small employers are also, by far, the least likely to provide any insurance at all. Whereas 98 percent of employers with more than 100 workers offer some health insurance (mostly through self-insurance), only about a third of employers with 25 or fewer workers purchase health insurance.[21] Market reformers argue that these destabilizing effects could be avoided or minimized if states were prevented from insisting that health insurance become even more comprehensive.

INCREASING PATIENT SENSITIVITY TO MEDICAL COSTS

Decreasing Coverage or Going Bare

Drawing on these economic insights, economists and other public policy analysts have developed a number of proposals to increase patient sensitivity to medical costs by decreasing the scope of health insurance. The simplest approach is to remove the tax distortion by counting as ordinary income any amounts that employers pay toward health insurance premiums. This move is viewed as politically infeasible, however, since this tax break, like that for interest on home mortgages, has wide popular appeal. Moreover, to be consistent, the same tax break would have to be removed from other fringe benefits, resulting in employees paying taxes for other implicit income such as on-site child care, health club memberships, and employee discounts. Some of the taxpayer discontent might be smoothed over, however, if the tax exclusion were replaced with a different, more equitable tax break such as a tax credit that is at least neutral with respect to income. In other words, everyone who purchases insurance would receive a tax break of the same dollar value rather than the highly regressive subsidy that presently gives much less relief to low-income taxpayers.

An alternative is to cap the size of the tax benefit at a level that more closely approximates the least expensive kind of insurance that many middle-income people would choose to buy out of pocket. Economists theorize that, without the tax subsidy, many people would buy what is known as "catastrophic coverage," that is, insurance that pays only for the very high costs of serious illness or injury. One common version of catastrophic coverage is to simply raise the deductible level in standard, comprehensive insurance to an amount that most people could afford (not without some pain) to pay out of ordinary earnings, say, $3000 a year for an average wage earner. This would require consumers to pay the full costs of routine or common items of care such as setting a broken leg, performing a minor surgical procedure, or seeing a doctor for a child's ear ache. Once the deductible threshold is met in a year, any remaining expenses would be covered at 100 percent.

Market reformers also call for the federal government to preempt states' authority to impose mandated benefits. Economists explain that it usually makes no sense to mandate or encourage insurance that many consumers are unwilling to buy. Insurance is often not desirable or feasible for services whose consumption is discretionary, and much of modern medicine consists of discretionary items. Some sectors of medicine have higher discretionary components than others; therefore, unregulated and unsubsidized markets may produce coverage options that are sharply reduced for pockets of service such as mental health, dental, infertility, alternative practitioners, and the like. Even though these areas contain many important and expensive services that are highly valued, either patients can afford them out of pocket or distorting incentives make it unworkable to insure them.

A good example is insurance for long-term nursing care.[22] Although there is a strong desire for this type of insurance, particularly among the elderly, it is not available from private insurers on very generous terms because only those people who have a high expectation of going to a nursing home choose to purchase; therefore, the premiums are so high that those who can afford them often can also afford simply to pay out of pocket when the need arises. Potential purchasers might also worry that having nursing home insurance makes it easier for family members to insist on institutional care instead of giving personal support at home. Consequently, for many consumers, it may produce a better allocation of resources in the long run to pay for some health care services entirely out of pocket, even though they may not be able to afford as much care as they might ideally want when the need arises. For somewhat different reasons, consumers might also wish to go entirely without any insurance for certain categories of very expensive mainstream medicine such as organ transplants or life-support when terminally ill, even though they will be entirely unable to pay when the need arises.

A third and more measured way to limit insurance is for consumers to contract for comprehensive insurance, perhaps with only modest deductibles, but employing a standard of care markedly lower than what prevails now in the highly subsidized market.[23] Thus, consumers might remain eligible for very expensive and high-tech life-saving procedures, as well as for more routine expensive diagnostic testing, but only where both need and potential benefit are compelling or demonstrably clear. No longer could endless amounts be spent pursuing ultimate certainty in diagnosis and safety, or on extreme long-shot chances at staving off near-certain death or disability. Insurance contracts would specify much more demanding criteria of medical urgency, leaving consumers to pay for more attenuated medical expenditures out of pocket.[24]

Market reformers see all of these kinds of limited health insurance as reasonable possibilities that might result from undistorted consumer choice. Where market advocates have the greatest division within their own ranks is over whether to tolerate the possibility of many people not purchasing any health insurance at all. They acknowledge that subsidies must be provided to those social classes that cannot be expected to afford even minimal insurance on their own, such as the poor, the disabled, and the elderly. But what about middle- or upper-class people who can afford insurance but foolishly or strategically choose not to buy? One reaction is that social mavericks are entitled to this freedom, just as they may choose to engage in risky behavior and suffer the consequences. They will be entitled to publicly supported care in the event of dire emergencies. Otherwise, the uninsured will have to make do on whatever they can afford out of pocket.

Other market reformers, however, envision a system in which everyone is covered by the private insurance of their choice. This would entail a mandate for employers or individuals to purchase insurance, but would leave them much wider discretion over what type of insurance to purchase. Consistent with other versions of market reform, this decision would not be influenced by a regressive tax subsidy. Instead, a system of tax credits would give everyone enough support to purchase a minimally decent catastrophic coverage plan, and leave to individuals the choice of whether to purchase additional coverage with after-tax dollars.

The result of any of these reforms is that patients will be subject to a much greater degree of cost sharing than at present, either because their comprehensive insurance has a much larger deductible or copayment or because the scope of insurance is significantly reduced.[25] This greatly increased exposure to medical costs will require consumers to shop more aggressively for the best buys in medical care and to question their physicians more closely over the necessity of recommended treatment. The type of market behavior that reformers envision is exemplified by cosmetic surgery, which is universally not insured. Active competition exists among cosmetic surgeons based on both quality and cost factors. As a result, cosmetic surgeons typically approach potential patients in a consumer-friendly fashion that allows them to carefully evaluate whether a particular service is worth the price and, if so, who provides the best value.[26] Most cosmetic patients receive plenty of opportunity to interview the doctor, learn of his past track record, obtain a fixed price, and acquire other relevant information.

In contrast, where market discipline is absent because consumers are not scrutinizing costs, providers engage in highly irrational pricing behavior. In one survey of Dallas hospitals, for instance, charges for common blood and urine tests varied threefold among area hospitals, and in a nationwide survey hospital prices for some common tests were found to vary tenfold.[27] These confusing and inconsistent pricing patterns, backed up by a cult of institutional secrecy, make it difficult if not impossible at present to learn the individual costs incurred during a hospital stay, even after discharge, let alone at the time the consumption decision is made. Economists believe that patients who pay more out of pocket will insist on much greater visibility of prices, thereby forcing prices down and reducing consumption of some services.

Empirical studies verify that patients subject to increased cost sharing spend dramatically less on health care than those who are fully insured. The RAND Health Insurance Experiment, which is discussed in detail below, found in a large controlled study that consumers with catastrophic coverage[28] cut their health care costs by one-third compared with those who have nearly free care.[29] This finding is confirmed by natural experiments that observe real-world market behavior when insurers suddenly raise or lower co-insurance amounts. Rather precipitous drops in spending have occurred when copayments were increased even modestly, and sharp increases in spending have resulted when cost-sharing requirements were relaxed.[30] These findings create at least a prima facie case for increased cost sharing resulting in more rational economic behavior. They have fueled the interest of Congress and the states in crafting a publicly acceptable way to encourage consumers to bear more responsibility for the costs of their medical treatment.

Medical Savings Accounts

Medical Savings Accounts (MSAs) are the most attractive version of health insurance that relies heavily on cost-sensitive patient decision making.[31] Although the details vary considerably, the gist of the MSA idea is to couple a catastrophic insurance policy with a forced-savings device that resembles an Individual Retirement Account.[32] This Medical Savings Account would be funded by employers (or consumers) with the money they save by purchasing insurance that has a much higher deductible. The most optimistic proposals assume that the premium savings from purchasing the catastrophic insurance will equal the subscriber's increased financial exposure as a result of the higher deductible. For instance, if conventional 80 percent coverage with a $500 deductible now costs $5500, a catastrophic coverage policy with a $3000 deductible would hopefully cost approximately $3500, and so the MSA could be funded at $2000, the difference between the two. This amount is sufficient to pay for all additional medical expenses that fall under the higher deductible.[33] Even if funding is not initially this generous, MSA funds not spent one year can roll over to the next. Therefore, for most subscribers it is only necessary to contribute the average amount of out-of-pocket spending each year in order to fully cover the deductible within a few years.[34]

If individuals or employers contribute more to their MSAs each year than their average yearly spending on out-of-pocket medical expenses, then MSAs will accumulate large life-time savings accounts. This nest egg can then be used to cover the expected burdens of old age: loss of earnings, increased medical costs (especially for chronic ailments), and the expense of long-term nursing care. Indeed, some proponents of MSAs see as one of the more attractive features their ability to relieve the government from a wide array of social welfare responsibilities. Government entitlement programs like social security and Medicare could be drastically scaled back by forcing or encouraging individuals to save in anticipation of their future needs rather than using the political system, as we now do, to transfer wealth from the young to the elderly.[35] For instance, Medicare might be replaced by a system where, upon retirement, individuals purchase a private lifetime health insurance policy of their choice from funds accumulated in their MSAs, much like they now create a source of retirement income by choosing how to invest and annuitize their private pension funds.[36]

Although a few employers have experimented with MSAs and catastrophic coverage, this attractive proposal has not come into widespread use primarily due to its disadvantaged status under income and payroll tax provisions. Tax protection now exists for the catastrophic insurance policy but not for funds put into an MSA to cover the deductible. Existing flexible spending accounts, which might be adapted to this purpose, require employees to forfeit any unspent funds at the year's end and therefore are unpopular or only lightly used. Otherwise, MSAs are legal, but when employers shift money from generous insurance coverage to funding MSAs, those monies become taxable as income to the employees and do not give rise to any tax breaks (unless the employee has other medical expenses that combined exceed the 7.5 percent of income necessary to claim a medical expense deduction). Under existing law, the shift to an MSA imposes a similar but somewhat lesser economic penalty on the employer's payroll tax bill.

In order to give MSAs a fair chance, most MSA proposals, unlike other market reforms, focus on extending rather than restricting the existing tax subsidy so that a level playing field exists for types of insurance that have more patient cost sharing. Some MSA proposals go further and affirmatively encourage the MSA approach, giving it a bigger tax break than normal insurance by exempting MSA investment earnings from any tax, either when the earnings accrue or when they are eventually spent. In this way, MSA proposals are often more generous than existing IRAs, in which both contributions and earnings are eventually taxed when they are withdrawn upon retirement.

One reason that MSAs have such fervent advocates is that the few existing experiments with them have generated such positive cost-savings results. Some employers have achieved savings of 30 percent over budgeted health care expenses, and others have experienced near-zero cost increases or even cost decreases over several years. Workers also appear happy with MSAs since, when offered, the great majority elect them despite the existing tax penalty, and in some work forces, plans similar to MSAs have produced year-end bonuses or rebates of $600–$800 per employee.[37]

Further evidence of their savings potential comes from the RAND Health Insurance Experiment discussed above. Its catastrophic plan operated much like an

MSA since the researchers gave the participants a cash advance to pay for costs that fell within the high-level deductible. The participants under the catastrophic-type coverage spent 15 percent less than those in the conventional fee-for-service arrangements and almost one-third less than those who received free care. Their total medical expenses were equivalent to those enrolled in the HMO plan.

THE CASE AGAINST PATIENT COST SHARING

Market reformers have made a powerful economic and moral case for increasing patients' sensitivity to the costs of medical care by diminishing the scope of insurance. This argument is not without serious flaws and limitations, however. Not even the most ardent market advocate envisions a world entirely without health insurance. And even when patients pay out of pocket, they will continue to rely to a considerable extent on the advice of their doctors—the very people who are being paid. Establishing the strength and scope of these inherent limits to patient-directed spending decisions requires a detailed critique of the case in favor of increased patient cost sharing. This critique is intended not so much to question the desirability as it is to question the feasibility of achieving the ends set by market reformers.[38] I do not mean to repel any notion of patients making their own spending decisions; instead, my aim is to better appreciate what additional decision-making mechanisms are necessary.

The following sections will make three basic points. (1) Because of the special attributes of medical care, consumers resist being exposed to the costs of treatment and therefore insurance will remain widespread despite market reforms. (2) Patients are not likely to make objectively correct decisions even when they do bear the costs of treatment. (3) Administrative complexities make it difficult to have a smoothly functioning market with widely varying types of insurance. For these many and substantial reasons, it is easy to conclude that increased patient cost sharing, despite its considerable merit, is inherently limited in its ability to address all, or even the bulk of, medical spending decisions. Because health care resources cannot be allocated entirely by individual patient decisions, some substantial role must remain for doctors to make cost-sensitive decisions at the bedside or for insurers or government officials to impose limits from outside the treatment relationship.

Consumers' Desire to Remain Oblivious to Cost

The Attraction of Insurance

Health care resources will never be allocated entirely or even mostly according to individual consumers' spending decisions because of the prominent role that insurance necessarily plays in medicine. During the first half of this century it was feasible to be without insurance, but now medicine is simply too effective and too expensive for us to ever expect large numbers of people to go without coverage. This point is so obvious that it is seldom explained, but articulating the many supporting reasons helps to fully appreciate its power.

Early in the century, it was not only possible but desirable to go without health insurance. Medicine simply had little to offer, and what it did offer was affordable out of pocket. It was only in the 1920s that surgical techniques began to develop rapidly, and only in the 1930s and 1940s that effective medications became widespread. Previously, doctors played mostly a palliative role in which they helped comfort patients and give them some hope while waiting for nature to take its course. Even after the advance of scientific developments, effective medical procedures were short, simple, and relatively affordable. It was only in the postwar period of the 1950s and 1960s that expensive, high-tech medicine such as X-rays and complex surgeries became widely available.

The development of lifesaving procedures outside the reach of most families' incomes spurred the market for health insurance, which spread rapidly during this same postwar period. For reasons that are too lengthy to explain here, however, the type of insurance that spread covered far more than these extraordinary expenses. In part due to the tax subsidy described above, comprehensive insurance covering nearly all medical expenses became the norm. This wide availability of insurance fueled a remarkable growth in medical technology that, despite its many flaws, now constitutes the most sophisticated, successful, and expensive health care system in the world, by far. Due to the capabilities of modern medicine, illness and injury can be catastrophically expensive, and due to the vagaries of nature, they often arise in a completely unpredictable fashion. Moderate injuries from a car accident, resulting in a hospital stay of only a few days, can quickly cost tens of thousands of dollars. Massive trauma or serious illness leading to extensive hospitalization can easily exceed $100,000. Examples include cancer or premature birth. Transplants for major organs such as the heart or liver cost over one-quarter of a million dollars including follow-up care. Serious illness entailing complex treatment that occurs over several years can total in the millions of dollars. Examples include recurrent cancers, repeated organ transplants, and multiple severe birth defects.

These conditions of massive expense and sudden, unexpected occurrence are the ideal setting for insurance.[39] These are the same conditions that make fire insurance and life insurance so popular. They are likely to be permanent conditions in medicine. Therefore, we can be confident that most people will continue to buy significant amounts of coverage even if all social subsidies are removed.

Catastrophic and Bare Bones Insurance

At the moment, we can only speculate, however, on the extent to which this is true. Conclusive evidence on the popularity of health insurance does not exist in an undistorted, unsubsidized market. The present popularity of health insurance is produced by the tax subsidy that attaches to employer-paid fringe benefits. After retirement, health insurance remains broadly popular with the elderly. Those in the middle- and upper-income groups almost universally choose to purchase private Medigap coverage to pay for the costs not covered by Medicare. But, as economists have explained, this choice is also highly subsidized because private Medigap policies pay only 20 percent of the costs of the extra treatment that results from full coverage; the remainder is covered by Medicare itself for free.[40]

Without these artificial stimulants, market reformers believe that consumers will purchase less comprehensive insurance than they now do—in particular, they assume a much higher deductible of, say, $2000, will be common. They observe that 80 percent of people never reach this level of spending in any year, and so most people will pay for all of their medical expenses entirely out of pocket.[41] This may be true, but it is deceptive. Although most people would pay all their medical expenses, the lion's share of medical spending is concentrated in the minority of patients with serious conditions whose spending far exceeds even catastrophic deductible levels. The great bulk of people who suffer from fairly minor and less expensive conditions account for only a small portion of health care spending. In any given year, the 10 percent of patients with the most severe conditions will account for about two-thirds of total health care expenditures, while the bottom two-thirds of patients account for only about 10 percent of total expenditures.[42] Therefore, even if market reforms caused everyone to purchase catastrophic insurance with a $2000 deductible, only about 20 percent of medical expenditures would be made entirely through individual patient purchasing decisions at the time of treatment. (A $3000 deductible would cover those who account for only about 25 percent of present spending and even a $5000 deductible would cover those who account for less than 40 percent of spending.) The rest would continue to be covered by catastrophic insurance and therefore not be subject to individual patient spending decisions.

The foregoing assumes that the form of insurance consumers will choose is comprehensive coverage with a high deductible. Instead, it is possible consumers will choose first-dollar coverage but only over a limited range of medicine. In other words, rather than cutting horizontally by eliminating the bottom $3000 of coverage from across the whole spectrum of medicine, consumers may cut vertically by chopping off all coverage for entire categories of conditions or treatments. For instance, they might choose not to cover high-cost organ transplants at all, or they may decide that it is not worth the extra premium expense to cover high-tech life-support when they are terminally ill or in a permanent coma. If so, as the argument goes, then limited insurance cannot help but save money since consumers would have decided in advance to forego entirely these items of expensive treatment.

There are two reasons why this speculation might not be entirely true. First, eliminating individual categories of treatment does not save nearly as much as people often assume. I will illustrate with the widely quoted statistic that almost one-third of Medicare spending occurs in the last year of life and 40 percent of this comes in the last month of life. This statistic suggests that there is lots of money to save on dying patients, but the difficulty is that often there is no way to know ahead of time which patients are in fact dying. Without this knowledge, it is only after treatment is attempted and fails that we learn for which patients treatment was useful or futile. Withdrawing expensive treatment only when we are certain that a patient is beyond recovery would save only 3 percent or less of all health care spending. A number of studies have been unable to document any savings from living wills and similar devices as they are currently used.[43]

Another example of the limited cost-savings potential for excluding entire items of treatment comes from the bitter controversy that is now raging over whether an experimental bone marrow transplant procedure should be used for cases of severe breast cancer.[44] Many insurers vehemently opposed paying for this expensive procedure ($150,000 and up) because they considered it unproven and potentially harmful. After losing many court battles and after a number of state legislatures required coverage, some major insurers are now beginning to include this coverage. To the surprise of many who witnessed the bitter and expensive fights that were waged to avoid this extra coverage, this new cancer procedure comes at a cost of less than $5 per month.

Naturally, these individual items begin to add up to significant savings after a while, but in order to produce major reductions in the price of insurance, the resulting coverage is so riddled with holes that few subscribers find it attractive. Over half the states have enacted so-called "bare bones" laws that allow insurers to sell stripped-down coverage to previously uninsured purchasers at greatly reduced prices. However, in most states these efforts have been a dismal failure and have produced only a modest response in the best circumstances. The mandated benefits most subject to criticism—such as for acupuncture and chiropractic services—add very little to the cost of insurance,[45] and the 10 percent savings produced by paring back most mandates[46] is not sufficient to attract a large number of new subscribers. Therefore, insurers have had to reduce prices by drastically limiting the scope of coverage using very low maximum payment limits. Some bare bones policies cover only 20 days of hospitalization or cap benefits at $50,000 annually. This produces an insurance package that is so unattractive few people wish to purchase it despite its reasonable price, even those who have no insurance at all. Most bare bones laws have resulted in sales of no more than a few hundred policies, and in several states only a few dozen or fewer people have purchased these plans.[47]

The final pot of cold water to throw on the cost-savings potential of greatly reduced insurance is that, once patients are exposed to the costs of treatment, they still may not act as aggressive consumers. Instead, given the fear instilled by illness and the awe in which many people hold their doctors, there is reason to question how much patients will significantly alter their behavior. Evidence from the impressive RAND Health Insurance Experiment suggests not as much as one might think. As discussed in more detail below, the RAND researchers found that patients who pay for almost all of the costs of treatment up to a catastrophic level cut back primarily on initial contacts with their doctors. Doctor visits are not where health spending is excessive in our country, however; the United States has fewer doctor visits per person than most European countries.[48] More important, once patients who pay out of pocket see a doctor, they continue to incur the same level of expense as patients with full insurance, suggesting that they follow their doctors' recommendations blindly regardless of the costs. The combination of this desire to remain well insured and the tendency to follow physicians' advice even when not insured led analysts at RAND to project that eliminating the tax subsidy for health insurance would reduce total health care spending only 2–4 percent.[49]

The Social Dimension of Health Insurance

Health insurance is attractive not only to us as individuals; it is also socially desirable. When people are in peril, our strong instinct is to come to their rescue. This humanitarian instinct is a second important feature of medicine that distinguishes it from other consumer goods and that makes insurance uniquely important. Our country values minimally decent health care as a basic social entitlement, and the only convenient way to meet this social obligation is through some public or private insurance mechanism. We are libertarians to the extent that we leave individuals free for the most part to engage in highly risky behavior, but our humanitarian and egalitarian values come to the forefront when we observe people who are actively suffering from whatever causes, including their own improvidence. Therefore, even when people are in distress due to their own foolish behavior—say, lung cancer caused by a lifetime of smoking or broken bones suffered in a hang-gliding accident—most of us are not content to simply watch them suffer.

This strong rescue ethic expresses itself in many ways that are fundamentally important in making resource allocation decisions.[50] Here, it means that our society will care for people in serious and obvious distress regardless of whether they can pay. This attitude is presently institutionalized in various laws that require even private, for-profit hospitals to accept emergency patients for free.[51] In addition to emergency treatment, most people believe that everyone regardless of poverty or improvidence should have a regular source of care for more routine and non-life-threatening ailments for which there is highly effective treatment, even when that treatment is expensive. For some conditions, universal access is desirable because it helps to contain the spread of contagious diseases; for other, purely individual, conditions, access is still desirable because we cringe at the thought that people may be suffering greatly from easily preventable illness. Many people have an even more expansive commitment to universal access that would make the same level of medical treatment available to everyone on an essentially equal basis regardless of income or health risk behavior, although this position is more controversial.[52]

The critical point for this discussion is that this rescue ethic and egalitarian viewpoint, at whatever level they are embraced, strongly invite a social insurance system of some sort. This is because the need for health care, unlike all other basic social obligations, varies so tremendously from one individual to another. It is possible with food, housing, education, and other similar necessities of life to distribute the basic social minimum in more or less equal increments through vouchers or by providing the service directly. We can all survive on about the same amount of food, none of us requires dramatically more living space than others for basic shelter, and it suffices to dole out educational services in roughly equally amounts. Even if individual needs in these other areas vary by a factor of severalfold, this is minuscule compared with the nearly infinite variation in individual needs for health care. Some people live almost their entire life without a single visit to the doctor; others are severely disabled from birth and require constant care; yet others have sudden and severe episodes of acute illness requiring intensive care.

These extraordinarily diverse medical needs cannot be met through any notion of equal or similar increments of service. Imagine the absurdity of giving each person a booklet of health care coupons to cash in when they are sick, as we do with food stamps. Some would never use their coupons, while others would quickly exhaust all of theirs. Due to this wide variability, the only way to meet our humanitarian commitment to a decent level of health care is to provide universal access to a basic system of support. This system could be supplied by well-staffed and -funded public clinics and hospitals, as it is in some parts of the country, but this system as it now exists is not universal and is woefully underfunded. Instead, we have chosen to rely on a financial reimbursement model that provides access to care in private facilities. This private provision of a social service with widely varying individual needs means that some form of universal insurance is a necessity.

In its present form, this social insurance system operates through the government-run insurance programs of Medicare and Medicaid. Instead of running its own insurance program, the government might also use a system of private insurance that is purchased with publicly funded vouchers. Either way, some form of insurance will remain a necessity for those who do not buy any on their own. And even without an explicit insurance program, the same cost-insulating effect results when people without coverage receive care for free from public or private facilities.

This point goes even further. Not only must everyone have some form of guaranteed coverage in order to satisfy the social obligation of minimal care, but those most in need must receive a type of coverage that insulates them the most from treatment costs. This is true even with the minimalist assumption that our social conscience kicks in only at the level of "catastrophic" coverage rather than demanding strictly equal treatment among all patients. Our sense of what constitutes catastrophe in the realm of health insurance is determined more by the financial consequences than the physical consequences. Health care expenses are catastrophic in relation to one's underlying wealth. Therefore, a minimal safety-net obligation cannot be met through the same type of catastrophic coverage that is purchased by the middle class. Catastrophic coverage for a poor person requires much more insurance than it does for a rich person. Someone who is well off can afford, say, $10,000 a year or more of out-of-pocket expenses whereas a poor person may not be able to afford even $1000 a year. To support the poor person at a catastrophic level requires almost as much insurance as does supporting her comprehensively.[53]

A similar point holds for the elderly and disabled. Although as a group they may be more financially well off than the poor, their average health care expenses are much higher. Therefore, catastrophic insurance would have to cover them for a much greater portion of their total medical expenditures than for the ordinary consumer. Consequently, the poor, the elderly, and the disabled—those presently covered by Medicaid and Medicare—are largely removed from the economizing incentives that market reformers intend to focus on discrete treatment decisions. For these populations, the chances are much greater that, in any given year, they will quickly exhaust their deductibles and fall into the fully insured zone. This is not just a minor abridgment of market reformers' vision. Although these groups constitute a minority of our population, they account for almost half of all treatment costs. On this ground alone, then, individual patients cannot make the bulk of resource allocation decisions for almost half of the potential market.

For patients under public-sponsored insurance, resource allocation decisions must be made either by the provider or by the government. If providers are required to supply the same standard of medical care to these patients as they do to their private patients, then it might be argued that the constraint imposed in the private market will be carried over to the public sector. A uniform standard of care would enforce in the public sector the same cost-sensitive spending decisions made by patients in the private sector. This would be true, however, only at the aggregate level. A broad legal or professional standard of care could never be tailored to the level of particular patients' desires and values that a pure market system is expected to accomplish.

Moreover, this equal standard of care approach is equivalent to embracing a strict egalitarian model for social support, which many market reformers (and others) do not advocate.[54] Instead, they envision that public-supported patients will receive an adequate but lower standard of care. A two-tiered system for public versus private patients is also justified by the pragmatic concern that making public insurance too attractive will deter people from obtaining their own private insurance. A different standard of care for public patients requires, however, some other mechanism for defining the norms of adequacy than simple reference to the existing private market. Necessarily, that nonmarket mechanism must rely on providers, government officials, or other third parties to make medical spending decisions, not the patients themselves who, for the most part, bear few of the costs of treatment.

At this point, it might be helpful to recapitulate the lengthy and complex argument in this section by stating as simply as possible its essential points:

- Our social conscience requires that no one suffer avoidable misery.
- The wide variability in medical needs means that, for health care, this social commitment must be met through some type of guaranteed access to a comprehensive range of services.
- For moral and pragmatic reasons, this public guarantee requires the adoption of a lower standard of care than that prevailing in the private market.
- Those who qualify for public programs cannot be made to bear much of the costs of their care, either due to their poverty or to the magnitude of their health problems.
- The only option, then, is to use nonmarket political, institutional, or professional mechanisms to set the appropriate standard of care.
- This point affects a substantial portion of the medical services rendered in our country.

The Phenomenology of Illness

I wish to return now to a further exploration of why patients find health insurance to be so attractive. So far, we have merely counted up the portion of spending decisions likely to be made without insurance, assuming that people respond to market reforms with the insurance-purchasing behavior that reformers theorize. I will now engage in a more qualitative exploration of whether this behavior is indeed likely or desirable by examining the reasons for patients' reluctance to consider costs in the face of illness. In this analysis, I will explain the phenomenology of illness and the power of healing in order to make the therapeutic case that patients may often recover faster and better if they avoid aggressive consumerism.[55]

Counting on individual patients to wisely allocate health care resources assumes (1) a fully informed and (2) autonomous adult patient (3) paying out of pocket who (4) decides at the time of treatment (5) whether particular items of treatment are worth their costs. This model can be critiqued on each of these assumptions and from a variety of perspectives. With reference to (3)–(5), we have just noted that, for most health care costs, patients in fact will not pay out of pocket since most health care spending occurs within the zone that is insulated even by catastrophic insurance. Further below, we examine with respect to (1) whether patients are actually fully informed. This section will critique the free-market model by questioning assumption (2): whether adult patients should be expected to act as rational and autonomous deliberators when they are ill and seeking treatment.

The Ontological Assault of Illness

The attitude market reformers take toward the effects of illness on patient responsibility is captured by the following passage from medical ethicist Haavi Morreim:

Even in the era of consumerism and informed consent, physicians continue to carry the brunt of the medical and moral responsibilities while patients enjoy freedoms and rights with little responsibility. This pattern needs to be changed. . . . [C]ompetent patients should generally be expected to make their own choices, . . . [i]n other words, patients should not expect physicians to be nannies. Physicians are not responsible for patients. They are responsible only for their own conduct. They should provide careful evaluations and recommendations, and carry out skillfully whatever treatment is mutually chosen. . . . But they are not obligated to out-guess silence, compensate for undisclosed noncompliance, or otherwise take on the neglected tasks of a responsible adult.[56]

This stern attitude is not unique to market reformers. It is shared by the more empathetic perspective that underlies the law of informed consent, which takes the view that patients should be involved in all significant aspects of treatment decision making.

This "hyperrational" vision of autonomous decision making is increasingly coming under attack, however, for ignoring the reality of how patients experience illness. According to Professor Carl Schneider, this autonomy view offers a "picture of human nature [that] is far too simple, far too disembodied . . . , a bloodless, flat, distant, abstract, depersonalized, impoverished view of the way people think, feel, and act."[57] A starkly different picture is painted by narrative accounts written by patients, physicians, and philosophers who are sensitive to the actual phenomenology of illness.[58]

Illness is frequently described as an "ontological assault." It undermines one's personal identity by attacking the fundamental unity of mind and body. In a state of health, our body is part of an integrated sense of self that responds instinctively to our will and serves our inner purposes almost effortlessly. When illness strikes, our body becomes an enemy of self. It does not respond as we wish and its frailties dominate our conscious thoughts. Illness undermines one of our most fundamental assumptions in everyday life—that we will continue to exist and function much as we have in the past. Serious illness shatters our "primordial sense of invulnerability."[59]

The profound incapacitating effect of this assault on our very being is much more debilitating than any of life's other major disruptions, whether they be divorce, incarceration, or impoverishment. Physician and philosopher Edmund Pellegrino observes correctly that

In no other deprivation is the dissolution of the person so intimate that it impairs the capacity to deal with all other deprivations. The poor man can still hope for a change of fortune, the prisoner for a reprieve, the lonely for a friend. But the ill person remains impaired even when freed of these other constraints on the free exercise of his humanity.[60]

Consider also this account by a philosopher and patient who herself suffers from a severe chronic illness, multiple sclerosis:

The most deeply held assumption of daily life is the assumption that I, personally, will continue to be alive and it is in light of this assumption that one engages in daily activities. The onset of illness, however, brings one concretely face-to-face with personal vulnerability. . . . Thus, the person who is ill . . . is unable readily to fit illness into the typified schema used to organize and interpret experience. . . . One finds oneself preoccupied with the demands of the here and now, confined to the present moment, unable effectively to project into the future.[61]

In addition to these profound internal effects, illness exerts powerful external constraints on individual autonomy. When ill we are often immobilized and confined to bed in a prone position and subjected to mind-altering medications. This compromises our physical ability to act and deliberate and places us in a psychological state of dependency. Treatment also compromises physical integrity and exposes us to singular vulnerability by giving physicians unprecedented access to our bodies and personal histories. Treatment requires us to expose every part of ourselves, down to our very blood and guts, while we remain prostrate or unconscious.

Typically, when ill, we do not resist what would otherwise be viewed as utterly repugnant invasions and vulnerabilities. Sickness returns us to an infantile state where our strongest desire is usually to be cared for and to be relieved of the responsibility and anxiety of deciding and acting.[62] "Such sick people . . . may plausibly prefer not to take on any kind of work, much less the fierce, foreign, and forbidding labor of medical decisions."[63] This is true even for the most knowledgeable of patients—physicians themselves. Franz Ingelfinger, M.D., long-time editor of the eminently prestigious *New England Journal of Medicine* and an expert in diseases of the esophagus, found himself in a dilemma over how best to treat his own difficult case of cancer of the esophagus. His doctors, respecting their patient's world-renowned expertise, were leaving this vexing decision to him:

As a result, not only I but my wife, my son and daughter-in-law (both doctors), and other family members became increasingly confused and emotionally distraught. Finally, when the pangs of indecision had become nearly intolerable, one wise physician friend said, "What you need is a doctor." . . . When that excellent advice was followed, my family and I sensed immediate and immense relief.[64]

Taking these stories to heart, many ethicists and theorists are beginning to question the extent to which ordinary adult patients actually desire to make their own medical decisions, even apart from financial considerations.[65] A variety of studies have documented that many patients, when asked, would rather not be forced to make important and difficult medical decisions on their own, when only medical risks and not money are at stake.[66] Although patients want to be informed of what is being done to them and why, and they want the opportunity to refuse treatment altogether, they often prefer that the physician decide which course of treatment is best, and they even more prefer not to be burdened with all the intricate technical decisions about how best to execute that decision. Additional studies have documented that attitudes about patient autonomy differ dramatically among cultural and ethnic groups.[67] Even if this reluctance to decide is only a minority point of view, it is a sensible and significant one. We can only assume that it would be intensified if financial responsibility were added to the medical risk.

It would we cruel in the extreme to force patients who do not want to do so to make their own medical spending decisions when suffering from the debilitation of illness. Hospitals and physician groups increasingly demand a reliable source of payment in advance of treatment rather than waiting afterward to settle up. Not having insurance therefore will force economics into the forefront of patients' deliberations over treatment. Even those who are financially able to assume full exposure to costs could hardly be faulted for being emotionally disabled. Paying for treatment out of pocket forces patients to trade off the chances of recovery against other uses of money for themselves and their families. The treatment option being presented may cut into a child's college education or deny a spouse a promised vacation. It may come at a time when finances are strapped and so result in incurring large debt at the very moment that the patient doubts his ability to continue productive work. Money's influence will not be gentle or kind.

To denigrate this scenario is not necessarily to condemn it as morally wrong; it is only to observe that there are obvious reasons patients might prefer to minimize financial concerns when they are sick, even if the consequence is higher health care costs. Bruce Vladeck, current administrator of Medicare and Medicaid, does a particularly good job of stating this point:

Consumers have sought the kinds of health insurance they have, not because they wish to act irrationally in the aggregate economic sense, but precisely because they don't wish to be forced to make rational trade-offs when they are confronted with medical care consumption decisions. No matter how we draw our curves or shape our abstract arguments, the elemental fact is that medical care is about living and dying, something considered by many to be of a rather different character from the purchase of tomatoes. The primary characteristic of most consumers of medical care most of the time is that they are scared. They are scared of dying, or disfigurement, or permanent disability; and these are serious matters. It is hardly fair to expect any of us to make rational decisions about matters of such import. As a society, we may be prepared to pay a substantial economic premium to insulate people from having to make such decisions.[68]

Advocates of patient decision making respond in two ways to this strong case for insulation from costs. First, they observe that much of medical spending is on elective care for nonurgent conditions that never even approach this level of gravity. But my description of the real experience of illness applies to simple and serious conditions alike. Sickness does not have to be life threatening for it to profoundly affect thinking and functioning. A bad flu bug, a relentless shooting pain, a case of food poisoning, an inconsolable child, or even an unexplained lump or a persistent bad cough can have these menacing and incapacitating effects at least to some degree. Even if this state of mind is the exception in medical treatment encounters, it nevertheless is the dominant explanation of why the medical system exists and why we want insurance. Medical ethics and health care policy should have its primary focus on the quintessential features of the treatment relationship even if those features account for only a fraction of spending decisions. Nor is it possible to craft a market-based scheme that relieves the burdens of decision making only in cases where these concerns are most serious. The cost of treatment has no predictable relationship to the areas of medicine where the psychological dimension is acute. This dimension can be present or absent in large measure both for patients with life-threatening illnesses treated with high-tech medicine and for patients with only temporary discomfort that is easily cured.[69]

Some of the intensity of immediate financial pressure can be tempered at the point of treatment with the Medical Savings Accounts (MSAs) described above. MSAs are a "forced"-savings device similar to pension funds that create a tax-sheltered source to draw on for uninsured medical expenses. Depending on the precise terms of the MSA arrangement, all medical spending decisions up to the deductible threshold of catastrophic insurance coverage would be made with MSA funds. This should relieve a great deal of the anxiety caused by the expense of serious illness and keep patients from making Faustian deals with medical fate. These funds are already set aside for medical treatment and are not immediately available for other uses. Accordingly, a patient will not be hampered by a short-term cash flow problem, bad credit history, or daily consumer temptations. But, to the extent that this is true, patients are not in fact making fully cost-sensitive decisions. The only way to relieve the anxiety of patient spending decisions is to lessen the stakes of the decision. An MSA is one way to lessen those stakes. Another is to purchase insurance that pays 80 percent of all costs. My purpose is not to assert that one way is clearly inferior to the other—only to demonstrate that, either way, patients have good reasons to avoid making fully cost-sensitive treatment decisions even under market-based reforms.

The Mystical Power of Healing

Were medicine an entirely scientific and mechanistic enterprise, the market reformer's vision of active consumerism might prevail, at least for less serious ailments. Then, a patient or family member could evaluate, based on the probabilities and costs, which of several treatment options best achieves the patient's mixed medical and nonmedical objectives. Much of medicine is of this rational quality, but an essential nonrational component of medicine might be destroyed if patients or their families were to assume the arm's-length, adversarial, negotiating stance that epitomizes market transactions. This essential component is the mystical power of healing: by this, I mean the hidden elements of the treatment encounter that result in healing through what might be termed charismatic or self-healing means. The power of healing I refer to is the dimension of doctoring that enables physicians to confer relief through spiritual or emotional means akin to those used by parents or priests.[70]

Before alienating the skeptical reader entirely, let me illustrate with an everyday example from my own experience. Last year when my six-year-old daughter was suffering from a common ear ache, her distress brought her to inconsolable tears while waiting more than an hour to be seen by the doctor. I convinced a nurse to take her temperature, give her an aspirin, and say a few kind words of reassurance. Instantaneously, my daughter felt much better, far quicker than any possible pharmacological effect could have taken hold. I was puzzled by this abrupt improvement until I had my own excruciating ear ache a few weeks later and experienced exactly the same sort of instantaneous relief as soon as the doctor examined me and wrote a prescription. Knowing that I was in the good hands of a trained professional who offered the prospect of relief produced in me a sense of exhilaration and a release of anxiety accompanied by a pronounced improvement of my symptoms. This instantaneous recovery might be attributed simply to excessive nerves or to a more complex type of placebo effect but, however labeled or explained, it was effective. The pain was not just more bearable; it went away.

Researchers and physicians have documented countless similar examples of mundane and miraculous relief caused by a largely nonscientific or "nonspecific" process of healing.[71] This placebo effect is not limited to purely psychological states, bizarre conditions, especially susceptible patients, or manipulative physicians. This effect has been documented in the treatment of diabetes, cancer, and heart disease, for instance, and without the physicians even intending to cause the effect. In one scientific study, two sets of patients were subjected to different surgical procedures to treat angina (chest pain): In one, the standard chest operation was performed; in the other, only a pretence of operating was made by cutting the skin under anesthesia. Both the sham and the real procedure produced equal relief of physical symptoms.[72] A review of other surgical and medical procedures once firmly believed to be effective but later discarded as entirely unfounded led one author to speculate that placebo healing effects may be present to a significant extent in 70 percent of all clinical encounters.[73]

Those who have studied this nonspecific healing effect conclude that it pervades medicine, both in modern times and in prescientific and primitive cultures.[74] This is because the effect is connected more to the intervention of the healer than it is to the particular therapeutic agent used. Put another way, the doctor himself is a therapeutic agent, regardless of the actual effectiveness of the particular drug or procedure.[75] In each culture and each era, there has been a prevailing theory of medical treatment, many of which are pure fantasy if not dangerous, yet remarkably few have been proven to be wholly without benefit. Doctors and healers have been universally respected throughout the ages and across primitive and advanced societies; we can only assume that most of them have offered some form of relief despite the now-apparent quackery they once practiced. Indeed, it has often been said that the history of medicine until this century has been the history of the placebo effect. Now that medicine has a firm scientific foundation, this mystical or charismatic element has been surpassed by technological skill, but it will never be entirely displaced. One of the prominent trends in modern medicine is the revival of both popular and scientific interest in these poorly understood domains of caring for patients through alternative or holistic schools of medicine.[76]

The best scientific explanation for this charismatic healing effect is that the process of treatment, and not its specific content, has universal benefit for many or most illnesses, regardless of the specific physiological effects of the treatment. The treatment process has this universal healing power by virtue of the archetypal characteristics that activate the patient's own healing mechanisms—mechanisms that are still largely undiscovered and unexplained. This is best demonstrated by the fact that the basic structure of the treatment encounter is remarkably the same across all systems of medicine, including Western, Eastern, religious, herbal, and primitive. In each of these belief systems, society recognizes the healing powers of a professional elite (physicians or shamans) that administers personally to the patient with physical touching and healing agents (drugs or herbs), often in a dramatic and cathartic ritualistic process (surgery or exorcism) performed in a setting specially designed for the purpose (hospital or bonfire). In this process, patients feel cared for (by nurses or mystics), they are given an explanation for their condition (diagnosis or demonization) that is consistent with their prevailing belief system (scientific medicine or spirit worship), and they are assigned tasks of self-care in which they take responsibility in part for their own improvement (dietary regimen or prayer).[77]

These many symbolic structural elements are thought to activate patients' internal healing powers through a variety of psychological channels. A patient who knows someone is devoted to caring for him is able to release the dread and anxiety that may be heightening discomfort and weakening the body's resistance. Believing in the power of the healer may enable the patient to regress to an earlier, more infantile state of mind that enhances this release and the resulting comfort. This confidence in the healer is elevated by the healer's status in society, by his invocation of methods consistent with that society's belief system, and by his offering an explanation of the otherwise-troubling and disorienting disease that makes sense to the patient. And this belief is further cemented by the ritualistic and dramatic elements of laying on of hands, taking of medication, climactic performance, and hallowed setting.

Interesting, you might say, but what does this have to do with patient cost sharing? The point is obviously not that paying for care out of pocket per se undermines these healing powers, for none of these systems of care other than scientific medicine has developed under comprehensive insurance. The point is this: When paying out of pocket, it is difficult for patients or families to act as aggressive and skeptical consumers if this mystical healing power is to be given its strongest effect. Critical to this healing power is the patient's confidence and trust in the healer. "The image of omnipotence is an essential component of the healer."[78]

The healer appears able to activate the patient's own healing mechanisms because the patient turns himself over both in mind and body to the healer. "A patient's hope and trust lead to a 'letting go' that counteracts stress and is often the key to getting well."[79] Psychiatrists, starting with Freud, have described this phenomenon as "transference," in which patients foist on their healers qualities they formerly attributed to their parents in infancy when parents were viewed as all-powerful and all-knowing. "Deep in patients' unconscious, physicians are viewed as miracle workers, patterned after the fantasied all-caring parents of infancy. Medicine, after all, was born in magic and religion, and the doctor-priest-magician-parent unity that persists in patients' unconscious cannot be broken."[80] It is plausible to assume, although we do not know for sure, that maintaining this unity requires relinquishing the skepticism, critical faculties, and other defense mechanisms used in ordinary consumer transactions.

Advocates of patient autonomy might respond that these limitations on decision-making capacity do not undermine their case because they merely justify the patient delegating his spending authority to a family member. Partial incapacity does not justify insulating both the patient and his family from all personal and financial responsibility. Indeed, this is the way that medical decision making has always been handled in most serious treatment situations. Physicians communicate just as actively with families as they do with patients, and these decisions are often made collectively within the family and communicated by family members. Therefore, the patient's reluctance to decide is beside the point. There is much truth to this rebuttal, but it is not wholly convincing. Many patients have no family members able or willing to assume this role. For those that do, the family also is anxious about the prospects for recovery, perhaps more so than the patient, and therefore they too long to place trust and responsibility in an authoritative practitioner. The family may be better situated than the patient to scrutinize the doctor's decisions, but they may also be equally reluctant to do so. I hasten to concede that none of these assertions is known with any degree of empirical confidence. We are forced into this highly speculative reading of anecdotal accounts from physicians, anthropologists, and enthnographic researchers since empirical testing of this nonspecific healing power is very difficult and has not been widely attempted.[81] Nevertheless, many informed observers and patients view the charismatic dimension of healing as fundamental to the treatment relationship. Most of these accounts do not address the precise question before us: the desirability of patients or families bargaining aggressively over price. Instead, others have analyzed what meaning the healer's charismatic power has for issues of medical ethics such as informed consent. They have concluded that this healing power does not absolve physicians from the obligation to talk with their patients.[82] However, these same commentators acknowledge that proper respect for the healing relationship limits patients' ability to aggressively scrutinize their doctors' decisions.

If this account of the therapeutic benefit inherent in all clinical encounters is plausible on its face, then patients and their families may have strong reasons not to act as adversarial consumers at the point of treatment decision making. Adopting this skeptical attitude could reduce an archetypal parent-like or priest-like relationship to a mechanistic craft that for many illnesses may nullify its most potent element. Even if the core benefit of medical encounters can be preserved in a more actively consumerist environment, these concerns raise serious questions about whether patients who are given the chance will actually choose to engage in the discrete cost/benefit reflections that economists assume. Patients' desires to turn the burdens of decision making over to a trained and trusted professional may cause them either to resist greater cost sharing or to resist making economic decisions even if they are bearing more of the costs. Either possibility would partially undermine the economic case for catastrophic insurance.

The Quality of Patients' Medical Spending Decisions

It is useful to distinguish between critiques of market reforms that are internal to market theory and critiques that are external. The prior discussion is an internal critique because it uses criteria taken from economics itself. The case for consumer-driven spending decisions is only so strong in economic terms—as is a consumer's own desire to be exposed to the costs of treatment. If patients in fact prefer to remain insulated from costs, it simply does not matter whether they might be capable of making better resource allocation decisions than doctors or third parties. They simply won't decide. This section adopts a different perspective. It assumes patients will be willing to make their own spending decisions but it questions the starting premise of economic theory—that the resulting allocation of health care resources will, on the whole, be superior to the allocation that would result if others were to decide for patients. This is an external critique of economic theory because it challenges the assumption that whatever informed consumers choose is by definition optimal. The following discussion counters this underlying premise with analysis of and evidence on whether patients in fact do better when they have more responsibility for the costs of their own treatment.

Penny Wise and Pound Foolish?

Hardly any consumers feel able to make intelligent health care spending decisions *entirely* on their own. Medical science is so complex and rapidly changing that even doctors usually are not confident about making treatment decisions for themselves or their families outside their area of specialization. Patients sometimes develop extraordinary expertise in their particular condition, especially when the ailment is chronic and so produces a long history of treatment encounters. But this surely is a small minority of patients. Most have no opportunity or inclination, to learn about all the factors that go into complex clinical judgment. Even well-educated people fail to think about medical issues in quasi-scientific terms.[83] One representative survey found that only 10 percent of Americans can provide a minimally correct explanation of what bacteria are, and only 20 percent know enough about DNA to understand a typical news story about it.[84] Carl Schneider comments that "the patient's vision will often . . . be clouded by the mass of unreliable medical information, folklore, and superstition most of us have assimilated over a lifetime of inattentive reading, careless listening, forgotten science, and outdated learning."[85]

Market advocates respond that this state of consumer ignorance is an artifact of the historical noncompetitiveness of the medical market. Patients lack the knowledge and experience required to make their own medical spending decisions because they have never been forced to do so. If insurance were structured so that patients bore the cost consequences of treatment decisions, they would have a strong motivation to acquire the necessary information, and providers would have the reciprocal incentive to supply that information. Other well-functioning markets are able to develop adequate sources of information on issues involving complex judgment. It is no more necessary for patients to go to medical school before making intelligent health care spending decisions than it is for them to have mechanical engineering degrees before buying a car. Both for medical and for transportation decisions, consumers can rely on comparative performance statistics, expert evaluations (for example, *Consumer Reports*), and general reputation and word of mouth. Indeed, impressive advances are occurring even now in the quality and quantity of medical information sources for consumers. Examples include interactive video explanations by former patients of the consequences of making certain difficult treatment decisions,[86] and "report cards" or other statistical profiles that compare the performance of different doctors, hospitals, and HMOs.

I have great enthusiasm for these innovations in giving patients much greater understanding of the medical spending decisions they face at the time of treatment. But, without empirical verification, it is difficult to know whether patients on the whole will make good spending decisions or whether they will be penny wise and pound foolish. Some strong empirical evidence does exist, but before examining it, it is helpful to explore this debate further at a conceptual level.

The argument that patients will acquire the ability to make better informed spending decisions is not fully convincing at a conceptual level because there are several reasons why health care decisions are entirely different from other complex consumer choices. These are reasons that go beyond the platitude that health care decisions are more important, although we should not lose sight of the force of that observation. The advantages of consumer decision making grow stronger as the stakes of the decision grow higher. So, too, we should have greater concern for deficits in consumer knowledge when death and disability are threatened. This observation alone does not distinguish medicine, though, because other consumer purchases also suffer from information deficits and also threaten life and limb, yet we still rely to a considerable extent on market allocation mechanisms.[87] Medicine, however, has several unique attributes that make the force of these antimarket arguments much stronger.

The primary difference between medicine and many other consumer goods is that most important medical decisions occur only once in a person's life and at a time of crisis. This means there is no opportunity to learn by repeated trial and error. Pure markets work best when each consumer makes immediate consumption decisions frequently over an extended period. Examples include consumables such as food, clothing, and entertainment. Even for major consumer purchases such as houses, cars, and computers, or other serious economic decisions such as job choices, there are several decision points and learning opportunities over the course of a lifetime. But most people who are afflicted with illness have only one bypass operation, one bout of cancer, or one bad car accident. Therefore, there is reason to believe they lack the information necessary to make correct decisions, where incorrect is defined as later coming to regret their decision.[88]

The second fundamental difference between health care and other market goods concerns outside sources of consumer information. For other goods, if information does not come from direct consumer experience, it is acquired through countless other sources such as word of mouth, surveys, and advertisements. Although these other sources are available for health care, it is unlikely they will ever displace patients' primary reliance on their personal physician. For most of us most of the time, we make our medical decisions based on the information presented by the same doctor who will either perform the treatment or who will choose the treating doctor to whom we are referred. As sociologist Paul Starr explains:

> when ill and in need of care, most patients cannot readily shop around comparing prices. They generally do not feel they know enough even to ask the right questions. When they first seek medical care, people usually are uncertain about what their treatment will ultimately involve, much less cost. And once they are in the middle of treatment, changing providers is often not feasible. Particularly when patients are hospitalized, decisions about treatment are in the hands of doctors and other professionals. For most patients in the midst of illness, therefore, price-conscious purchasing is literally impossible.[89]

Bodenheimer and Grumbach make this point somewhat facetiously:

> [A patient] develops acute abdominal pain and goes to the hospital to purchase a remedy for her pain. The physician tells her that she has acute cholecystitis or a perforated ulcer and recommends hospitalization, abdominal sonogram, and upper endoscopy. Will [a patient], lying on a gurney in the emergency department and clutching her abdomen with one hand, use her other hand to leaf through her *Textbook of Internal Medicine* to determine whether she really needs these services, and should she have brought along a copy of *Consumer Reports* to learn where to purchase them at the cheapest price?"[90]

The possibility of second opinions always exists, but they are infrequently obtained. Most patients are content to rely on their physicians' discretion so long as they are told what decision the doctor is making and why.[91] Other, more self-reliant, patients like to have a menu of options presented to them and sufficient explanation in order to make their own selection, but even then many want to know which choice their doctor would make if it were her decision, and few are willing to disagree with the doctor's recommendation.

Naturally, this reliance on expert opinion improves the quality of decision making over what would occur if patients made their own, ill-informed medical decisions. But this still is not the economist's ideal because there is no easy way for consumers to evaluate the quality of their physicians' recommendations. There are several reasons apart from the physician's technical competence to question whether doctors make optimal spending recommendations. Physicians are paid to perform the treatment chosen and their recommendation is economically biased by the method of payment. Depending on the type of payment and type of physician, the bias might be toward more, less, or different treatment than the patient ideally would desire.[92] Physicians also have a professional stake in treatment decisions. Their intellectual curiosity, desire to develop new skills, and interest in advancing medical science may cause them to lean one way or the other for reasons not strictly in accord with an individual patient's value system.[93] As a consequence, medical decisions made by treating physicians will differ predictably from what patients would make on their own if fully informed.

For these reasons, it is not feasible to expect a viable consumer-driven market to develop for discrete treatment decisions, similar to the one that exists, for instance, in car *repairs*. Instead, the market that seems natural for health care is similar to the one that exists for the *purchase* of new or used automobiles. In theory, a market for auto purchases could exist that required the purchaser to specify the precise mechanical components of the car, much like we now assemble unique configurations for entertainment centers or for IBM-clone computers. But instead we purchase cars according to the manufacturers' general reputation and the performance statistics of a limited number of models. Similarly, even if all artificial distortions, subsidies, and regulations were removed from the market in health care, the form of decision making that is likely to take hold is not one where consumers deliberate over the cost-effectiveness of individual items of treatment. Instead, consumers are likely to want to make informed choices over more manageable bundles of decisions, namely, by choosing among providers or insurance plans based on general reputation or overall performance statistics.

A cost-conscious market in the choice of physicians or insurers may be all that most market reformers have in mind, but this is not the system of patient-made spending decisions described at the outset of this chapter. Instead, the market-driven choice of doctor or insurer assigns spending authority to one of the other allocation systems discussed in the remainder of this book. *Managed care* is the name given these other systems, and it is managed care that advocates of patient cost sharing view as the antithesis of their ideal. To describe a properly functioning market in terms of the informed choice of physicians and insurers, then, is to concede that, for a large portion of medicine, patients should not make their own discrete spending decisions.

These limits on consumer knowledge and judgment are so apparent that they are hardly remarked upon in the existing medical market. The economist's argument that consumer scrutiny of physician behavior will intensify when market forces become more dominant loses sight of the fact that an extremely active market has long existed in medicine. It is a market in the quality of care. For the very reason that conventional insurance is so excessive, patients have strong incentives and unconstrained ability to shop aggressively over the quality of care. But these strong market forces express themselves for the most part only in the careful evaluation and selection of physicians and hospitals, not in detailed scrutiny of individual treatment decisions. Few people would argue now, when for the most part only medical risk is at stake and not economic costs, that patients would be well served if they made their own treatment decisions.

Physicians are much more than skilled craftsmen. Patients would be foolish to relegate their physicians to the perfunctory role of merely executing the instructions given to them, like some barber who is told where and how much to cut. It is unrealistic to expect any fundamentally different role for patient decision making to emerge from market reform. Although the introduction of strong cost considerations would dramatically alter the substance of medical decision making, there is no reason to expect that costs will alter the basic structure of decision-making authority. Instead, the sources of information and the contours of patient involvement will almost certainly remain about the same, only the decisions will now be more informed by their cost consequences.

Because the optimal shape of a market in health care appears to be one where patients rely heavily on their doctors' advice, two conclusions can be drawn: either (1) market reforms will not in fact cause most patients most of the time to make their own spending decisions at the level of individual treatment choices, or (2) if patients do make such decisions, the decisions will not be as good as those that would be made if patients deferred to their physicians. Remarkably, both of these possibilities have been shown to exist simultaneously in an extraordinary social science study known as the RAND Health Insurance Experiment.

The RAND Health Insurance Experiment

It is rare to be able to turn to rigorous empirical science to help resolve conceptual debates like the ones in this chapter. But just such an opportunity exists by virtue of the massive social experiment in health insurance conducted by The RAND Corporation, a nonprofit research think tank. The RAND Health Insurance Experiment is one of the largest controlled experiments ever conducted in any field of social inquiry and human behavior.[94] What makes this research so remarkable is that, unlike most social science work, it was not merely the study of naturally occurring behavior. Instead, these researchers designed a controlled experiment that enabled them to draw much more powerful conclusions than is normally possible. A controlled experiment is much better than observing natural events because it creates much greater confidence that any observed differences in behavior are caused by the specific factors introduced into the experiment. In a natural, uncontrolled setting, the risk is much greater that observed behavior is caused by hidden factors that are impossible to measure.

The RAND experiment randomly assigned 2000 families throughout the country to 14 different health insurance policies for three-to-five-year periods and then observed the resulting patterns of treatment, spending, and health outcomes. This experiment has produced a rich source of evidence on many of the most important questions in health care public policy.[95] Our focus here is on the consequences of patients paying for more of their treatment out of pocket. The experimental insurance plans differed primarily according to the amount of coinsurance required of participants. The "free care" plans required participants to pay none or only 5 percent of the costs of treatment, whereas the catastrophic plan required them to pay for 95 percent of the costs, up to an annual maximum of $1000 or a percentage of their income, whichever was less.[96] In between these extremes, other participants were enrolled in plans with 25 percent and 50 percent coinsurance, subject to the same or similar annual maximums ($1000 or 5–15 percent of income). Patients were allowed to see any doctor they wanted, and providers were paid their normal charges on a fee-for-service basis (except for the one HMO plan discussed in Chapter 4).

The RAND researchers then collected hordes of information about health status and patient satisfaction from lengthy questionnaires and extensive diaries kept by the participants, as well as from direct medical examinations. This information was used to develop a variety of measures for participants' general mental and physical health status, physical and social functioning, specific diseases, personal attitudes, health habits, and risk of dying.[97] The researchers also evaluated the appropriateness of discrete treatment encounters by having a panel of independent expert physicians review selected medical records.

The RAND researchers made several findings of critical importance to our inquiry. Under some measures of health status, participants were demonstrably worse off as a result of greatly increased cost sharing, although not to a very dramatic extent. People with free care had lower blood pressure, better corrected vision, and a lower risk of dying from poor health or health behaviors. More troubling, however, is that these effects where more pronounced for low-income participants (those with income up to two times the federal poverty level), even though much of the impact of cost sharing was dampened by limiting their financial exposure to a percentage of their income.[98]

These findings are supported by other, less revealing studies that establish that people without any insurance or with limited insurance are in worse health than those with full insurance. For instance, people without any insurance have a 20–50 percent greater risk of death than those with private insurance, and uninsured patients have three times greater chance of having a poor outcome during a hospital stay.[99] What these uncontrolled research studies fail to reveal is whether paying out of pocket causes the worsened health status, whether people in bad health cannot obtain full insurance, or whether some third factor such as age, employment, location, or income causes both poor health and worse insurance.

So far, these are findings on the *aggregate* effects of cost sharing on spending and health. These aggregate findings are amplified by the RAND study's analysis of individual treatment encounters. To evaluate the appropriateness of treatment, independent expert physicians reviewed selected medical records in detail to determine whether patients who avoided treatment costs as a result of cost sharing made objectively good treatment decisions. There were two surprising findings, both of which are troubling for market reformers. First, patients did not use good judgment about whether to consult a physician at the outset. Those who paid more out of pocket cut back on physician visits and hospitalizations across the board—both for conditions where treatment would be highly effective and those where treatment would likely be ineffective.[100] Again, this detrimental response was much more pronounced for low-income participants. Even when the decision to see a doctor involved their children, low-income participants were much more likely to forego highly effective care than were other participants, despite the lower financial exposure to low-income participants (due to the percentage-of-income cap).

On the other hand, once patients sought treatment, they received the same level of care regardless of how much they had to pay out of pocket.[101] This is strong evidence confirming the speculation above that patients are both not capable of making good individual treatment decisions on their own and that they rely heavily on their physicians' recommendations even when they are paying out of pocket. At the point of deciding whether or not to go to the doctor, RAND patients who paid out of pocket were unable to selectively reduce predominantly ineffective visits, but once they went to the doctor, they received treatment to the same extent as those who did not have to pay.

These findings confirm that increased cost sharing will lower health care spending, but they cast considerable doubt on whether catastrophic insurance alone will result in improved cost effectiveness. Efficiency entails not just saving money but choosing wisely how to spend it. The dilemma is that in the nonideal settings in which most medicine is practiced, patients rely primarily on physician advice to know what to do, and physicians' judgments are affected by how they are paid and what they know about their patients. The RAND study did not evaluate changes in physician payment, nor can it be used to demonstrate the more systemic effects that would occur when market reforms are wide spread. Physicians might be much more responsive to cost constraints if all, not just a small portion, of their patients were paying substantial amounts out of pocket. Even though this is doubtlessly true, it would mean that resource allocation would occur more through expert physician judgment than through patients just saying no. This only confirms that, if cost savings are to be achieved at the same time that the quality of decision making is improved, some method must be found to influence the behavior of physicians, not just patients, at the point of treatment. That influence might be the loss of business from patients who are not satisfied, but it also might come from the manner in which physicians are paid, or how their work is supervised by insurers or regulators—the decision making mechanisms explored in Chapters 3 and 4.

Inherent and Practical Complexities

There is one more line of attack on market reforms that place the primary responsibility for health care spending decisions on individual patients. It is to examine the intricate details needed to implement such a scheme in the complexities of the real world. In the abstract, it is a simple proposition for patients to pay more of the costs of their treatment out of pocket; all that is required is to make insurance less comprehensive. In practice, however, this is not so easily accomplished. I will use the proposal for medical savings accounts (MSAs) outlined above as the primary example to illustrate this point, but the same points apply with varying force to virtually any market reform proposal.[102]

MSAs allow consumers to place the money they save by purchasing cheaper insurance in a tax-protected savings account they can draw from to pay for their increased out-of-pocket medical costs. The main difficulty in implementing the MSA proposal as a vehicle for increased patient cost sharing is to make MSAs attractive enough in comparison with existing, highly subsidized comprehensive insurance such that consumers will voluntarily opt for them. MSA proposals confront this difficulty because it would be contrary to market theory to force consumers into any particular form of insurance they did not voluntarily choose, but it is politically infeasible to eliminate the tax subsidy that makes comprehensive insurance so attractive at present. Therefore, if MSAs are not made attractive enough, they will have little impact simply because few people will choose them. Witness the low level of enthusiasm for existing flexible spending accounts, which are offered by fewer than 10 percent of employers and are elected by only a small minority of employees even when available.[103]

If MSAs are made too attractive, however, their cost-savings potential will be severely dampened, thereby undercutting their very purpose. Some proposals make MSAs attractive by extending the existing tax subsidy so that it covers the out-of-pocket payments that previously were not insured and therefore that were paid for with after-tax dollars. This would encourage subscribers to overfund their MSAs, making them even more willing to incur medical expenses than at present. Thus, depending on how MSAs are constructed, at the extreme they may well result in patients giving almost no thought to the costs of any of their treatment, both below and above the high deductible level, with the result that MSAs could make the cost-insulating effect of insurance even more extensive than it now is.

To illustrate, a typical subscriber now pays for the first $500 of medical costs entirely out of pocket and 20 percent thereafter with after-tax (nonsubsidized) dollars. Under most MSA proposals, all spending below the deductible is wrapped into the MSA and receives a tax subsidy proportionate to the patient's federal tax bracket, which ranges from about 15 to 40 percent for most people. If costs remain low or if the deductible is not raised, then consumers are better off with MSAs than with conventional insurance, since 100 percent of $500 dollars (under conventional insurance) is a worse hit than 60 percent of $500 (under tax-subsidized MSAs). The MSA imposes more individual cost sharing only when medical spending exceeds about $800 for someone in a 40 percent bracket.[104]

Even costs above this break-even level may have little actual impact on patients' spending deliberations if patients do not perceive that the money taken from MSA accounts is available for other medical or nonmedical uses. True, most MSA proposals allow unspent funds to be rolled forward for medical expenses in future years, and eventually to be "cashed out" upon retirement, perhaps as pure income or perhaps to pay for long-term nursing care. But it is unconvincing to assert that the possibility of saving for these potential future uses will have as strong a cautionary effect on present spending as does having the cash immediately in hand. Indeed, it is this very suppression of the immediacy of the financial carrot/stick that is viewed as one of the advantages of the MSA version of catastrophic insurance, but this advantage works to the disadvantage of the proposal's cost-savings goal. To economists, money in the bank may be equivalent to money in the pocket, but for many people, pocket money burns a hole while invested money is easily forgotten.

What is most dysfunctional about the MSA proposal is not that it strikes the wrong balance between the two competing concerns of excessive versus anemic cost consciousness; rather, it is that this balance is left entirely to bureaucratic, centralized decision making instead of to market forces.[105] Because the MSA device relies heavily on tax subsidies for its implementation, whether it will be viewed as attractive to the rational subscriber depends much more on that subscriber's individual tax situation and his perceived immediate medical needs than on the subscriber's more general attitude about bearing risk versus shifting risk. Therefore, some subscribers who, in a subsidy-neutral environment would otherwise prefer less insurance and more individual responsibility might opt out of MSAs because of restrictions on how these savings accounts are accumulated and spent, whereas others who might prefer more insulation from cost and would be willing to pay the price for regular, unsubsidized insurance will be seduced into MSAs by their too-generous tax breaks.

Just as market theory says that only the market can determine the optimal level of health care spending, so this theory must hold that only the undistorted market can determine the optimal types and amounts of insurance coverage. For just this reason, managed care advocate Mark Pauly has teamed up with MSA advocate John Goodman to propose a tax credit that equally encourages the purchase of any type of health insurance.[106] While leveling the tax playing field might make the existing market distortions less severe, the resulting scheme will still involve the government in a great degree of social engineering just to set the terms of the contest among insurance types. For MSAs, the government must establish the highest acceptable deductible level, the components of a minimum benefits package, the size of tax subsidy needed to induce optimal participation, exactly how money in the account can be spent, what uses can be made of unspent funds carried forward, how large the account can eventually be allowed to grow, and whether accumulated sums can ever be cashed out for nonmedical needs such as retirement income. These complex design issues mean that the government must make many of the same social policy decisions as if the government were to subsidize health spending directly.

The degree of government intervention needed to make markets behave properly is also seen in other features of MSAs that cause potential market dislocations of various sorts. For instance, aggressive public subsidies for MSAs would hamper the emerging market in comprehensive managed care plans. This is because MSAs are designed to fit with catastrophic insurance, which is typically sold only in a conventional fee-for-service form. The clearest sign of this is that MSAs are being touted most aggressively by smaller "niche" insurers who do not typically offer any managed care products because they lack the market concentration and capital to assemble competitive managed care networks.[107]

MSAs are incompatible with managed care because the portion below the deductible threshold is intended to be spent freely from the MSA without even the forms of utilization review that are typical in fee-for-service insurance. After all, it's the patient's own money, so she should be free to spend it on anything she wants. Amounts above the MSA deductible are likewise subjected to only minimal managed care oversight since it would be very cumbersome to require patients to enter an HMO treatment setting only when their spending exceeds a threshold in a certain year. Moreover, these higher amounts are expected to carry no cost-sharing responsibility from the patient, not even the typical 20 percent, because they occur above a catastrophic, stop-loss level. Although it is possible to alter these various features so that MSAs fit better with managed care insurance, doing so may require additional government intervention.

The risk that MSAs will destabilize rather than improve the health insurance market is also seen in their potential for creating biased or adverse selection. Biased selection results when one type of insurance, because of its particular attributes, attracts subscribers whose health risk differs from a cross section of the population. An insurance plan that attracts healthier subscribers experiences favorable selection; one that attracts sicker subscribers experiences adverse selection. It is obvious that subscribers who expect few or no medical expenses will find catastrophic policies coupled with MSAs to be more attractive than the more expensive conventional comprehensive insurance, and just the opposite will be true for chronically ill subscribers.[108] Once this pattern sets into place, it could snowball to an extent that the comprehensive insurance option becomes economically unviable because it attracts only the sickest patients. This would result if the price of comprehensive insurance begins to spiral up as healthier patients leave for MSAs, making comprehensive insurance so expensive that virtually no one finds it attractive. Short of this extreme, biased selection can result in the price of MSA insurance being artificially low and that of comprehensive insurance being artificially high.[109] This may make some of the perceived savings from MSAs purely illusory; in other words, they may not really be reducing medical expenditures, but only shifting them onto other companies. Of more serious theoretical concern, these artificial price distortions can result in people being forced into MSAs who do not prefer this increased risk exposure.[110]

The magnitude of this biased selection effect will depend on the structure of the market and the array of choices consumers face. Of critical importance are whether the purchase of *any* insurance is mandatory or optional; how many insurance options each consumer faces or whether the choice is made by the employer for the whole group; and the degree of difference among the choices. For the most part, empirical findings are largely anecdotal. Within the Federal Employee Health Benefits Program (covering all federal workers), adverse selection resulted in the high-option (low deductible) fee-for-service plan in one area attracting risks that were 50 percent higher than the plan's actuarial value based on standard risks, whereas the low-option (high deductible) version of the same plan attracted risks that were about 40 percent lower than the plan's value based on standard risks.[111] Another study found that an insurer offering two different plans with the same actuarial value attracted subscribers with 79 percent higher claims to one than to the other.[112] As a consequence of these adverse selection problems, several fee-for-service plans and dozens of HMOs withdrew from the federal employee system during the late 1980s. Similar problems have plagued the California Public Employees Retirement System[113] as well as large private employers offering multiple options. In one study, a high-option plan attracted enrollees that were as much as four times more expensive than those who chose the low-option plan from the same employer.[114]

Correcting for these possible market dislocations requires complex mechanisms and formulae for measuring and adjusting the relative risk differentials among insurance pools. A full treatment of this topic is beyond the scope of this book, but suffice it to say that we are still a number of years away from having sophisticated and validated risk adjustment measures. Even were they available, their construction and application would once again involve government regulators in making centralized policy decisions, thereby displacing a significant portion of the value judgments that MSA proponents intend the market to make. For instance, if risk adjustment gave credit for being overweight, smoking, or having three drinks a night—all valid indicators of likely medical costs—then subscribers would be sent an economic signal that these costs and behaviors are of no concern to the community, but if these factors were not given credit, then we would be adopting a social policy that penalized people for perfectly legal lifestyle choices while not penalizing others, such as those who parachute for a hobby, have high-risk occupations, or are in child-bearing years. There is no consensus on which social policy is correct, but some decision must be made in order to have a smoothly operating market that offers greater consumer choice.

These administrative complexities are not unique to the particular attributes of MSAs. Similar complications arise under virtually any market reform proposal that seeks to impose greater patient cost sharing. For instance, simple unadorned catastrophic insurance would better meet the economic ideal if the deductible were adjusted to the level of the subscriber's income rather than being fixed for everyone. The goal of catastrophic coverage is to expose patients to the full cost of treatment up to amounts they can afford and to reserve insurance for amounts that would expose them to serious hardship or denial. This make-or-break level obviously differs widely among individuals. However, to vary the deductible is also to vary the value of the insurance. Accordingly, a sliding-scale form of catastrophic insurance would require variable rather than fixed subsidies. But how rapidly this income adjustment should be phased in and how graduated the deductible should be are questions of social engineering that only the government can decide.

Similarly, proposals to remove all subsidies and government controls from the insurance market incorrectly suggest that markets can be left entirely alone. Although economist Mark Pauly and his colleagues do not go quite that far, they do advocate abolishing the tax subsidy that attaches to employer-purchased group insurance and requiring individuals to purchase insurance on their own, with the support of an individual tax credit.[115] This switch from group to individual insurance would cause the variation in individual prices to dramatically increase, however, since healthier and sicker subscribers would no longer be pooled together in employer groups. Pauly argues that the cost-spreading function performed by group insurance can be replaced with vouchers that are adjusted for each subscriber's risk classification. That is, older or sicker people would receive a more valuable voucher since they would face a higher price in the unregulated market. But how much more valuable is a question for social policy decision making, not one that the market can make on its own. If the government were simply to pay a percentage of the cost of any insurance selected, it would be reintroducing close to the same subsidy that exists now in the tax laws. But for the government instead to independently set a fixed voucher amount that varies by objective measures of age and health status, it must have a system for valuing age and for measuring health status.

The point of this section, simply put, is that no proposal for market reform in health care can eliminate the government from making substantive decisions that affect resource allocation. The government's role can be minimized, but not exterminated. How far in the background the government should remain is of course an issue that produces considerable disagreement, which I have not attempted to resolve here. My purpose is only to establish yet another reason why it is facile to assume that we can allocate health care resources entirely, or even predominantly, through spending decisions made exclusively by individual patients at the time of treatment. Instead, we must continue to explore the proper role for cost-sensitive decision making by physicians, insurers, and the government.

CONCLUSION

On balance, increased patient cost sharing is an attractive mechanism for allocating a portion of health care spending. Even though patients have very good reasons for not wanting to be fully exposed to the economic consequences of their treatment decisions, existing tax law and market structures provide them too much shelter. Medical Savings Accounts are a particularly appealing way to implement market-based insurance reform because they create a vehicle for making the purchase of catastrophic insurance more attractive than at present. MSAs encourage employers to contribute to employees the money they save from switching to high-deductible insurance by neutralizing the tax penalty that would otherwise result from this shift.

Patient cost sharing can carry us only so far, however. Even when tax subsidies are removed or equalized, consumers will still choose to purchase a considerable amount of insurance, which means that a large majority of health care spending will still be controlled by physicians, insurers, or the government. The need for insurance is even greater for those who cannot reasonably afford much of their medical care on their own: the poor, elderly, and disabled. Since these groups account for a major portion of all health care spending, the potential for patient cost sharing is even further reduced.

Even if patient cost sharing is successful in holding down spending, there are grounds for serious concern about the quality of decision making that will result. Patients lack the information and capacity to make their own treatment decisions, and when forced to do so, their health may suffer. Optimal patient care, and patients' own preferences, appear to require delegating substantial authority to physicians, even when patients are exposed to financial risk.

Finally, the complexities of designing a workable market in real-world settings require us to depart from the market ideal. Government controls are necessary to keep the introduction of a radically different form of insurance from exacerbating adverse selection in a manner that might render other, desirable forms of insurance unavailable or less affordable. Of particular concern is that MSAs appear incompatible with tightly managed systems of health care delivery such as HMOs, even though these are at least equally effective at containing costs and satisfying consumers.

Therefore, it is easy to conclude that, despite the many positive features of patient cost sharing, it is does not comprise the complete and final solution for health care resource allocation. Indeed, there are grounds for debating whether some proposals such as MSAs that offer only an incremental improvement over the status quo are worth the effort. Certainly, MSAs should not be banned or discouraged, but no one has yet made a convincing case that they should be the uniquely favored form of insurance.

Whatever the resolution of the existing public policy debate over MSAs and other market reforms, it is clear that they do not adequately resolve most health care spending decisions through pure market mechanisms. Most health care spending will continue to occur through the vehicle of insurance, and patients who pay out of pocket will continue to rely to a considerable extent on their physicians' expert advice. Therefore, even the purest forms of market competition result in only a limited range of spending decisions made directly by patients. Although consumer decisions may dominate the choice of insurance and the choice of physician, these decisions create agency relationships in which patients delegate authority to others. This inevitability of insurance means that we must examine directly the merits and drawbacks of these other mechanisms for making health care spending decisions.

Notes

1. Moffit 1994, at 473.
2. Goodman and Musgrave 1992, at x–xi.
3. Ibid. at 29–30.
4. Epstein 1992.
5. Enthoven 1980.
6. Schuck 1994.
7. Cobbs v. Grant, 502 P.2d 1, 9–10 (Cal. 1972).
8. Informed consent as it relates to refusals of treatment is discussed in much greater detail in Chapter 6.
9. Further elaboration can be found in Chapter 7.
10. The consensus on this point is reflected in President's Commission 1982. See also Blumstein 1981.
11. See, e.g., Pauly 1980; Goodman and Musgrave 1992, at Chapter 9.
12. Donahue 1994.
13. Goodman and Musgrave 1992, at 266.
14. See ibid. at 234–40. This example is based on premiums charged by Golden Rule Insurance Co. to families of average health in cities with average health care costs. Even more extreme examples can be generated with data from high-cost locations or for high-risk subscribers.
15. Ibid. at 43.
16. Brook 1989.
17. This is true even though about 15 percent of people have no insurance and about 10 percent of hospital and 20 percent of physician revenues come from out-of-pocket

payments. People without insurance often receive their care for free through public hospitals and emergency rooms. A good portion of out-of-pocket payments are the co-insurance amounts from people who are insured. Therefore, only a small percentage of health care services are paid for entirely out of pocket, either by those without insurance or by those with insurance who have not yet exhausted their deductible amounts.

18. Sislowitz 1988, at 23.

19. Newsweek, Jan. 26, 1987, at 44, col. 3.

20. Jensen 1993; Gabel and Jensen 1989.

21. Hall 1994b, at 16–25.

22. Pauly 1990.

23. For a comprehensive and largely convincing treatment of these ideas, see Havighurst 1995.

24. Various mechanisms are available for defining and enforcing this higher threshold of insurance coverage: detailed treatment rules, financial incentives to physicians, or generic standards of appropriateness. Each of these is the subject of other chapters in this book. The focus here is not on which contracting method is best for defining care that is covered but on how much of the treatment costs below the threshold consumers should be exposed to. In other words, this chapter examines how *high* to set the threshold; later chapters examine the mechanics of defining and enforcing the threshold.

25. Marquis and Buchanan 1994 (projecting that, if the tax subsidy were removed, the number of consumers who buy the least expensive form of insurance would double). See also Morrisey 1992; Monheit and Harvey 1993.

26. Goodman and Musgrave 1992.

27. Ibid. at 174–76.

28. In the RAND experiment, catastrophic coverage required patients to pay 95 percent of the health care costs, up to the lesser of $1000 or a percentage of their income. The income limit ranged from 5 to 15 percent for different experimental groups. The experiment was conducted mostly in the 1970s, so the $1000 limit functioned essentially like the higher deductible does now in conventional catastrophic coverage.

29. Keeler and Rolph 1983.

30. For instance, a new 25 percent co-insurance requirement by one employer reduced the use of physician services about 25 percent, and an HMO that imposed a five-dollar copayment for outpatient visits experienced a 10–20 percent decline in visits. A comprehensive review of the evidence can be found in Rice and Morrison 1994; and in Morrisey 1992. Observe also that Medicare patients who purchase Medigap policies that cover most deductibles and co-insurance use the hospital one-quarter to one-third more.

31. The most vocal proponent of MSAs from the public policy community is John Goodman, who writes on behalf of The Cato Institute. Goodman and Musgrave 1992, at Chapters 8 and 15; Goodman and Musgrave 1994, at Chapter 5. One of the staunchest Congressional advocates is Senator Phil Gramm. Gramm 1994. See also Jensen and Morlock 1994.

32. For a general description, in addition to the sources in the previous note, see Tweed 1994, at 40.

33. Here is the math: Take the difference between the two deductibles and multiply by 80 percent, which is the amount the conventional insurance would have reimbursed for the increment that is now subject to the higher deductible. The resulting $2000 is the amount needed in one year to put the subscriber in the same economic position as before.

34. See Goodman and Musgrave 1992, at Chapters 5 and 8.

35. Singapore is an example of a country that uses the MSA device to create forced savings for a wide range of expected welfare needs. Ibid. at Chapter 19.

36. Ibid. at Chapter 15.

37. Tweed 1994, at 40–46; Jensen and Morlock 1994, at 17; Goodman and Musgrave 1992. For a contrasting view, see Hsiao 1995, who reports that MSAs have failed to control spending in Singapore, where they were first used as the basis for system-wide reform.

38. For a trenchant attack on the goals of market reform, see Frankford 1992.

39. The seminal work explaining the economic necessity of health insurance is Arrow 1963.

40. In other words, private Medigap coverage, by eliminating the copayment obligation under Medicare, increases the use of Medicare services but absorbs only 20 percent of the cost of this increase. At the margin, then, Medigap coverage receives an 80 percent subsidy from Medicare. See Pauly, Eisenberg and Radany et al. 1992, at 56–57.

41. Jensen and Morlock 1994, at 15.

42. Berk and Monheit 1992, at 145–149.

43. Emanuel and Emanuel 1994.

44. See Hall and Anderson 1992.

45. U.S. Government Accounting Office 1992, at 32.

46. It is not possible to eliminate all mandates since some—such as guaranteed renewability and continuity of coverage laws and requiring family policies to cover newborns despite their preexisting congenital defects—are highly desirable and promote the goal of market reform.

47. See generally Families USA 1993; Laudicina 1992; Butler 1992. These demonstrations are revealing, however, only for voluntary purchase by people presently without insurance. They do not show whether people who presently have comprehensive insurance will find bare bones coverage more attractive once the tax subsidy is removed.

48. Rasell 1995.

49. Marquis and Buchanan 1994.

50. See generally Morreim 1994c; Hadorn 1991a; Calabresi and Bobbitt 1978; Blumstein 1981.

51. For a survey, see Curran, Hall, and Kaye 1990, at 518–53.

52. For a thorough analysis, see Churchill 1994.

53. For additional discussion of income adjustments to cost-sharing requirements, see Rice and Thorpe 1993.

54. See, e.g., Blumstein 1981. An admirable attempt to reconcile market theory with a single-tier system can be found, however, in Elhauge 1994, who argues for universal entitlement to a middle-class standard of health insurance based on a mix of moral and pragmatic grounds. The essence of Professor Elhauge's argument is that our basic moral instinct for all goods is an egalitarian standard, which nevertheless we often refuse to honor because of the uncontrollable incentive effects of offering a free ride. Health care is different because it suffers much less from the "moral hazard" problems encountered by other social guarantees since sickness is unpleasant enough that few people are encouraged by generous insurance to neglect their health. One can respond, though, that health behaviors are indeed sensitive to costs, and that health insurance creates moral hazard concerns not only for the incidence of sickness but also for the costs of treatment. See Hall 1994a.

55. This analysis is broadly consistent with the intellectual development in legal analysis know as "therapeutic jurisprudence," which argues that law and public policy in the medical arena should be more consciously aware of the actual effects on patients' welfare and less concerned with abstract principles drawn from nonmedical contexts. See generally Wexler and Winnick 1991.

56. Morreim 1994a, at 96–7, 103.

57. Schneider 1994, at 1080. See also Schneider 1996, for a more extensive development of this critique of hyperrationalism.

58. In addition to the sources cited in the following notes, see Pellegrino 1979; Pellegrino and Thomasma 1981; Cassell 1982; Cassell 1985; Kleinman 1988.

59. Silberman 1991.

60. Pellegrino 1982, at 159.

61. Toombs 1992, at 21, 69. For another gripping account, see the discussion in Bovbjerg et al. 1987 of the difficulty kidney disease patients have in making mixed economic and medical decisions when they are first diagnosed.

62. On this regression to infancy caused by sickness, see Burt 1979; Somers and Somers 1961, at 459–60.

63. Schneider 1996, at 171.

64. Ingelfinger 1980.

65. Schneider 1996; Schneider 1994; Schuck 1994; Dworkin 1993.

66. See, for example, Strull et al. 1984; Lidz et al. 1983; Ende et al. 1980; Vertinsky et al. 1974. For general reviews, see Schneider 1996; Schneider 1994; Meisel and Roth 1983.

67. For example, Carrese and Rhodes 1995; Blackhall et al. 1995; Ventres and Nichter et al. 1993. See Levine 1991.

68. Vladeck 1981, at 211–12.

69. Brody 1987a, at 29.

70. On the prevalence of the image of physician as parent or priest, see May 1983.

71. In addition to the sources in the following notes, see Spiro 1986; Brody 1980.

72. Beecher 1961.

73. Roberts et al. 1993; Roberts 1995.

74. Turner et al., 1994; Moerman 1983; Brody 1980.

75. Suchman and Matthews 1988; Houston 1938.

76. Cohen 1995; O'Connor 1995; Moyers 1993; Frohoch 1992; Siegel 1990; Cousins 1979; Siegel 1986.

77. The leading work developing this explanation is Frank 1973. See also Brody 1992; Novack 1987; Spiro 1986.

78. Cassell 1985, at 141. See also Cassell 1991.

79. Siegel 1986.

80. Katz 1984, at 142–47, 192. See also Burt 1979.

81. There are some scattered scientific studies demonstrating the placebo effect and the effect of certain of these healing rituals, but no scientific studies exploring what ingredients make this process work, and especially no studies on whether forcing a more consumer-oriented role on patients is counterproductive to healing. It is noteworthy, though, that patients themselves are more reluctant to make their own medical decisions the sicker they are, whereas the assumption of the dominant autonomy paradigm would lead one to just the opposite conclusion that patient control is more important the more critical the decision is. See Schneider 1994, at 1091.

82. E.g., Brody 1992; Katz 1984; Burt 1979.

83. This general point is amplified in the context of MSAs in Minnesota Department of Health 1994. See also, Stacy 1994.

84. Russell 1994.

85. Schneider 1996, at 137.

86. See, for example, Kasper et al. 1992.

87. It is noteworthy, however, that where safety concerns are the highest, such as in home construction, automobile design, and workplace safety precautions, our society

relies to a much greater extent on regulatory intervention than it does for other consumer goods.

88. Chapter 4 develops this thought further in the context of the myth of Ulysses and the Sirens. There, I take a more accommodating attitude toward these infirmities in patients' decision-making capacity. However, the issue there is different. It concerns the capacity to choose a doctor or an insurance plan, not individual items of treatment, and it asks whether such decisions are so flawed as to be entirely unenforceable, not, as here, whether they are so flawless as to be optimal.

89. Starr 1993, at 1668.

90. Bodenheimer and Grumbach 1994, at 634.

91. See Strull et al. 1984; Lidz et al. 1983; Ende et al. 1980; Vertinsky et al. 1974. For general reviews, see Schneider 1994; Meisel and Roth 1983.

92. See Chapter 5 for elaboration.

93. Veatch 1990.

94. In present dollars, it cost the government $200 million. For a general review and analysis of the experiment, see Rice and Morrison 1994; U.S. Congress 1993.

95. Findings from the experiment are contained in hundreds of different publications. The most comprehensive single report is Newhouse et al. 1993.

96. The income maximums ranged from 5 to 15 percent. Some participants received their maximum out-of-pocket limits in side payments as compensation for enrolling in the experiment if the terms of this insurance were less generous than the insurance they had prior to the experiment. Because this side payment was made monthly and regardless of whether treatment expenses were incurred, it presumably had the same effect as a modest increase in wages and was not viewed as a change in the terms of the insurance. See generally, Newhouse et al. 1993, Chapter 2.

97. Newhouse et al. 1993, Chapter 6.

98. Rasell 1995.

99. Sorlie, Johnson, Backlund, and Bradham 1994; Hadley, Steinberg, and Feder 1991. For a comprehensive summary and critique of this body of evidence, see U.S. Congress 1992b.

100. Lohr, Brook, and Kamberg et al. 1986; Siu et al. 1986.

101. Keeler and Rolph 1983. See Newhouse et al. 1993, Chapters 4 and 5. On the other hand, increased cost-sharing for the use of emergency room services has been shown to result in patients selectively reducing nonemergent use of hospital services. Selby et al. 1996.

102. For instance, compare the complexities involved in market reform proposals aimed at comprehensive insurance. Hall 1994b.

103. Pauly 1994.

104. See Pauly 1994 for a thorough demonstration of these points. See also Keeler et al. 1996.

105. This point comes from Pauly 1994.

106. Pauly and Goodman 1995. A tax credit provides the same tax subsidy to each insurance purchaser regardless of their income or how much their insurance costs. Therefore, it avoids the distortions created by the existing tax deduction, which gives a greater tax subsidy to people who spend more and to people with higher incomes.

107. For example, see Rooney 1992; Council for Affordable Health Insurance 1993. See Tweed 1994, at 42. Golden Rule Insurance Company, one of the leading advocates of MSAs, is a substantial company at a national level, but does not (to my knowledge) have a large share of many individual local markets. Managed care networks are based in local, not national markets.

108. This may explain in part why existing catastrophic insurance policies appear to be such a good buy. Their price advantage may not reflect so much their economizing incentives as it does their ability to attract healthier-than-average subscribers to the insurance pool.

109. For a general discussion of adverse selection in the market for health care insurance, see Hall 1994b, at 40–41 and sources cited therein. For a description of its effect on MSAs and catastrophic coverage, see Jensen and Morlock 1994; Nichols 1995. The Congressional Budget Office concluded in an analysis of one of the Republican MSA plans introduced during the 103d Congress that, if they were widely offered, MSAs would sharply raise the price of standard coverage, undermine broad community pooling, and eventually lead to a two-tiered system of sick versus healthy subscribers. See Tweed 1994, at 42; Meyer 1994, at 3, 10. See also Keeler et al. 1996.

110. For a clear and thorough development of these points, see Pauly 1994.

111. Although the risk-neutral value of the high-option plan was only 42 percent greater than the low-option plan, the actual costs for subscribers in the high-option plan were 264 percent higher (as measured by the experience-based premiums that were charged). Institute of Medicine 1993, at 176.

112. Ibid. See also, Marquis 1992.

113. Luft et al. 1985, at 197–229.

114. Ellis 1985.

115. Pauly et al. 1992. Employers would be allowed to continue purchasing insurance for their workers, but would not be encouraged to do so.

3

Third-Party Rules

The previous chapter argues that it is an unappealing solution to the health care spending problem to force unwilling patients to pay for most of their own medical costs out of pocket. Fortunately, there is no compelling need to adopt this extreme position. The medical–industrial complex has no shortage of other institutions perfectly willing to set spending limits for consumers. The principal contenders are insurance companies, government agencies, and employers—those who pay for the treatment. I classify these as "third-party," "centralized," or "external" decision makers. They are third-party or external authorities because they are outside of the primary doctor/patient relationship. They are centralized because, by and large, they make uniform decisions for everyone under their authority. Third-party authorities also include the courts and innovative institutions such as citizen committees or physician overseers. This chapter addresses anyone who makes medical spending decisions other than the doctor or patient who is directly involved in the particular treatment affected by the decision. If either of these parties to the treatment relationship feels bound by an explicit resource constraint on a treatment option, then a third-party spending decision has been imposed.

It may not appear very attractive to give profit-making insurance companies and bureaucratic regulators authority to set cost-sensitive limits on medical choices, but this is in fact the direction that our country is presently headed. Medical journals and physician conversations are peppered with references to the growing "managerial-review process in which armies of claims clerks, administrators, auditors, form processors, peer reviewers, functionaries, and technocrats of every description insinuate themselves into a complex system that authorizes, pays for and delivers medical care."[1] Witness the outrage in the following physician's letter to the editor:

To call myself a vascular surgeon, I had to do well in college, then spend the next 12 years working grueling hours, depriving myself of most of the joys of young adulthood and immersing myself in other people's worst misery. . . . I now have an army of vindictive bureaucrats and largely untrained reviewers nipping at my heels, and must spend many hours a week defending myself against their overwhelmingly wrongheaded second-guessing of clinical decisions.[2]

In contrast with these vitriolic objections by physicians, many prominent medical ethicists believe that external authority of some type is the only morally appropriate mechanism for making resource allocation decisions, or is at least morally superior to physicians or patients making their own rationing decisions at the bedside.[3]

This chapter will examine this debate first by undertaking the fairly easy task of critiquing the most bureaucratic forms of external rationing mechanisms. I will then analyze more appealing versions of third-party rationing that rely either on legalistic processes or on technocratic authority. The chapter then examines the most idealistic version of democratic or collective decision making, and it concludes by discussing a proposed hybrid between physician discretion and third-party rules: third-party physician discretion. This progression from the actual to the possible should remind us that criticism of existing imperfect institutions is all too easy. But it is also facile to ignore these flaws by positing purely ideal solutions to real world problems. Only by taking a hard look at how good ideas function in concrete settings can we know their full potential and limits.

BUREAUCRATIC AND LEGALISTIC MECHANISMS

Rationing by Insurers and Regulators

The Unpopularity of Bureaucratic Rationing

As reflected in the previous quotations, almost no one has a kind word to say about bureaucratic rationing. Despite the attempts of employers and insurers to sugar-coat third-party authority as sound medical management ("managed care," "case managers," "quality assurance," etc.), most people see bureaucrats as "enemies of patients."[4] Accordingly, popular sentiment is overwhelmingly opposed to making medical spending decisions through either governmental or commercial institutions. A nationwide survey by Northwestern National Life Insurance Company found that 50 percent of people would most trust a national panel of medical professionals to make rationing decisions for them. A panel of consumers came in a distant second, at 18 percent. Elected officials and the U.S. court system were left choking on dust at 3 and 5 percent, respectively.[5] A different poll conducted by the Employee Benefit Research Institute found that 35 percent of those surveyed would prefer their family doctor to set any necessary limits on health care services, 35 percent would chose a local panel of medical professionals, and only 9 percent would favor insurers or employers setting limits.[6] A third nationwide survey, conducted by Louis Harris, found that 34 percent of people think a committee of other patients should decide what procedures are covered by insurance, 32 percent think doctors should make this decision, but only 6, 4, and 3 percent, respectively, believed that government, employers, or insurers should have this authority.[7]

This hostility to bureaucratic rationing exists for good reason. We have no basis to expect that those who exercise bureaucratic power will either know or incorporate the values of those they affect by their decisions. Claims processors for private insurance companies often have only minimal education or experience in health care,[8] and they work within a corporate culture that emphasizes bottom-line economic performance. Nearly everyone has had some maddening experience with the red tape entailed in obtaining reimbursement for everyday medical expenses. Because of the massive number of individual claims that insurers must process, and because of the antagonistic legal environment in which they operate, insurers can make wildly inconsistent coverage decisions even within the same company.[9] Although competitive market constraints and legal oversight serve to hold insurers somewhat accountable,[10] the public continues to hold a strongly negative view of the insurance industry's motives and actions.

The picture within government insurance programs is not much more attractive, perhaps because they are structured just like conventional insurance. Medicare, the largest government program, is actually run in its day-to-day dealings by private insurance companies. In order to appease hospitals and doctors, in the 1960s the federal government structured Medicare in a fashion that delegates to private insurers the tasks of front-line claims administration. This was done at a time when the dominant insurers were Blue Cross/Blue Shield plans controlled by doctors and hospitals, and so when insurers exercised very little oversight of medical judgment. Now, however, medical providers view the insurance industry, including the Blues, as a hostile force that threatens clinical autonomy. Doctors consider the Medicare program to be the single largest source of mindless bureaucratic intervention into their daily lives,[11] but they are also feeling overwhelmed by the tide of managed care that is sweeping the private market.

The Unwillingness of Bureaucrats to Ration
The unpopularity of bureaucratic rationing is not simply a matter of public and professional sentiment. It is expressed through social institutions that handicap regulators and insurers in their ability to make tough resource allocation decisions. A prime example is the repeated spectacle of highly visible media and grassroots campaigns orchestrated by desperate families when a government or private insurer

threatens to deny a life-saving organ transplant.[12] Under the glare of public scrutiny, government bureaucratic rationing suffers from the weakness of the political will.[13] As political scientist James Morone observes, "what rationer would relish the prospect of facing an aroused American Association of Retired People . . . or, for that matter, the Children's Defense Fund?"[14] We may admire the regulator who is moved by sympathy for a patient near death, but regulators also succumb to lobbying pressure by special interest groups. This tends to favor more cohesive, highly mobilized, and better financed elements of society such as providers and drug manufacturers who have very large stakes in these spending decisions.

One effect of this interest group politics is that Medicaid, which covers the poor, has received woefully insufficient funding while Medicare, which covers the elderly, a large and politically mobilized group, has historically received far more ample allotments.[15] Similarly, in Oregon, political scientist Larry Brown excoriates the "distasteful and transparent coalition-building strategy" used to pass its supposedly "bold" rationing plan (discussed below). The plan targets only the most politically and socially vulnerable components of the Medicaid population—indigent single mothers—leaving untouched the elderly and disabled, as well as the general population. In Brown's view, "The state's vaunted 'hard choices' . . . turned out to be all too easy: the most needy, vulnerable, and disorganized, those least equipped to squeak, got the castor oil."[16] In contrast, the groups Oregon consulted to gauge the quality-of-life factors used in its rationing scheme were composed largely of health professionals and white, college educated, upper-middle-class people.[17]

Even in England, where health care rationing is among the most severe in the industrialized nations, government regulators have a difficult time making overt rationing decisions. According to one survey, "only 12 of 114 health authorities stated that they would either not buy or limit the availability of specific forms of treatment," and even then most of the services they mentioned were items such as tattoo removal, breast augmentation, and in vitro fertilization. "Clearly, this is rationing at the margins; . . . these decisions represent symbolic gestures . . . rather than a serious attempt to address the issues."[18]

Private insurers are also handicapped by popular opinion in their ability to set and enforce limits on medical spending. Despite the perception that insurers ruthlessly deny coverage in order to save money, the reality is that they have been extremely reluctant, on the whole, to engage in any form of explicit resource allocation. This is because, historically, courts have been unreceptive or outright hostile to insurers' attempts to interfere in clinical discretion for any reason, including safety and effectiveness concerns, let alone on account of cost/benefit tradeoffs. Instead, courts have traditionally insisted on total deference to practicing physicians. One extreme example is *Duncan v. J.C. Penney Life Insurance Co.*,[19] where the court required coverage for two three-week periods of hospitalization for a husband and wife for bruises and sprains, under facts that "strongly indicate[d] a motive on the part of the Duncans . . . to reap financial gain."[20] The court ordered the insurer to pay even though the Duncans's doctor admitted that the care could have been administered at home and five other doctors agreed that hospitalization was not medically necessary. Other examples come from cases where insurers were required to pay for alternative cancer therapies such as laetrile and "immuno-augmentative" treatment that were outlawed in the United States but delivered in Mexican and Caribbean clinics.[21] These decisions are based on the view that, in deciding what is "medically necessary" or "experimental," the treating doctor's judgment is far more reliable than that of a corporate insurer whose profit margin is affected by the decision.[22]

This difficulty of enforcing payment denials for inappropriate care has made insurers notoriously submissive. At first, insurance policies contained no explicit limitations on the appropriateness of treatment for which they paid. Instead, they covered, within defined monetary and service limits, all care ordered by any physician.[23] Insurance then began to limit coverage to medically necessary and nonexperimental treatment, but insurers still have been willing to defend their denials of coverage only at the outer extremes of medical practice.

There are three basic levels at which medical procedures, drugs, and devices can be evaluated. They can be found (1) safe and effective, (2) cost effective, and/ or (3) cost beneficial. The first level, which is employed by the Food and Drug Administration (FDA) to evaluate all new drugs and devices, asks only whether, on balance, the procedure's medical benefits outweigh its medical risks. The second level asks whether this medical benefit is superior to what can be achieved by other procedures at equal or lesser cost. Only the third level asks whether a net increase in medical benefit is worth the cost.[24]

Health insurers have historically operated only at the first level, seeking to justify their coverage denials primarily as a means to protect patients from harmful or fraudulent care.[25] They have not even asked whether a beneficial result might be obtained more cheaply, let alone whether a marginally increased benefit is simply too expensive to be worth the cost. They have asked only that some medical benefit be demonstrated, however slight, leaving the choice of less versus more effective and less versus more expensive modalities to the doctor and patient.[26] Government insurers have been similarly reluctant to engage in open and systematic resource allocation. A proposal to introduce cost-effectiveness review (the second tier) into Medicare coverage decisions has remained unadopted for over seven years.[27]

Even with their current greater resolve, insurers deny only 1–2 percent of claims reviewed,[28] despite the growing body of literature suggesting that a much greater portion of medical practice currently being covered, perhaps 25 percent, is inappropriate. Although insurers are considering incorporating economic cost in their assessments of medical effectiveness, this means only that they might move to the second tier of assessment, not that they are taking on the much more controversial role of paying for services only if the benefits exceed the costs. Whether they can make even this modest move depends, of course, on how successful they have been in the first tier.

To gauge the extent to which courts will allow insurers to assess medical effectiveness, I led a research team that conducted a comprehensive review of all published judicial opinions on health insurance for the last 35 years that involved an issue of medical appropriateness. This study coded and analyzed statistically a multitude of factors that might influence the outcome of these legal decisions. We found, first, that both public and private insurers, despite their inherent caution, lose almost 60 percent of the coverage denials they seek to defend in court. This statistic holds up across most categories of health insurance and most types of treatment. Very few factors were found to alter insurers' chance of success. They were equally likely to lose whether they relied on scientific evidence from prestigious research institutes, whether they based their decision on an ad hoc literature review, or whether they had no supporting scientific evidence at all. More important than the quality of the evidence were procedural or legal technicalities such as whether the case arose under the federal law known as ERISA, which governs employment-based insurance. Insurers win 55 percent of cases under ERISA. This is largely because this body of law gives more credence to contractual language that assigns to the insurer the authority to determine the meaning of ambiguous contract language. Curiously, though, insurers do not fare substantially better simply because their contracts specifically exclude the treatment in question. Unless the contract gives the insurer explicit authority to interpret its terms, courts simply find ways to declare even treatment-specific language ambiguous or to interpret the language so it does not fit the precise clinical circumstances of the case.[29]

These findings document the reluctance of judges and juries to honor insurers' assessment of medical appropriateness using only safety and effectiveness norms. Although insurers may be finding somewhat more success in federal court under certain contract terms, our research found no evidence that courts will be more deferential if insurers begin to base their decisions on economic as well as scientific criteria. To the contrary, judicial review is most stringent when economic motivation is detected. Few courts are willing to recognize that insurers who try to save money act in the interest of the entire subscriber pool. Instead, courts see a profit-making insurer who has already received its premium refusing to honor reasonable treatment requests by a sick patient. In this context, economic motivation appears to be an unconscionable conflict of interest. With this predictable judicial reaction, it is certain that insurers' cost-containment efforts will continue to be cautious and muted at best.

Judges and Juries

Private and government insurers are not only legally handicapped in their ability to engage in systematic resource allocation, they are not trusted to do so by either the public, the medical profession, or the courts. Therefore, another option worth considering is the judicial system itself. If judges and juries, expressing popular sentiment, will not honor bureaucratic rationing, they might be expected themselves to make acceptable medical spending decisions when they decide disputes between patients and public or private insurers over the terms of health insurance coverage. Viewed simply, a potential insurance purchaser is faced with a Hobbesian choice: a treating physician with an incentive for ordering too much and a reviewing insurer with an incentive to pay for too little. Judicial resolution of these competing conflicts superficially appears to be an attractive solution to an intractable choice between these imperfect decision makers. Additional reflection reveals, however, that we all might view it in our best mutual interests to keep these decisions out of the courts as well.

The most obvious reason is that the judicial system is ill-suited to decide scientific questions.[30] Lay judges and juries must rely on expert testimony, and the adversarial setting in which this evidence is presented tends to distort its accuracy. In contrast to scientific processes, litigants in the adversarial system carefully choose their witnesses with tactical advantages in mind. Witnesses that are opinionated and dogmatic are favored over those that have a more balanced view of the competing merits.[31] Moreover, because winning, not truth-finding, is the ultimate objective, litigants resort to tactics that actively undermine truthfulness from a scientific perspective, such as exploiting the demeanor of the opposing scientists and launching ad hominem attacks on their personal credibility. In this adversarial climate, it is difficult for judges and juries to divine scientific fact from science fiction.[32]

A second structural obstacle to effective resource allocation by courts is the constitutional limitation that they can only decide the issues that are brought to them in concrete disputes. Unlike legislatures or administrative agencies, courts may not issue sweeping pronouncements with binding legal force beyond the context of the cases immediately before them. Courts are limited to those disputes that private parties decide are worth the costs of litigation. Because lawyers are expensive and litigation is time-consuming, courts are likely to see only a small and biased sampling out of the entire range of medical practice—those with very high costs or where the patient is in very serious condition. A comprehensive review of all published judicial opinions on health insurance involving an issue of medical appropriateness was able to find only 203 cases decided between 1960 and 1994. On average, these cases took two and a half years to resolve (median = 2), and involved treatment costing about $50,000 (median = $10,000–$50,000). Due to this expense and delay, only 20 published cases per year are being decided in the 1990s, and even this small number is far more than were being decided in prior decades.

It is true that these few decisions establish precedents that influence how countless other disputes are resolved out of court, but the range of precedential effect is not very great. Medical appropriateness decisions, by their nature, are highly sensitive to the particular facts of each case. The influence of one case on another is qualified not only by the patient's individual condition but also by the specific wording of the contract, the negotiations leading up to the contract, and the particular behavior of the parties leading up to the dispute.[33] Therefore, a prior judicial decision may be of only marginal relevance to a new dispute even if it involves precisely the same treatment. The inability of courts to be at the bedside of every patient keeps them from playing a primary role in medical spending decisions throughout society.

Even if litigation were much less cumbersome and decisions were rendered by specialized clinically trained judges with access to all the relevant data, there is another reason why we might not prefer judges and juries to make medical spending decisions. The courts, when faced with the dire condition of an individual patient who has purchased insurance, are prone to minimize the social costs of treatment. As law professor Einer Elhauge explains:

It is one thing to reject the absolutist claim [that costs should have no role] in the abstract; it is quite another to face a real flesh and blood person who would benefit from health care and deny it to them because it costs too much. The point is not one of mere public relations, but of the predictable problems that befall such a legal or institutional framing for resource allocation. Actual human beings, forced to make actual decisions framed as health versus money, find themselves seeming and feeling inhumane. And they resort to just about any mechanisms of self-denial or short-term spending measures to avoid or postpone facing the reality of scarcity.[34]

Superficially, this humane response seems correct since individualized consideration is a hallmark of our justice system,[35] but further reflection reveals that it is wrong to neglect the broader perspective. This conflict in perspectives can be illuminated using three interrelated conceptual principles: (1) insurability versus medical necessity as the decision norm; (2) the ex ante versus the ex post perspective; and (3) adjudicative versus legislative facts.

Resource allocation disputes are most appropriately viewed as an insurance-purchasing decision by a pool of subscribers, not a medical treatment decision made by an individual patient. Where the parties leave the scope of coverage ill-defined, a particular case is rationally decided by asking what range of treatment options the purchasers would have chosen to insure at the time they signed up, not what treatment they want to receive now that the insurance has been paid for and their illness is manifest.[36]

In the case of experimental treatment for cancer, for instance, the relevant question is not whether a terminally ill patient for whom all other therapies have failed would want to pull out all the stops; the relevant question is whether a cross section of mostly healthy subscribers would pay their share of the cost of these last-gasp treatments to provide for the unlikely event of personally being in the same situation. It is not always the preference of subscribers to insure for all health care that provides any benefit, or even for all health care that proves to be cost beneficial. As explained in Chapter 2, some very beneficial care may be well worth paying for out-of-pocket at the time of illness but may not be efficient to insure for in advance.

This insurance-purchasing perspective is especially appropriate in the context of interpreting the insurance exclusion of "experimental" treatment. When this term is applied to new therapies for terminally ill patients, courts have ruled that any possibility of success makes the procedure medically appropriate because the patient is sure to die and all other therapies have proven ineffective.[37] But medical appropriateness is not the sole reason for excluding coverage of experimental treatment. There are serious concerns about the insurability of experimental care simply because it constitutes new, unanticipated treatment not reflected in the actuarial data used to price the insurance policy. Although purchasers of health insurance might choose to pay an extra premium to cover rapidly evolving medical technologies, they may also determine that the price is not worth the insurance benefit. The newest technologies are expensive to insure, not only because of their costs but more so because their costs are so uncertain. By definition, experimental treatment lacks a well-documented track record, and, given the pace of medical advances, some such treatments that patients might seek do not even exist at the time the insurance premium is set. It is expensive to insure against risks that cannot be accurately quantified, and it is particularly difficult to insure against the cost of something that is entirely unknown.

It can be argued in response that experimental therapies for terminally ill patients are the very type of risks that are the most insurable, in the sense that insurance is most appropriate for high-cost, low-incidence events with catastrophic consequences. This is true, but the market is capable of striking a balance between the insurable and uninsurable elements of experimental care. Thus, an insurance product might state that it excludes experimental therapy except in cases of life-threatening illness.[38] Other consumers may decide they are better off bearing this risk themselves (even if this means forgoing new treatments altogether) until new technologies are in sufficiently widespread use that their actual effect on the pooled health care risks can be known with greater certainty and incorporated into actuarial projections more precisely.[39]

Courts are institutionally ill-suited to apply this insurability perspective to coverage disputes. By the very nature of the adjudicative process, they are presented with an individual sick patient who is already insured, not a pool of healthy people deciding what insurance to purchase. Economists, who label these opposing views the ex post versus the ex ante perspectives, observe that efficient legal rules and contractual arrangements cannot be generated from the ex post litigation perspective:[40]

[S]table insurance requires unemotional assessment of risk and disbursement of payments, with the temperament of an actuary and a bookkeeper, treating people as statistics. The driving force in the law today is sympathy and emotion in the individual case. Legal rules rooted in a spirit of compulsion, and applied emotionally case by case, are profoundly inimical to insurance.[41]

This inherent judicial myopia is demonstrated by the results in Medicaid coverage disputes, where the group perspective should be much more evident due to extremely limited funding for the poor. Despite the obvious misallocation of resources caused by ordering coverage for expensive and questionable services, some courts (notably, the Eighth Circuit) nevertheless consistently rule in favor of treatment for extreme procedures such as sex-change operations and multiple-organ transplants.[42] The potential for judicial distortion is most apparent in the extreme case of a terminally ill patient. From the ex post perspective imposed by case-specific judicial review, potentially an infinite amount of money is worth even an infinitesimally small chance of recovery because without the treatment the patient will not be around to enjoy whatever is saved by forgoing treatment. This perspective loses sight of the ex ante view that such an attitude would make insurance so expensive that other terminally ill patients might not be able to afford it at all once this attitude is anticipated by the insurer.

Legal scholars underscore the institutional limits of case-specific adjudication by using the more academic terms of "legislative facts" or "polycentrism." Adjudication is best suited for disputes in which all affected parties can be brought into a single arena and the relevant facts relate to those parties as individuals. A simple automobile accident or a property dispute are prime examples. Typically, disputes between two parties to a contract are also ideal subjects for adjudication. Health insurance disputes differ, however, because, unlike other kinds of insurance with more defined benefits, these disputes turn on broad questions of what is medically effective and socially appropriate. When these sorts of issues are presented to public regulators, administrative law scholars have labeled them "legislative" rather than "adjudicative" issues and have advocated the use of non-adversarial processes for their resolution.[43] The same notion is captured by Lon Fuller's concept of "polycentrism," as applied to private disputes. In his seminal article *The Forms and Limits of Adjudication*,[44] Professor Fuller identified as the principal limitation to adjudication those polycentric disputes whose resolution is akin to building a bridge:[45]

There are rational principles for building bridges of structural steel. But there is no rational principle which states, for example, that the angle between girder A and girder B must always be 45 degrees. This depends on the bridge as a whole. One cannot construct a bridge by conducting successive separate arguments concerning the proper angle for every pair of intersecting girders. One must deal with the whole structure.[46]

The cost/benefit trade-offs and the principles of insurability that underlie medical spending decisions partake heavily of these same aspects of polycentrism.

To recognize these limits is not to say that courts lack all authority to decide insurance coverage disputes. When presented with a legitimate dispute, a court must decide. But, in so doing, the proper role of the court is to enforce the insurance contract or statute faithfully as written. Some judges, especially in the federal courts, are beginning to enforce these institutional limits by expressing reluctance to second-guess the resource allocation decisions made by the market or the political process. One recent opinion stated: "Unfortunately, this case presents an issue which this court as an institution is ill-equipped to handle. The court must confine itself to the narrow legal question presented and leave public policy and social reform to the other branches of government. Cases of this nature present compelling social questions which go well beyond the limits of this court."[47] Another court issued the following heart-felt explanation of its judicial restraint:

> Despite rumors to the contrary, those who wear judicial robes are human beings, and as persons, are inspired and motivated by compassion as anyone would be. Consequently, we often must remind ourselves that in our official capacities, we have authority only to issue rulings within the narrow parameters of the law and the facts before us. The temptation to go about, doing good where we see fit, and to make things less difficult for those who come before us, regardless of the law, is strong. But the law, without which judges are nothing, abjures such unlicensed formulation of unauthorized social policy by the judiciary. Plaintiff . . . well deserves, and in a perfect world would be entitled to, all known medical treatments to control the horrid disease from which she suffers. In ruling as this court must, no personal satisfaction is taken, but that the law was followed. The court will have to live with the haunting thought that [plaintiff], and perhaps others insured by . . . similar plans, may not ultimately receive the treatment they need and deserve.[48]

This leaves us on the horns of a dilemma: (1) Either judges recognize that they lack the capacity to make informed resource allocation decisions, thereby placing patients at the mercy of bureaucratic rationers, or (2) judges intervene, thereby systematically making decisions that informed subscribers might not approve at the time they select their insurance. Courts appear ill-equipped to stake a middle ground between doing nothing to check insurers and doing too much to protect individual patients. Therefore, we must continue our search for a more appealing, nonbureaucratic and nonlegalistic option for making medical spending decisions.

TECHNOCRATIC RESOURCE ALLOCATION AND THE EMERGING ROLE OF SCIENCE

The analysis so far might be criticized for its excessive focus on the minute defects of existing, imperfect institutions, to the neglect of numerous possibilities for improving these institutional blemishes. Private insurers may in fact act from the wrong motive, and government regulators and the courts may now lack the proper expertise and perspective, but we should not be blind to the potential for reforming these institutions or creating new ones that contain the proper combination of motivation and expertise.

One of the most promising possibilities is to either augment or replace these existing institutions with ones composed of disinterested scientists and physicians.

These technocratic experts might be capable of allocating wisely through cost-sensitive rules based on careful empirical research. Our society holds tremendous respect for technocratic solutions to complex social problems. Throughout countless walks of life, we turn to computers, number crunchers, and scientists for guidance on important allocation decisions. Engineers tell us how strong to build bridges, economists control inflation by tweaking interest rates, and chemists warn of environmental dangers and toxic exposures. Medicine is currently undergoing a similar explosion of interest in technocratic solutions to its resource allocation dilemmas.[49]

In medicine, this arena of activity is known by various names, such as the outcomes and effectiveness movement, medical technology assessment, or health services research. Its driving force is the realization that, for far too long, most of medical practice has evolved without the benefit of systematic measurement and reflection. Historically, the vast bulk of our nation's considerable investment in medical research has occurred only at the stage of determining whether innovations in treatment provide an advance over conventional methods. Little effort has gone into either weeding out discredited techniques, comparing different versions of accepted techniques, or measuring the costs of advances against their incremental benefits. As a result, according to commonly quoted estimates, fewer than one-quarter of existing medical procedures, perhaps only 10 percent, have been subject to thorough evaluation.

The call for better evaluation of new and existing medical technologies resulted in the creation in 1989 of the federal Agency for Health Care Policy and Research and in the flowering of health services research in academic and industry settings. Private think tanks like the RAND Corporation, professional medical societies like the American Medical Association (AMA), individual hospitals and HMOs, and even drug manufacturers have all jumped on the outcomes and effectiveness research bandwagon.[50] The final product of this emerging science is a practical decision tool known as a practice protocol or clinical pathway, which specifies for a given condition or medical application the precise indicators for each step in a detailed sequence of treatment decisions. Other products of this systematic assessment activity are not as prescriptive. Practice guidelines or practice parameters offer more general or discursive guidance by summarizing existing knowledge and marking the outer bounds of acceptable practice. For instance, a practice guideline might state that coronary angiography is appropriate for a patient with nonspecific chest pains and a positive treadmill test but inappropriate for a patient with only stable mild angina, whereas a practice protocol might specify much more concretely the quantitative test results and the conditions under which chest pain are experienced. In either event, the net effect is a substantial restriction in the latitude of discretion enjoyed by individual clinicians.

These tools can be used in reimbursement settings that raise the prospect of resource allocation. Although few developers of practice guidelines or protocols openly incorporate cost considerations into their deliberations, it is clear that prudent use of resources is the primary motivation for Congress having created the Agency for Health Care Policy and Research and for the considerable interest that insurers have in supporting this activity. Even if resource allocation is not now a dominant consideration in the scientific/technocratic community, the pieces are all in place for costs to play a much larger role in future years as resource constraints become more severe.

Two versions of how this might occur in actual insurance contracts and legal disputes have been developed, one by law professor Clark Havighurst using practice protocols, and the other by myself and economist Gerard Anderson using more general assessment criteria.[51] Professor Havighurst advocates using multiple competing sets of detailed practice protocols to express alternative standards of medical appropriateness in insurance contracts.[52] He reasons that parties to the contract can refer to existing sets of protocols as a way of overcoming the past difficulties they experienced with very general terms such as "medically necessary."

Anderson and I propose a more complex use of general language.[53] We sketch a taxonomy that specifies hierarchical categories of technology assessment relating to each of five dimensions: (1) safety, (2) effectiveness, (3) cost, (4) level of confidence in empirical findings, and (5) the outcome measures to be used in evaluating each of these. Using this scheme, one might limit treatment options to those that are demonstrably safe and are at least as effective as the available alternatives, with effectiveness defined in terms of outcome measures such as quality-adjusted life years (QALYs) and costing no more than $50,000 per QALY gained.[54] The key to our proposal is not the exact substance of the terms used to express medical effectiveness, but the fact that whatever terms are chosen are precisely the same terms used by the research community to express its findings on effectiveness. A tight fit between the contract language and the supporting evidence in a particular case provides greater assurance that courts will honor the resource allocation decisions made in the contract. This assurance increases if the contract itself specifies the independent scientific agencies whose findings are deemed binding on the parties.

These proposals might well succeed in overcoming the legal obstacles surveyed above that have inhibited more robust cost containment efforts by insurers and government regulators. Taking the decisions away from self-interested insurers and giving them to technical experts may convince the courts to honor statutory and contractual resource limitations more forthrightly. Nevertheless, there are a number of reasons why we may not be fully satisfied with the resulting allocation decisions or the processes that lead up to them. The remainder of this section catalogues a host of such reasons, exploring the most important ones in some detail.

This counterpoint is explained primarily in reference to the Oregon rationing plan, which is the most extensive effort at third-party technocratic rationing to date. In the early 1990s, Oregon decided to expand the number of people it could afford to enroll in Medicaid by limiting the medical procedures covered to those that produce the most medical benefit. This form of rationing contrasts with that in other states, which cover most medically necessary procedures but deny eligibility to over half the people in poverty. Details of Oregon's rationing scheme will emerge throughout the discussion below, but the essentials can be stated briefly as follows. Oregon ranks over 700 condition–treatment pairs (for example, surgery for appendicitis) according to the degree of medical benefit produced. The state legislature then determines how much it can afford to fund Medicaid in the aggregate, and actuaries tell the state how far down the list it can afford to go in order to maintain coverage for all eligible recipients below the poverty guideline. In forming this ranking, Oregon first employed a strict cost/effectiveness assessment, but due to severe criticism, the second ranking employed a looser evaluative process that combined effectiveness ratings with consumer preferences for quality-of-life factors.[55] This led to the additional criticism that the ranking entailed disability discrimination, so the final ranking eliminated quality-of-life factors and focused almost exclusively on medical effectiveness.[56]

A more recent effort to create a comprehensive set of resource rules is the six volumes of clinical guidelines developed by the insurance consulting firm Milliman & Robertson. These guidelines are widely used by HMOs, employers, and large managed care insurers to determine medical necessity under private insurance contracts. Referring to examples such as the Oregon list and the "M & R" guidelines might be considered going after easy prey, given their well-known flaws, many of which are correctable at least in theory. However, Oregon and other precedents tell us how technocratic rationing occurs in actual practice, and they help to illustrate that some flaws are endemic to any such effort, however thoroughly revised it might be.

THE FLAWS OF RULE-BASED RATIONING

The central flaw of technocratic resource allocation is that it must rely on a centralized rule-based system to enforce its decisions, in contrast with the individualized judgment that now characterizes most medical practice. The use of rules is both a practical necessity and one of the factors that make the technocratic solution appealing. The argument of the technology assessment community is that science produces an answer that is objectively correct. When we know the truth, it is wrong and unjust not to do what is right for everyone, and the only way to do that is through mandatory, categorical standards. Rules are necessary to technocratic rationing because scientific research teams cannot be assembled at the bedside of each patient. Because scientific knowledge tends to speak in generalities and probabilities, its expressions naturally emanate in a rule-based form.[57]

The contrasting version of decision making is individualized professional discretion, in which an expert knowledgeable in medical science decides what is best in each particular case. This does not qualify as technocratic resource allocation because the research community does not make the decision; it only supplies background information. The decision is made at the bedside by the doctor in consultation with the individual patient, considering all the factors they view as relevant to the decision. Technocratic, rule-based rationing says feed a fever and starve a cold (or is it the other way around?), whereas professional, discretionary rationing says do what's best for this patient, knowing what has and has not worked well for prior patients.

Whether rationing should occur through technocratic mechanisms therefore turns in large part on whether, for medicine in general, centralized rule-based decisions are preferable to individualized discretionary ones. This comparative analysis bears also on the other major forms of third-party resource allocation— bureaucratic and democratic—since they too usually operate through rules. I will therefore undertake an extensive analysis of the competing merits of rules versus discretion, looking at this issue first in general terms, and then as it applies more particularly to medical decisions.

Rules versus Discretion Generally

Quite a lot of thought has been devoted in recent years to analyzing the comparative advantages and disadvantages of using general rules versus individualized discretion to address various social problems. Although these theorists diverge considerably in their points of emphasis, there is broad consensus that neither mechanism in its pure form is universally preferred over the other.[58] Almost all social systems will employ a mix of the two. Although this uncontroversial assertion hardly needs defense, it bears considerable thought. An expanded explanation helps us better understand the proper domain of rules versus discretion and therefore assists in crafting the best mix in each social sphere

Rules have the following major advantages.

1. They save time. This is because they minimize the need to consult first principles in each instance. Rules accumulate, instantiate, and propagate past wisdom and experience in a manner that is impossible for any one individual to replicate instantaneously. Rules are like doing math by calculator rather than by long division; just punch in the data and out pops the answer.
2. Rules embody a collection of process attributes which enhance their value regardless of their actual effects on people. These "process values" include even-handedness, visibility, predictability, and participation.[59] These attributes help to legitimize the resulting decision in a way that individual authority cannot. Rules foster a sense of justice by treating like cases alike. Because they are announced in advance of the decision, they give prior notice, which allows planning. Basing a decision on rules also makes more visible the reason or

justification for action. Moreover, because rules reflect the views of a broad array of people, they foster a sense of participation in the decision, especially where the person affected by the rule was involved in its development or was represented by others who were.

Rules have the following major disadvantages:

1. Because they generalize, they are inaccurate. Even the most specific and detailed rules necessarily generalize to some degree; it is the essence of their quality as rules that they classify cases according to a limited (even if extensive) set of factors. The complexity of human affairs dictates that a limited set of factors will rarely, if ever, capture perfectly the background justification that motivates the rule. Therefore, rules will always be both underinclusive and overinclusive, to at least some degree. Unanticipated circumstances will always arise that call out for exceptions or amendments, but deciding strictly by rule prevents such an instantaneous adjustment. The exceptional case can form the basis for subsequent amendment of the rule, but to deviate on the spot is to exercise discretion, not rule-based authority.
2. Rulemakers can suffer from biases, limitations in their knowledge, and ordinary mistakes and misjudgments, just as can discretionary decision makers. When these errors occur, they affect many more people than the errors of a single practitioner.
3. To decide by rule means that the rule itself serves as the sole justification for the decision. Therefore, rules foreclose access to the justifications underlying the rule. This is essential to their efficiency advantage, but it blunts the sense of responsibility when mistakes occur. Mistakes under discretionary decisions are clearly identified as such and attributable to the one who made the decision. Mistakes under rules are not clearly seen as such, because the rule itself tends to define the norm. Therefore, if the rule is followed, an appeal to the ideal norm that lies behind the rule may be considered irrelevant. Even if recognized, the defect in a rule is attributable to the rule designer and not the rule implementer. This insulation from responsibility may cause officials who face tough decisions to place too much reliance on rules designed by someone else.

Discretionary decision making enjoys and suffers a complementary list of pros and cons. On the positive side:

1. Discretionary decisions, because they are case-specific, have the potential to perfectly reflect the underlying substantive concerns that motivate action. A discretionary decision maker has direct access to fundamental principles and purposes, and complete freedom to individualize his actions according to every nuance of each individual case. Ralph Waldo Emerson reminds us that "A fool-

ish consistency is the hobgoblin of little minds, adored by statesmen and philosophers and divines."[60] Discretion avoids the mistake of disregarding relevant differences.

2. This quality of discretionary judgment promotes not only the potential for greater accuracy, but also a somewhat different set of process or dignitary values. Rules promote equality by treating like cases alike, whereas individualized discretion treats different cases differently. This individualized attention—being able to plead one's case to the ultimate authority—is just as strong an aspect of our sense of justice as is the principle of equality fostered by rules. This notion is captured in the aphorism that "The worse the society, the more law there will be. In Hell there will be nothing but law, and due process will be meticulously observed."[61]

Discretionary decisions are subject to the following negatives:

1. They offer ample opportunity for bias, dishonesty, and mistakes by the decision maker.
2. Arriving at the best possible decision in each case is expensive and time consuming.
3. The bases for discretionary decisions are often hidden, which prevents people from planning for, objecting to, or even knowing about important decisions that affect them.

These and other competing attributes are succinctly summarized in Table 3–1, adapted from Professor Duncan Kennedy.[62]

Rules versus Discretion In Medical Settings

Based on these many powerful negative and positive traits, no social sphere is likely to be dominated exclusively by either rules or by discretion. From what I've said so far, though, it might appear that rules are especially unsuited for the medical arena. The following description by political theorist Fred Schauer of the defects of rules in general seems as if it is aimed directly at medical decision making:

The choice of the appropriate degree of rule-based [decision making] . . . is necessarily a function of the purpose a decision-making environment is thought to serve. Some decision-making environments . . . focus on the richness and uniqueness of immediate experience. Their sights are set on . . . the importance of getting *this* decision just right. In such environments the decision-makers will ordinarily have the freedom to explore every possible fact or argument that might bear on making the best decision in *this* instance, for it is precisely the *thisness* of the event that is most vital. At its extreme, such a system might, and arguably should, deny the relevance of mandatory rules entirely. The virtues of stability would bow to the desire to get things right, and in such a framework rules *qua* rules ought to have little if any force.[63]

Table 3–1. Good and bad aspects of decision-making by rules versus discretion

Rules		Discretion	
Good	Bad	Bad	Good
Neutrality	Rigidity	Bias	Flexibility
Uniformity	Conformity	Favoritism	Individualization
Precision	Anality	Sloppiness	Creativity
Certainty	Compulsiveness	Uncertainty	Spontaneity
Autonomy	Alienation	Totalitarianism	Participation
Rights	Vested Interests	Tyranny	Community
Privacy	Isolation	Intrusiveness	Concern
Efficiency	Indifference	Sentimentality	Equity
Order	Reaction	Chaos	Evolution
Exactingness	Punitiveness	Permissiveness	Tolerance
Self-reliance	Stinginess	Romanticism	Generosity
Boundaries	Walls	Invasion	Empathy
Stability	Sclerosis	Disintegration	Progress
Security	Threatenedness	Dependence	Trust

Legal theorist Carl Schneider also summarizes the comparative advantages of discretion over rules in terms that seem fully applicable to medicine:

Sometimes rule-makers fail to anticipate all the problems a rule is written to solve. Discretion can fill gaps in rules. Sometimes two or more rules simultaneously apply but dictate conflicting results. Discretion can permit the decision-maker to resolve the conflict in ways that best accommodate all the interests involved. Sometimes a rule will, applied to a particular case, produce a result that conflicts with the rule's purpose . . . or that conflicts with our understanding of what justice demands. Discretion can let the decision-maker do justice. And sometimes the circumstances in which a rule must be applied will be so complex that no effective rule can be written. Discretion frees the decision-maker to deal with that complexity.[64]

In contrast with the apparent negatives of rules in the medical arena, the positive attributes of rules have their greatest force in political, legal, and commercial arenas. These are where the process values inherent in rules come most strongly to the fore. The greatest need exists in commercial transactions for certainty and predictability in order to have a smoothly functioning economy. Public arenas are where we have the greatest concern about strict evenhandedness. When the government is doling out benefits or imposing social burdens, we are more willing to tolerate broad generalities that produce somewhat inaccurate allocations in order to ensure no improper favoritism or antagonism.

Discretion abounds even in these public spheres, however. Discretionary judgment dominates some of the most critical aspects of our legal system, including damages awards in civil litigation, child custody disputes, decisions to prosecute criminal cases, and the very question of guilt or innocence decided by juries in criminal trials. The extent of debate and commentary on this issue by administrative law scholars demonstrates that there is room for discretion in even the most bureaucratic of legal arenas. Excessive use of rules in welfare administration has been decried for the effects on the professionalism of case workers and the resulting attitudes of beneficiaries.[65] Disability income regulations have also been criticized for their rigidity.[66] In recent years, the most visible and intense debate has been over the federal criminal sentencing guidelines, which remove virtually all of the judge's traditional discretion over the length of imprisonment.[67] Critics attack this attempt at "foolish consistency" for failing to consider sufficiently the exact circumstances of the crime, the personality and past history of the defendant, and local community attitudes and mores.

The Case in Favor of Rules

I stress the controversial nature of rules in the legal arena—one generally thought to be the best suited for rules—in order, by contrast, to emphasize the even more difficult case one faces in justifying rule-based decision making in medicine. Before articulating all of the many deficiencies of medical rules, however, let me stress their positive aspects, for my position certainly is not that practice guidelines and other forms of structured decision making have no place in medicine. The argument over the choice of rationing mechanisms too often falsely pits unchannelled incentives against inflexible standards. This is not a winner-take-all contest; the ideal will certainly fall within a range of acceptable mixtures of the two.[68] Rules might best establish which treatments are entirely excluded, when dramatic and high-stakes treatment can be withheld, and what the broad parameters are for ordinary items of care. Where little disagreement exists and where the science is clear, detailed practice guidelines might prescribe some forms of treatment in a precise, cookbook fashion. The undefined spheres of medicine or those where patient values vary widely could then be shaped by financial, professional, and liability incentives, in combination with physicians' conversations with their patients. This is merely general speculation, however. We will never know which mixes and what forms of rules and incentives are acceptable until the merits and flaws of each approach and their proper domains receive rigorous empirical inquiry and analytical debate.

My argument here will not do justice to rule-based medicine since the strongest case in favor is not the positive one directly on the merits of rules but is the negative one that articulates the defects of the leading contenders to rules. Because the proper place for medical rules is based on this second-best or "least worst" rationale, full appreciation of rules can be had only after considering the competing analysis in the next chapter of the many serious concerns about physicians rationing care at the bedside. It is necessary, however, to respond here at least partially to these concerns.

The strongest response to the obvious flaws in physician discretion is that we have always relied predominantly on physician discretion despite these flaws. Precisely the same arguments now being raised in favor of rule-based *cost*/benefit tradeoffs could also be made in favor of using rules to make *medical risk*/benefit calculations. Nevertheless, for questions of medical benefit, society strongly prefers individualized professional judgment, shaped by financial and liability incentives. It is only in the era of limited health care resources that we hear of the many corrupting biases that infect physicians' bedside judgment. But choosing the *medically* optimal course of treatment is also subject to personal bias and professional idiosyncracies. Despite the widespread calls for explicit clinical guidelines to improve the quality of care and reduce the unexplained variation in physician practice patterns, no one is naive enough to believe that, while we wait for perfection on these matters, we should determine the intricacies of medical benefit entirely by binding rules. We have little more basis for taking comfort in this solution when costs are factored into the equation. For both risk/benefit and cost/benefit calculations, there is every reason to believe that a rule-based approach would neither be uniformly superior to physician judgment, nor that it would be capable of entirely displacing physician discretion.

The shift in focus from medical benefits to medical costs does have some significance for the relative importance of rules, however. The prior section explains that the "process values" fostered by rules increase in force in proportion to how public the arena is in which decision making occurs. At some point, we are willing to sacrifice an increment of accuracy and individuality in order to achieve greater predictability and uniformity, where the latter have important symbolic and social value. In medicine, this shift in perspective from private benefits to public costs occurs, at least to some degree, by virtue of the communal nature of health insurance. If we each paid for our medical costs individually, we could insist on "designer medicine" perfectly tailored to each of our individual circumstances. Where the issue is how best to maximize medical benefit for each patient, no issue of fairness exists as *among* patients. The focus is entirely individual, and so the answer turns largely on issues of technical accuracy. But when we pool our resources to create health insurance, our medical decisions are necessarily paid for by someone else. Therefore, others have a right to insist that some limits be set, and others have the right to insist on equal treatment. Equal treatment within the same insurance pool can be guaranteed only through external, rule-based authority enforcing uniform standards. This justification for uniformity is even greater under public insurance programs such as Medicare and Medicaid.

The shift in focus from benefits to costs introduces fairness considerations that strengthen the case for rules. When the question becomes whether medical benefits are worth their costs, the decision implicitly or explicitly seeks to maximize medical benefit across a population of patients by sacrificing one patient's benefit for another's. The most dramatic instances of this dilemma are allocations of scarce life-saving organ transplants among multiple potential recipients. The pressing need to legitimize the loss of life suffered by some patients causes both physicians and society to strongly oppose distributing life-saving organs by ad hoc discretion. Because any hint of corruption or favoritism in this situation is intolerable, a uniform rule, even one as blunt and arbitrary as a simple lottery, is preferable to individual doctors advocating for their own patients.[69] As political and social theorist Jon Elster observes, "it seems to hold quite generally that people are more willing to accept bad outcomes if they are the unintended result of anonymous social processes than if they are the intended result of deliberate intervention."[70]

Rule-based medicine is also consistent with the *contractual* underpinnings of private health care financing and delivery systems. Legislators and public policy analysts increasingly seek to resolve difficult regulatory and social policy dilemmas by offering consumers options at the point of insurance enrollment. This is the fundamental premise of managed competition, and it is the foundation for reform proposals that I make later in this book and that are developed by other scholars.[71] The more resource allocation work that we require insurance contracts to perform, the more explicit must our allocation rules be so that consumers are well informed when they commit themselves to a rationing scheme. It is unfair to use contractual principles to foreclose treatment options if these consequences cannot be made clear at the time of enrollment, and they cannot be made clear without treatment protocols of sufficient precision. Consider, for instance, the story told by a former general counsel for the Sloan Kettering Cancer Institute who tried to learn whether each of six competing HMOs in the New York market would allow her to continue her specialist treatment for breast cancer. Despite her considerable expertise and persistence, she was unable to learn this simple fact from five of the six HMOs. One claimed that it "had 'no policy on breast cancer.'" "[B]ecause approvals are given on a case-by-case basis, a patient really couldn't know what coverage is available before selecting a plan. As PruCare's representative volunteered, 'You don't know until you actually hand in that claim form.'"[72] Explicit and binding resource allocation rules are necessary to overcome this critical limitation in essential consumer information.

Finally, rationing rules have the advantage of insulating physicians from responsibility for resource allocation. In part, this is desirable, because otherwise the prospect of physicians sacrificing individual medical benefit on account of costs might undermine the profound level of trust that patients must have in their doctors in order to submit to invasive procedures, and in order for healing processes to work optimally. This point, which is pursued at much greater length in the Chapter 5, is potentially the strongest basis for favoring rules over discretion.

The Case Against Rules

These process values of trustworthiness, uniformity, publicity, and predictability must nevertheless be weighed against the substantive values of accuracy and individuality that are sacrificed by rules. The principal objection to medical rules is that the nature of human mental and biological functioning and the state of medical science are such that no set of rules could possibly be detailed enough to capture all of the nuanced and judgmental aspects of medical decision making. Rule-based resource allocation epitomizes the mythical Procrustean bed in more than simply the usual metaphorical way. Fitting patients into preset categories for which their clinical circumstances and individual values are not perfectly suited might literally result in their legs being chopped off to accommodate the shape of the rule. There are many other expressions of the same opinion, more eloquent and informed than my own:

To be medically justified, rationing decisions have to be personalized, because no two patients are exactly the same and the anticipated benefits of a given procedure vary from patient to patient. . . . With each procedure, the cost-benefit assessment depends so heavily on individual circumstances that it is almost impossible to devise medically sound rules applicable to all patients. In fact, the task is so formidable that no one has yet offered a practical suggestion about how personalized rationing might be carried out systematically and on a wide scale.[73]

[Centralized rule-making] is too distant from the realistic contingencies of disease, the complexities of comorbidity, and the diversity of personal and family situations, to extend to specific clinical decisions under the conditions of uncertainty that characterize much of medical care. In a large and culturally heterogeneous society it is especially difficult to anticipate the varying needs, expectations and tastes of patients and their families.[74]

The processes of administrative decision-making are too crude and rigid to accommodate adequately to the detailed complexities of sickness, the contingencies of people's lives, and the uncertainties of human transactions that span a community as culturally diverse as our own.[75]

[W]hen care is provided in . . . a caring, continuous, committed physician-patient relationship, [t]he mutual decision making . . . can never be adequately covered in formal "practice guidelines," treatment algorithms, or rigidly defined contracts because they cannot possibly include either the distinct and profound specificity of the patient and physician as persons or the shared experiences and meanings that develop between them over time.[76]

The scientific basis of modern medicine might appear to argue in favor of heavy reliance on rules, since as noted above science lends itself to generalizable knowledge and systematized practice. But there is fundamental truth in the overused cliche that medicine is more art than science. The art metaphor is meant to capture the notion that medicine is a professional discipline involving the differential application of background scientific knowledge (as well as other sources of knowledge) to the circumstances of particular patients, much like an artist uses technical skills and visual observation to fashion a unique creation.[77] The reason medical practice cannot be wholly systematized is that biological, social, and human factors are far too numerous and complex in their variety and combinations to ever be reduced entirely to a comprehensive and binding set of treatment protocols. As the argument is frequently put: "One cannot practice good medicine by committee or cookbook or computer. A person or group reviewing summaries of information cannot possibly appreciate all the clinical factors that make each situation different—and it is these judgments that make medicine such a complex, demanding profession."[78]

The inability to adequately capture all of medical practice in a set of comprehensive rules is amply borne out by the Oregon Medicaid proposal, which is the most notable attempt to date to impose comprehensive, rule-based rationing. Aaron and Schwartz aptly describe the Oregon list as a "meat-ax" approach to rationing. All items above the funding line are entirely covered, no matter how mild the condition is or how marginal the necessity is for the medical intervention, while conditions below the line are not covered at all, no matter how severe or how great the potential is for improvement.[79] "Patients with incapacitating lumbar disk disease are grouped with patients whose disease is barely symptomatic."[80] For breast cancer, "no distinction is made among different stages, cell types, or other factors likely to influence the choice of treatment and expected outcomes, nor are different treatments distinguished (e.g., chemotherapy, radiation therapy, immunotherapy, or surgery)."[81] Despite the considerable sophistication of Oregon's methodology and the years of effort behind its rankings, over half specify only medical or surgical treatment generically, making no distinction for the different steps that might be used in treating a particular condition, and the rankings take no account at all for diagnostic steps.[82]

The Milliman & Robertson guidelines widely used by HMOs and other private insurers are equally blunt. They prescribe just one day of hospitalization for normal childbirth and only two days for a C-section. For a mastectomy, they specify no hospitalization at all, under the view that outpatient surgery is usually sufficient. These guidelines provide little clinical detail for determining when these norms do not apply to a more serious or complex case, leaving that issue to individual physician discretion.[83]

While it is possible to vastly improve on these examples, the practical barriers are formidable. A complete and empirically valid set of rationing rules would require rigorous scientific information on each of the almost 10,000 diagnostic entries in the World Health Organization's *International Classification of Diseases* (9th ed. 1991) (known as "ICD-9") and for each of the 10,000 medical interventions listed in the AMA's *Common Procedural Terminology* (known as "CPT" codes).[84] Medical-effectiveness researchers Robert Dubois and Robert Brook explain that, for just one category of illness (such as heart disease) involving only ten comorbidities and ten complications, a complete protocol would have to account for 10 billion different clinical scenarios, since each of the 20 conditions would have to be assessed not only in all possible combinations with each other, but also with all possible sequences.[85] For rules to be complete, each of these billions of clinical pathways would have to be accounted for within each major and minor disease category. Even without this degree of utter completeness, David Eddy, another prominent medical effectiveness researcher, explains that:

for any patient condition there are dozens of procedures that can be ordered, in any combination, at any time. The list of procedures that might be included in a workup of chest pain or hypertension would take more than a page, spanning the spectrum from simply asking questions, to blood studies, to x-rays. Even for highly specific diagnostic problems, there can be a large choice of procedures. For example, if a woman presents with a breast mass and her physician wants to know its approximate size and architecture, the physician might contemplate an imaging procedure. The choice could include mammography, ultrasonography, thermography, diaphanography, computed tomography, lymphography, Mammoscan, and nuclear magnetic resonance imaging. A physician who chose mammography would still have to decide between xeromammography and film mammography, with several brands being available for the latter. There are about a dozen procedures that apply the principles of thermography. And why should a diagnostic workup be limited to one test? Why not follow a negative mammogram with a computed tomogram (or vice versa)? For the detection of colorectal cancer, a physician can choose any combination of fecal occult blood tests (and there are more than a dozen brands), digital examination, rigid sigmoidoscopy, flexible 30 cm sigmoidoscopy, flexible 60 cm sigmoidoscopy, barium enema (either plain or air contrast), and colonoscopy. These choices are not trivial. Most procedures have different mechanisms of action and a long list of pros and cons. Different brands of fecal occult blood tests have very different sensitivities and specificities, and film mammography and xeromammography differ in their radiation exposure by a factor of about four. These procedures are for relatively well-defined diseases; imagine the problems of selecting procedures to evaluate symptoms like fatigue, headache, or fever that can have about a dozen causes.[86]

To gauge the magnitude of even a greatly abbreviated version of this monumental task, compare the performance of the Agency for Health Care Policy and Research (AHCPR), which after six years of sustained effort costing tens of millions of dollars has produced only about 15 practice guidelines.[87] Most of these guidelines are in areas where numerous clinical studies already exist, so before they could be replicated for all conditions and treatments, unimaginably vast resources would have to be devoted to producing rigorous experimental data on clinical effectiveness, patient outcomes, and cost/benefit information for each possible medical intervention. Ted Marmor and Jan Blustein explain that, "[i]deally, [such] research involves systematic and painstaking testing of therapies through randomized controlled clinical trials. But these experiments . . . are events of epic proportion, lasting for years, costing millions of dollars, involving thousands of patients, facing monumental bureaucratic barriers, and raising serious ethical issues.

Often, by the time clinical trials are completed, the technology they studied is outmoded."[88] David Eddy elaborates: "Some diseases are so rare that, in order to conduct the ideal clinical trials, it would be necessary to collect tens of thousands, if not hundreds of thousands, of participants. A good example concerns the frequency of the Pap smear. One might wonder why the merits of a three-year versus one-year frequency cannot be settled by a randomized controlled trial. Because of the low frequency of cervical cancer, and the small difference in outcomes expected for the two frequencies, almost one million women would be required for such a study."[89]

At present, the United States appears to lack the financial and political will to undertake even a greatly scaled back version of this massive effort. The National Institutes of Health (NIH) sees as its primary mission developing and assessing new medical technologies, largely through "bench" or "pure" science, as opposed to clinical trials of existing medical practices. Moreover, anecdotes abound in the health services research community about the hostility within NIH review committees to introducing cost dimensions into scientific research studies. The AHCPR is the agency with primary authority over assessing medical cost effectiveness. It receives only about 1 percent of the funding that goes to the NIH. Even the fledgling effort at AHCPR is threatened. It is on the Republican chopping block of agencies whose funding is being reduced in the effort to balance the federal budget and reduce taxes.[90] Previous Republican proposals would have eliminated the AHCPR altogether, just like its predecessor, the National Center for Health Care Technology, which, having received a similar mandate in 1978, was axed after only three short years, during the Reagan-era spate of antigovernment fervor, as the result of heavy lobbying by medical professional and industry groups who felt threatened by the agency's scrutiny.[91] The AHCPR similarly has abandoned its guideline development activity in response to political pressure and budget reductions. In short, the public and private research communities appear far from undertaking the unprecedented effort necessary to evaluate rigorously all existing medical procedures on an ongoing basis.

Even with such an effort, it is not at all clear that the information produced would be capable of expression in executable algorithms that are meaningful to clinical judgment. As Sandra Tanenbaum explains, effectiveness research "is not . . . a new foundation for clinical medicine; it is raw material for the artful practitioner."[92] The findings of scientific medical research are usually expressed in terms of probabilities and rarely in terms of certainties. When scientific medicine is certain, it speaks in terms of condition-specific certainties, not patient-specific ones. Where scientific knowledge is less certain, rule-based medical decisions face even greater difficulty. If all we know from scientific research is that procedure X is bad or of no use for 60 percent of patients but does help 40 percent, a regime that required rule-based decisions might deny the treatment to everyone. Traditionally, the art of clinical medicine is to attempt to discern through trial, error, and intuition which patients fall into the 60 percent and which into the 40 percent. Some freedom from rules is necessary in order for medical knowledge to advance in this fashion.

Rigorous scientific findings consider only one or a limited number of clinical categories, not the full, rich texture of human possibilities. This is best illustrated by the use of randomized controlled trials (RCT), which are considered the gold standard of medical research. The central purpose of RCT methodology is to exclude all the messy complications that might cloud the findings with respect to the critical factor or intervention under study, so as to obtain a definitive answer on whether that single factor or intervention makes a difference. This form of study results in the generalized, albeit certain, truth that, "all other factors being equal," X matters or does not matter (within accepted ranges of statistical probability). The difficulty, of course, is that all things rarely are the same. Patient A is different in many respects from the model patient, and some of these differences may affect the scientific finding in ways that we lack any scientific knowledge of, much less rigorous proof about. Analyzing and incorporating these differences through intuitive judgment, developed both through scientific study and through clinical experience, is the work of medical professionals.

Physicians make these judgments either through a type of gestalt pattern-recognition process that they are not able fully to articulate (much like one recognizes a familiar face without being able to explain its features) or by constructing in their minds a narrative, cause-and-effect explanation of what is happening to each patient and the physiology of the proposed intervention.[93] Clinical protocols that operate as definitive rules eliminate any role for this aspect of clinical professionalism. Both the intuitive and the narrative approaches to treatment are at odds with a rule's bald directive, which commands only *what* to do, with little explanation of or opportunity to consider *why*.

Consistency with Medical and Social Values

If sufficiently rigorous and detailed treatment protocols were technically feasible, the question would still remain: Are they desirable? Physical and mental health are matters riddled with personal value preferences that are difficult to sufficiently accommodate in a set of uniform rules. As sociologist David Mechanic explains, "People . . . differ in their personal agendas, their preferences for care, their tolerance for pain and discomfort, indeed their desire to live when deathly ill. These are matters better left to health professionals and patients to negotiate than to public polling or bureaucratic mandates."[94] Rene Dubos agrees that

health cannot be defined in the absolute, because different persons expect such different things from life. A Wall Street executive, a lumberjack in the Canadian Rockies, a newspaper boy at a crowded street corner, a steeplechase jockey, a cloistered monk, and the pilot of a supersonic combat plane have various physical and mental needs. The imperfections and limitations of the flesh and of the mind do not have equal importance to them. Their goals [and personalities] determine the kind of vigor and resistance required for success in their own lives.[95]

Strangers to the treatment relationship have no opportunity to appreciate the value preferences of individual patients. Collective decision making, whether it wants to or not, necessarily pursues a reductionist logic that sacrifices individual preferences for communal welfare.[96] For instance, in valuing different health outcomes, the original (but not the final) Oregon methodology equated one year of normal life with 10 years of life at one-tenth capacity, and it equated one life saved for 10 years with 10 lives saved for one year each.[97] This utilitarian logic is fundamental to all dominant methods of assessing the comparative effectiveness of medical treatments.[98] It assumes that everyone attaches the same value to a given health state, and it allows increments in those values to be summed and traded off across individuals. This approach to resource allocation is deeply disturbing and counterintuitive. As Philosopher John Taurek observes in his classic essay ("Should the Numbers Count?"), "The discomfort of each of a large number of individuals experiencing a minor headache does not add up to anyone's experiencing a migraine."[99] Although the absurdities of this extreme can be avoided, a rule-based system can never avoid the fundamental reductionist tendency to attribute similar preferences to everyone with a similar condition.

Externally imposed rationing rules are also inconsistent with values of medical professionalism. Medical sociologist David Mechanic explains that

> Explicit rationing is the mode of control most resented by working professionals since it intrudes on their practicing autonomy and discretion in a direct way. Administrative authority frequently becomes insensitive to the human dilemmas and variabilities so obvious at the clinical level. . . . Physicians and patients seek to manipulate and evade rules they view as irrational, and often such adaptive responses bring about subterfuge, perverse outcomes, and inequities in distribution.[100]

Physicians are especially notorious for their ability to rationalize their noncompliance with any authority that contravenes their clinical judgment. Ends-justify-means thinking is rampant among doctors.[101] Based on their past behavior, we can expect physicians to easily manipulate the letter of rationing rules they disagree with in spirit.

Moving onto a higher plane, rule-based medicine can also be attacked as inconsistent with the healing relationship that underlies many treatment encounters. The previous chapter describes the powerful nonscientific element that potentially exists in any treatment relationship by virtue of a doctor's charismatic power to put the patient's mind at ease and convince him of the possibility of cure, even where none may appear to exist. Although we lack much hard evidence about this phenomenon, something in this relationship of power, authority, and dependency between doctor and patient appears to relieve internal distress and activate self-healing mechanisms that produce results that modern science is now only able to classify as anomalous (or miraculous).

Because we do not know very much about this nonspecific healing power, it is difficult to speak with confidence about how it would be affected by increased reliance on rules. It is possible that physicians' use of clinical protocols would have no effect, or that greater prominence of scientific rules might enhance patients' confidence and trust in their treatment. It is also possible, though, to see external control as undermining the charismatic healing dimension of the treatment relationship. Those who describe this phenomenon speak of the intimacy between doctor and patient forming the basis for the physician's power.[102] Others see the debate over rules versus discretion as a power struggle, one that attempts to wrest authority from individual professional judgment and corral it within centralized institutional bureaucracies.[103] In this manner, the technocratic movement is considered by some to be part and parcel of the shift in medicine from an intimate relationship with a personal physician to a service delivery contract generated by an anonymous market institution—in Professor Frankford's words, the shift from humanism to "scientism and economism."[104]

Another negative value dimension of medical rules has to do with personal responsibility. Rules tend to insulate the provider from a claim of responsibility or liability made by the injured patient. In rule-based medicine, physicians are not held accountable for the content of rules or the outcome of treatment so long as they accurately follow the rules. Following rules, it is all too convenient to respond: "I was only doing what the insurance company, government agency, or professional association said I must do." Rule-based rationing therefore has the potential to promote in physicians a crass attitude of expendability toward their patients' welfare. As David Mechanic explains, "Centralized authority, however benevolent, is isolated from the pain, worry, uncertainty, and disruption that characterize serious illness. It too easily loses touch with the feelings of participants and the tone of interaction. The result is often perverse."[105]

This possibility is suggested by the atrocities committed by German physicians under Nazi rule. It is also suggested by a classic social science experiment, Stanley Milgram's electric shock deception, in which Milgram had his subjects administer fake electric shocks to actors who pretended to experience extreme pain. Milgram deceived the subjects into believing that the object of the study was to test each actor's ability to memorize random word associations.[106] By exerting the authority of science and the demands of the experimental design, the researchers were able to prod the subjects to administer shocks they believed to be not only intolerably painful, but in a few cases, lethal. "[T]he subjects acted as if their choice-making self was 'not there.' . . . [The] subjects achieved their compliance by conceiving themselves . . . as objects ruled by extrinsic forces beyond their personal control."[107] "Milgram concluded that when people complied with what was apparently an inhumane order, it was because their sense of responsibility had been diminished or altered: they were 'only following orders.'"[108] Similarly, physicians relieved of the responsibility for making their own decisions may go too far in enforcing inhumane applications of superficially acceptable rationing rules.

A final assault on exclusive, or even primary, reliance on rule-based rationing is the realization that, whether or not collective rules are preferable in principle, some measure of bedside discretion is a practical necessity in practice, since it will be practicing physicians who interpret, apply, and implement these rules. Even clinically precise rules will retain considerable room for physician discretion. Assume, for instance, that an HMO adopts a rule that it is appropriate to perform coronary angiography for a patient with nonspecific chest pain and a positive tread-mill test, but this procedure is inappropriate for a patient with only stable mild angina.[109] This is not a rule at all; it is merely a guideline. Because there is no metric of pain, stability, and severity of angina, in many if not most cases the treating physician cannot effectively be second-guessed except by the exercise of another physician's discretionary judgment. Therefore, it is not possible to deny treatment even under this very precise rule without some reliance on individual discretion.

The vast majority of practice guidelines in existence now have discretionary wording similar to this example.[110] If the AMA were to have its way, all guidelines would "include a disclaimer stating that they are not intended to displace the physician's discretion to conform treatment to the particular clinical circumstances of the individual patient."[111] Medical sociologist Eliot Freidson notes that "this opportunity [to deviate from treatment protocols] is provided to physicians in every review context with which I am now familiar. The rank and file practitioner thus has virtually statutory opportunity to use discretion in following standardized procedures and to deviate from them."[112]

Inevitably, then, treatment directives have only a limited potential for determining the actual course of medical care. At present, there are far too few in existence to control a significant portion of medical spending decisions. This state of affairs is likely to continue for quite some time given the Herculean effort required to produce the scientific findings necessary to formulate acceptable rules. And if scientifically valid clinical rules were widely adopted, there would be strong pressure to keep them flexible and discretionary in order to accommodate widely varying patient preferences and circumstances. Even conceding, then, that rule-based rationing is the preferable course to follow wherever possible, it would still be necessary to employ physician discretion at least at the residual level of filling in the cracks between the rules and encouraging faithfulness in the interpretation and application of the rules to particular cases.

IDEAL DEMOCRATIC PROCESSES

Realizing the many flaws and limitations in both bureaucratic and technocratic rationing, several thoughtful commentators have advocated ideal democratic processes for making the tough value judgments entailed in medical spending decisions. Medical ethicist Leonard Fleck advocates resource allocation through an "informed democratic consensus model" in which "rationing principles and protocols . . . will be freely self-imposed, explicit, consistently applied to all in that community, and a product of a shared conception of health care justice that will emerge from a conversation among undominated equals."[113] Philosopher Daniel Callahan envisions "democratically established standards, open to public debate" and "reflective of community values."[114] Fleck is heading an ambitious project called "Just Caring" to empanel groups of 50 citizens in each of 25 locations to discuss resource allocation problems.[115] He advocates replicating this grassroots democratic consensus approach in each Congressional district by empaneling representative citizen groups that would deliberate on discrete medical cost/benefit trade-off problems within the range where legitimate public disagreement exists.[116]

Fleck observes that the need for such a social resolution process will always be very large given the competing theories of justice in our liberal society, the deeply felt individual values that attach to medical decisions, and the continuing lack of conclusive evidence on technical questions. Since no permanent set of ordered principles will ever be capable of resolving the numerous controversial issues in medicine, we must resort to widely accepted *processes* rather than settled *principles* in order to arrive at any workable substantive decisions.

Fleck and others advocate community-based deliberation as the ideal process for several reasons. First, because democratic processes are representative, it can be said that the solutions they advance are chosen by the affected community rather than being imposed on it. Therefore, this process does not sacrifice patient autonomy to the extent of other third-party rationing mechanisms. Second, democratic deliberations are open for public observation and discussion, in contrast to other forms of resource allocation that are invisible or hard to discover. On this score, technocratic processes stand in sharp contrast because, by their very nature, they obscure the basis for decision from common understanding. Their quasi-scientific garb hides the underlying value conflicts from people lacking technical sophistication. Third, democratic processes are more likely than some other mechanisms to produce substantive rules that are applied evenhandedly without regard to social class, ethnic status, or random chance. Therefore, they help to embody egalitarian values and a sense of fairness and social justice.

Tentative and partial implementation of these ideals have appeared in several guises in recent years. The initial Oregon rationing list was based in large part on quality-of-life ratings provided by citizen polls and focus-group discussions that inquired into how ordinary people rate various physical conditions. HMOs are required by state law, and encouraged by federal law, to empanel grievance and review committees containing a large representation of ordinary subscribers. One of their functions is to determine the appropriateness of disputed items of treatment. Health insurance plans sponsored by labor unions frequently contain the same jury-of-peers component that asks other subscribers how to resolve disputes over coverage for the group. Physician ethicist Ezekiel Emanuel draws from these precedents to construct a communitarian model for moral deliberation within individual health plans. Most health plan members would be expected to participate directly, not just by representation, in setting the group's resource allocation policies.[117] Leonard Fleck advocates forming a "national health congress" composed of representatives from local citizen panels in each Congressional district.[118]

Overruling Deliberators

The democratic consensus ideal, despite its many appealing virtues, suffers from several debilitating moral and practical limitations. Chief among these is the very lack of technical expertise possessed by ordinary citizens. True, it is not necessary for the deliberators to personally possess this expertise, since expert consultants can provide advice and information to the deliberators as needed. But this advice might simply be ignored or so severely misunderstood that we will sometimes want to overrule the choices made. Consider some of the value choices made by Oregon's citizens in constructing their Medicaid rationing list. The first draft listed cheap office visits for ailments such as thumb-sucking and tooth capping much higher than expensive life-saving surgeries for conditions such as appendicitis and ectopic pregnancy.[119] The second listing avoided most of these absurdities after much hand tinkering,[120] but similar absurdities plagued the underlying quality-of-life assessments derived from public opinion surveys. For instance, the disabling complication of "trouble speaking" was applied equally to conditions that range from a mild lisp to mutism, and "burn over large areas of the body" was ranked the same as an "upset stomach."[121]

These embarrassments might be avoided if truly deliberative techniques were used rather than random telephone surveys. But, even then, we are likely to disagree with many of the value choices made, for the very reason that people hold widely divergent deeply felt views on the fundamental issues presented. Philosopher Norman Daniels describes this predictable lack of confidence in our fellow citizens' judgment as "the democracy problem." The bizarre or selfish decisions they are likely to sometimes reach create the need to somehow screen public opinion for plausible rationality and to prevent invidious bias. But, to accomplish this critical task, we must resort to some other, less democratic mechanism than citizen deliberation.[122] Daniels correctly observes the difficulty this presents for grassroots solutions to health care rationing problems: If we are to sometimes overrule group decisions, how are we to do so—according to what process, and under whose authority?[123] Answering these questions requires us to resort to a higher-level process or a set of principles that themselves may or may not be grounded in participatory democracy. In Oregon, some of the absurdities of casual public opinion were corrected in the third, revised list that ultimately was enacted, but this was only accomplished by either ignoring the public surveys completely or by using technocratic authority to overrule the choices made by ordinary citizens.[124]

I am not simply making the elitist argument that only experts are capable of deciding fairly and rationally. I am, after observing the outcome of actual citizen-group deliberations and public opinion polls, making the realistic argument that we are strongly inclined to exercise oversight in some form to prevent the most obvious irrationalities and biases. Taking seriously the argument in favor of public opinion, those who advocate democratic mechanisms are defeated by the logic of their own position if people, as a whole, would prefer not to be bound by the judgment of their peers. In this regard, consider the public opinion polls cited at the beginning of this chapter, which indicate overwhelming preference for professional rather than lay or bureaucratic mechanisms for health care resource allocation.[125]

This distrust of populist democracy does not condescend; a healthy dose of skepticism can be found at the very pinnacle of democratic structures. The American Constitution exists in large part to prevent the worst excesses of legislative deliberations on questions of social justice involving the distribution of benefits and burdens within society. We must recognize, as did our Founding Fathers, that majority rule can be tyrannical and oppressive from the perspective of those in the minority. Rationing has received its blackest eye from a citizen group referred to as the Seattle "God Squad" that apportioned the limited renal dialysis slots when this expensive procedure was first available to treat fatal kidney disease. One member of the committee recounts "voting against a young woman who was a known prostitute . . . [and] against a young man who . . . had been a ne'er-do-well, a real playboy," in favor of middle-class, suburbanite patients.[126]

These concerns leave us with the following dilemma, however: If we do not have a safeguarding process or a settled hierarchy of rationing principles by which to judge the results of citizen group deliberations, we may be unable to place life-and-death decisions at the mercy of public opinion. But if we did possess these backstop processes or principles, the very need for consulting the public in the first place would not be so pressing; we could simply consult the safeguard principles directly and use public opinion only as a backstop.

The Willingness to Deliberate

Another practical and theoretical problem with heavy reliance on citizen-group deliberations is that group members themselves, understanding their own limits in rationality and expertise, may not *want* the primary responsibility for deciding tough resource allocation questions. The very process of careful deliberation is one that does not come easily to every ordinary citizen. Critiquing diametrically opposed moral positions in the face of contradictory technical arguments (scientists disagree, too) can create an intense sense of unease among those who are not used to exercising these mental faculties, especially when life and death are at stake. Accordingly, citizen deliberators may not take their tasks seriously, or if they do, they may prefer delegating tough decisions—both their technical and their moral value components—to experts.

This speculation is backed by considerable anecdotal support. Consider living wills, through which potential patients are asked to make dramatic and difficult decisions concerning their own medical fates. Despite massive publicity and ample assistance, the vast majority of people still lack an advance medical directive. In my personal experience with recalcitrant family members and friends, this is due in considerable part to a simple unwillingness to confront or an inability to decide extremely difficult and troubling issues. Even the significant minority who make these decisions are not always willing to be strictly bound by them. In one fascinating study, researchers questioned dialysis patients who had executed advance directives about whether to stop treatment in the event they developed advanced Alzheimer's disease. They found that over half would still want their physicians to have some or complete leeway to override the directive with their best interests in mind.[127] Consider also the following account, which comes directly from the immediate context of citizen groups deliberating over rationing rules:

At the meeting in Vermont, run by the Vermont Ethics Network, participants were asked to . . . choose one of four new technologies to add to the plan, for the state can afford to pay for only one; improved arthritis treatment, an intensive monitored exercise program for heart attack patients, an experimental system for helping premature newborns breathe or expanded mammography services. The technologies are equally expensive, but they help a different number of people in different age groups. . . . The idea of making such life-and-death choices made many of the participants squirm in their folding chairs. "I don't like this; this is giving me a stomachache," said Betty Smith, after voting for the newborn resuscitation because, she said, it would save the lives of society's newest members. In the end, only 8 of the 15 participants were willing to choose, and each option ended up with two votes.[128]

We gain a deeper understanding of this fundamental unease from Guido Calabresi and Philip Bobbit's classic analysis of the "tragic choice" entailed when any sacrifice of lifesaving or prevention effort is necessitated by scarce resources.[129] Calabresi and Bobbit observe that rationing decisions are not easily amenable to rational public deliberation; therefore, rationing is more successful when it is hidden or implicit. We stint on mine safety but devote huge resources to futile attempts to rescue miners when they are trapped.[130] David Hadorn labels this phenomenon the "rule of rescue." "There is a fact about the human psyche . . . : people cannot stand idly by when an identified person's life is visibly threatened if effective rescue measures are available."[131]

Others describe this as the paradox of statistical versus identifiable lives.[132] We are more distressed by the visible loss of specific, identified lives than when a group of people face an uncertain risk, because then the loss is not directly apparent. Society frequently sacrifices safety for a pittance when the extra effort only increases the odds of avoiding a catastrophe, because then no actual person is in imminent danger, but after disaster strikes our psychic connection with the personality of the victim compels us to do everything we can, beyond the point of futility.

This emotional response may be irrational, but it is not without social meaning. Michael Shapiro explains that public policy toward medical treatment often has the consequence of expressing and consecrating important social values:

For example, treating access to scarce medical resources as a matter of entitlement rather than as a matter of contingent market transactions may communicate an implied proposition about the value of life and the worth and nonfungibility of individual persons. . . . Other things being equal, . . . treating disease (or person) X and not disease (or person) Y seems unprincipled and incomprehensible. The taint of irrationality casts the value of life in doubt. If life is lost because of irrelevant differences, lifesaving choices seem contingent and arbitrary and thus unimportant. . . . It is thus possible that, despite contrary appearances, the regulatory system is efficient with respect to *overall* societal goals, including the transmitting of lifesaving preferences.[133]

James Nelson illustrates these points with the following everyday example:

I will risk my life on the roads to do nothing more than secure a bag of potato chips, not to mention take the risk of eating them simply for fleeting gustatory sensations. But should I come up short in the potato chips v. life lottery, and suffer either a car or a cardiovascular accident, I do not expect society to respond by saying, "Well, tough luck, but you made an open-eyed trade-off here." No, I expect EMTs to rush to the scene and pound on my chest and speed me to the hospital in reckless disregard of the laws set down to reduce the risk faced by other travelers in search of potato chips and other goods. This social response, I am suggesting, can be seen as a way of marking the fact that our lives are shot through with incommensurable values, and that we have to wind our way through them in a way that does its best to acknowledge their separate significance.[134]

One consequence of the public values attached to lifesaving actions, in the view of Calabresi and Bobbit, is the unsettling realization that there is a social virtue in the hidden nature of tragic choices. "By making the result seem necessary, unavoidable, rather than chosen, . . . [e]vasion, disguise, temporizing, deception are all ways by which artfully chosen allocation methods can avoid the appearance of failing to reconcile values in conflict. . . . Averting the eyes enables us to save some lives even when we will not save all."[135] Bringing rationing decisions into the full light of public deliberation will only heighten their tragic nature. This will either disable us from making them or inflict greater social grief in the process. Thus, the more forthright method may not be the more socially desirable one.

Fleck and others have observed that this argument for dishonesty carries no moral weight since honesty is a preeminent moral principle.[136] But the argument is more subtle than advocating crass mendacity out of fiscal necessity. The point is this. When tragic choices are exposed, we correctly shy away from overt sacrifice of life just to save money. Publicity therefore imposes a social cost, which, if it were extended to every resource consumption decision, would cripple our ability to act. Consequently, we have reason to be cautious in selecting social mechanisms that heighten this awareness. This response certainly is not driven by morality, but neither is it immoral. An undisclosed truth is not a lie. To leave a book unread on the shelf is not to disguise its contents; it is to remain in purposeful ignorance. It is rational and morally defensible to not want to know, even if, once we know, we can no longer pretend we don't.

We must recognize that exposing morally acceptable compromises to the light of day may cause us to abandon these hidden compromises in a way that might actually heighten social injustice. The same scrutiny that reveals unfair *patterns* in the distribution of scarce resources may also reveal completely *random* inequities, which, because they are random, are not unjust. But once exposed we may no longer be able to tolerate either form of inequity, forcing us to accept an even more problematic compromise. The impossible pursuit of moral perfection may require us either to eliminate the treatment in question for everyone in order to ensure that no injustice occurs or to abandon the attempt at resource allocation altogether, thereby forcing the spending cuts on to some other as-yet-unscrutinized region of medicine or social welfare. This is essentially what has happened under Medicare. Public exposure of rationing kidney dialysis in the 1960s prompted Congress to fund the full costs of treatment for everyone with kidney failure. The resulting explosion in costs has deterred Congress from ever again funding any "single-disease" programs and is thought to have caused a decade of delay in bringing lifesaving heart transplantation into the Medicare program.[137]

The fact that some of the hidden facts of resource allocation may be morally disturbing is an excellent reason to explore them, and once exposed, to resolve the dilemma as best we can. But it is naive to assume that exposure will always or usually result in fairer or more equitable distribution. This is not only because of the obvious flaws in human and social institutions, but also because, even within ideal institutions, we lack a clear sense of what a just outcome would be. Invisible rationing, then, does not necessarily hide inequitable results. It sometimes hides the fact of rationing for the very reason that we lack the ability to decide what would be equitable.[138]

Representation, Bias, and Democracy

A further line of objection to citizen deliberators is that, even if they are willing to decide these tough issues, others may not feel bound by their decisions. This objection goes to the problem of representativeness. We obviously engage in a degree of fictitious characterization in saying that any particular panel of selected deliberators represents the views of those not on the panel.[139] This point holds true in varying degrees for national, local, and even neighborhood groups. Consider, for instance, a woman dying from breast cancer who is told that she may not have a new expensive procedure that would use massive doses of chemotherapy. She is denied this last-chance shot at life, despite its reported success in a number of trials, because the citizen panel in her district decided that its benefits were not sufficiently proven (considering the risks of the procedure) to warrant the large expense.

If the panel that made this decision were chosen through popular election, such a woman might register the following objections: (1) I voted, but not for a single person who was ultimately elected, or not for a majority of the panel, or not for all of the panel. (2) I didn't vote. (3) I voted, but didn't have good information on who was running because the insurance industry launched a massive publicity campaign for its hand-picked candidates. (4) I made an informed vote, but my preferred candidates weren't on the ballot (due to the onerous ballot qualification requirements). (5) All my candidates were elected, but I never dreamed then that I would be in this condition now; if I only knew then what I know now, I would definitely have voted for someone else.

Naturally, all of these flaws exist in spades with respect to the market-based decision mechanisms considered elsewhere in the book that rely on decisions made by employers or insurers, so I am not faulting only democratic mechanisms for these failings. My point is simply to observe that the claim to a higher level of autonomous choice breaks down under closer scrutiny of the real-world constraints on how citizen panels are selected. After careful attention to these imperfections, citizen panels begin to look almost as biased as the bureaucratic mechanisms so pilloried at the outset of the chapter.

Viewed another way, employers and government agencies have almost the same claim to representative status as do citizen groups. After all, my selection of a job could be taken as a ratification of the benefits package chosen by the employer, and government regulators are appointed by elected officials. In contrast, grassroots or populist organizations elsewhere in society are hardly free from taint, influence, or ineffectiveness. Consider the jaundiced view sometimes taken of how labor unions, large shareholders' meetings, and California juries function.

Suppose we avoid these problems of viewpoint bias by selecting panel members randomly—or, once an ideally formed panel is created, by making it self-perpetuating. Then it is insulated from the corrupting influences of mass-appeal politics. Nevertheless, it will be infected by numerous other biases that undermine popular acceptance of its pronouncements. What is the proper mix on an ideally composed panel, not just with respect to ordinary socioeconomic factors, but more importantly with respect to the members' own personal experiences with illness? A panel composed of mainly healthy wage earners and taxpayers is going to take a markedly different view of resource allocation than one composed of elderly, disabled, and chronically ill members. And, among the infirm, those who have experienced the particular disease at issue will view the trade-offs differently than others. The only panel that is fully representative of all of society *is* all of society.

The problem of representativeness and bias is especially acute for medical decisions due to the multiple value dimensions entailed in even a single decision. Consider the earlier breast cancer example. A panel would be viewed as biased if it had on it only those who have survived the condition in the past or those with family members who have died from it. But, so would one that had no such members. The original Oregon list was struck down as being in violation of the Americans with Disabilities Act for the very reason that the ranking formula placed too much weight on the diminished quality of life of patients who do not fully recover, as judged by people who are presently healthy. But what is the proper health-status mix of deliberators? Beyond health status, what about demographics? Would it be proper to have the breast cancer issue decided by a panel composed only of women? There is no obvious correct answer to these basic questions, which go to the fundamental fairness and representativeness of the process. It is not being facetious to observe that we are stuck with asking another panel how to compose the deliberating panel, and then wondering how that superpanel should be composed.

Further difficulties lurk around the next curve as well.[140] Even with the proper mix of deliberators willing to tackle the tough questions, how shall we present those questions to them? One possibility is the bottom-line economic question of whether they would be willing to pay the extra premium or taxes required to cover a specified incremental medical benefit they personally may never receive. This might be thought too economically crass, so instead we might ask the panel how they would rank different medical needs that have similar costs, that is, how they would choose among similar medical interventions that address different health problems. The latter is not just a less pocketbook-sensitive version of the same question; these are fundamentally different questions.[141] The first places the medical purchasing decision in opposition to spending outside the system, in a manner that invokes the deliberators' own economic self-interest. The other assumes a closed system where, presumably, no more money can be added, but the money saved from not doing one procedure is devoted to another medical use. Work by cognitive psychologists reveals that these "framing effects" have enormous influence on our collective intuitions about the correct answers.[142] This also holds true for practiced professionals; even doctors take markedly different views of proper medicine when asked about treating patients individually versus in groups.[143] The problem that this framing effect presents for citizen deliberation is that there is no uncontroversial way to decide which form of a question is correct. As with empaneling these groups, we would have to resort to other mechanisms, perhaps bureaucratic or technocratic ones, to resolve these fundamental procedural issues. In doing so we may be tempted to structure the procedure to obtain a result that we believe, for independent and nondemocratic reasons, to be the correct one.

Practical Feasibility

To overcome all of these obstacles, we would need to create panels of citizen deliberators who are actually willing to make the tough decisions about the correct questions—decisions most people are willing, in principle, to be bound by. If this were possible, would we then be pleased with the results? Not necessarily, for panels can operate only via rules, and therefore are subject to most of the criticisms leveled at technocratic processes.

Panels cannot be at the bedside of every patient facing a treatment decision with debatable cost/benefit trade-offs, for such trade-offs exist in the vast bulk of treatment encounters. It is a huge misconception to think that most of the tough questions cluster around relatively few high-profile treatments and that they can be made in an all-or-nothing fashion. Fleck makes this mistake when he argues that the deliberative task is manageable because there is a "very large core of health services for which we would have a very high degree of consensus" that benefits are worth the costs.[144] Actually, virtually any treatment in common use is capable of being extended to the point where benefits are debatable. Cheap lifesaving antibiotics are commonly overprescribed. Caesarian sections are still done far more than is recommended, and we perform heart bypass operations at a rate that other countries consider absurd. Almost every diagnostic test has uses that are absolutely essential and those that are completely marginal. MRI scans are only the latest tip of this slippery-sloped iceberg.

Effective resource allocation by democratic consensus would have to address in microscopic detail each of the same tens of thousands of condition–treatment pairings for which the technocrats are working to develop practice guidelines. And, for each of these, the citizen panel would have to express its views through categorical rules which, however specific, would inevitably fail to capture the nuances of clinical variations and individual value preferences. Where the panel is evenly split or has strongly held but differing views, there is no easy way to strike an acceptable compromise. Despite the complexity of the problem and the polarization of views, the visibility and authority of public representation compel deliberative groups to adopt a single solution.

Consider, for instance, the types of questions typically asked of the public in recent opinion polls that inquire into attitudes about resource allocation. One Louis Harris poll asked people which treatment they would choose for a health plan to fund if it could afford only one: a new screening test that would diagnose certain cancers one year earlier, thereby giving one person ten more years of life, or artificial electronic hands for ten people who had lost theirs in accidents. Responses were split 46 percent to 40 percent in favor of the cancer screening test. But, under the rules of this deliberation, a bare plurality vote dictates a single decision for everyone.[145] Some ethicists suggest the use of random selection when such "incommensurate" or irreconcilable values come into conflict,[146] but such an arbitrary resolution is clearly inferior to one that would tailor resource allocation decisions to the differing preferences that individuals actually have.

This catalogue of objections is not intended to rule out any role for public deliberation on medical resource allocation. To the contrary, I view this as one of the most appealing mechanisms for asserting external influence over medical spending. However, the limitations of public opinion, and the comparative strengths of technocratic and professional authorities, counsel a more advisory and informational role for citizen panels. As Jonathan Moreno argues, consensus panels should deliberate, not legislate.[147] Even without giving citizen panels the power to decide conclusively, there is certainly much wisdom in seeking their views on selected or wide-ranging issues that are the most troubling and controversial. The public could be invited in a sustained and formalized fashion to articulate general principles that others use to decide individual cases or to monitor the performance of the professional and technocratic communities. The public could also be called on to disapprove decisions or mechanisms they disagree with. In this fashion, resource allocation decisions can be reached through more of a dialectic than a democratic process.

PHYSICIAN OVERSEERS

The physician overseer model is a final mechanism for external control of doctor–patient spending decisions. This model is one in which an experienced clinician other than the treating physician exercises case-specific authority over allowable treatment options. This model is a bridge into the next chapter because it combines the bedside discretion discussed in that chapter with the notion of third-party decision making analyzed in this chapter. Each of the models of third-party authority discussed so far—bureaucratic, technocratic, and democratic—suffers the principal flaw of operating through categorical rules rather than case-specific discretion, a characteristic that is particularly unsuited to medical decision making. This characteristic is not absolutely essential to the exercise of third-party authority, however. The only reason it pervades most of this chapter is the practical limitation that the primary vehicles for centralized decision making—government agencies, insurance companies, and citizen panels—cannot conveniently operate at this individualized level across the entire range of medical encounters.[148]

One solution to this practical limitation is to create a new institutional structure that has this capacity. Medical ethicist Robert Veatch proposes just such an institutional innovation in the form of "medically trained agents" who mediate the conflict between treating physicians pushing for every conceivable medical benefit and insurance administrators constantly trying to pinch pennies.[149] These intermediate agents would probably be physicians but perhaps also nurse practitioners. They would be charged with determining which treatment limitations are consistent with general coverage principles in the insurance contract and with medical prudence in the individual patient's case. This is a role that calls for the application of case-specific medical expertise by someone other than the treating physician.

This proposal has a striking resemblance to the growing phenomenon of case management that presently exists within managed care practices. Insurance companies increasingly are hiring medical professionals such as nurses to communicate directly with physicians and patients about treatment choices and options in order to minimize costs for the most expensive episodes of care. The essence of this proposal is also captured in the now-commonplace role of an HMO medical director, who is called upon to mix medical and financial considerations in deciding on requests by fellow physicians to approve hospital admissions, expensive diagnostic testing, and nonstandard courses of medication. This role is increasingly being assumed as well by medical directors of independent medical groups that contract with HMOs on a capitated basis.[150]

Robert Veatch's proposal modifies these examples by insulating the physician overseer position somewhat from the insurance institution. His medical agents would be chosen by and accountable to the patient population, not the corporate entity or the physician group. They would be subject to a new professional ethic that calls on them to exercise independent judgment in a fashion that balances the interests of individual patients with those of the subscriber pool.

Unlike more conventional mechanisms of utilization review, these innovations involve experienced professionals making decisions based on extensive case review and after live contact with patients or treating physicians. Thus, this proposal would seem to capture the best of all possible worlds: setting enforceable limits while retaining the individualized expertise and personal attention of practicing physicians and without the compromises in professional ethics discussed in the next chapter. Recalling the earlier discussion of rules versus discretion, this might be characterized as "rule-sensitive particularism."[151] These physician overseers would apply categorical rules in a presumptive, not conclusive, fashion by exercising discretionary authority to interpret or override a rule in a particular case (not just to revise the rule for subsequent refinement), based on clinical judgment and the patient's unique characteristics.

The problem with this attractive solution is that it is almost too perfect. No existing role or institution embodies such ideal clinical mediators. Although they can be imagined, they are not in fact available and may be prohibitively expensive, since they entail a brand new layer of medical professionals. Physician overseers may be the best conceivable solution, but they are not the *only* conceivable solution. The question becomes, then, whether the institutional advantages of this proposal are worth its institutional costs. This proposal certainly appears much more preferable than a resource allocation mechanism that is entirely rule bound or removed from the clinical setting. Whether it is equally attractive compared to resource allocation by treating physicians must await further discussion of that alternative in the next chapter.

It is worth observing at this point, however, that these clinical mediators would possess much the same status as treating physicians. To have the requisite clinical knowledge and skill, they would need to be licensed as physicians. And to have sufficient knowledge of the individual case, they would need substantial patient contact, either directly or through the treating physician. Therefore, they would have all the attributes of an actual attending physician, including the authority to diagnose and prescribe, excluding only the authority to administer treatment.

One must ask, then, if these ideal physician overseers may exercise rationing authority, why is it not possible for actual treating physicians to exercise the same authority within existing, nonideal institutions? One possible answer is that patient trust is much more critical to the success of the treatment function than it is to the performance of the diagnosing and prescribing functions. This may be so because of the role that trust plays in patients' willingness to submit to treatment and in the psychological mechanisms that activate patients' hidden abilities to heal themselves, abilities that are now only dimly understood as the placebo effect.[152] This speculation depends on many unmeasured, and even unobserved, aspects of trust and healing, but if it is true, then it justifies imposing a somewhat different and perhaps more stringent ethic on hands-on treating physicians than on physicians with only the power to issue binding treatment directives. On the other hand, Howard Brody, the physician ethicist who has given these issues the most thought, holds the following contrary opinion:

> The power to make trade-offs among patients (based, one hopes, on sound judgments of relative likelihood of benefit) is a power that is inherent in medicine as generally practiced. The idea that we should somehow eliminate that power because it can be misused to the patient's detriment is unrealistic. It is not illogical but it would impose such radical changes on medical practice as to be utterly impractical. Therefore the division-of-labor model [such as assigning different functions to different doctors], which suggests that that power can and ought to be eliminated, is either an unrealistic call for utopian reform of medicine or (more likely) a mere verbal formula to preserve the fantasy of moral purity while ignoring the inconvenient realities.[153]

In conclusion, regardless of whether physician overseers are a necessary or a feasible solution, they underscore that there clearly is an irreducible intuitive core to medical practice, one that cannot be captured adequately in even an idealized set of standardized rules or a perfect version of bureaucratic or democratic authority. Undoubtedly, the domain of medicine that belongs to art rather than science has been artificially inflated in order to preserve physician prerogative.[154] It is certainly possible and desirable to bring greater definition and consistency to much of medical practice. But the centralized mechanisms that now exist will never function as a wholly satisfactory system for resource allocation. The best we can hope for is that treatment protocols will serve a useful purpose simply as a presumptive rule that forces physicians to think more carefully about the costs of their treatment decisions. By setting a baseline to which physicians must refer in formulating and justifying their treatment plans, protocols can influence the informal heuristics that are central to physicians' judgmental thought processes. Critical to this role, though, is the limitation that treatment directives must be non-binding. Some other influence—whether financial, educational, or professional—must be brought to bear on physician judgment both to reinforce external authority and to introduce resource sensitivity into the aspects of clinical judgment that cannot be reached by centralized rules. How these bedside spending decisions would and should be made is the subject to which we now turn.

Notes

1. Grumet 1989, at 608. See also Ellman 1989, at 721; American Society of Internal Medicine 1990, at 1–32.
2. Leonard 1992, at A16.
3. E.g., Callahan 1989, at 362; Leape 1995.
4. Macklin 1993.
5. Northwestern National Life Insurance Co. 1990.
6. Employee Benefit Research Institute 1992.
7. Medica Foundation 1994. These findings are confirmed by other more localized or nonscientific surveys. One that questioned magazine readers found that half favor some form of rationing and three-quarters of these believe doctors, not lawyers or insurance companies, should be the ones to decide which treatments to ration. "Should We Deny Some Kinds of Health Care?," Glamour Magazine, March 1994, at 149. A survey in Illinois found that only 10 percent of those questioned would opt for insurance companies over their personal physicians to decide standards of medical practice. 3 Health Care Daily (BNA) d8 (July 13, 1994).
8. Mitka 1993.
9. Peters and Rogers 1994; Pear 1994.
10. Hall and Anderson 1992, at 1668–1673.
11. Ellman 1989, at 721; American Society of Internal Medicine 1990, at 1–32.
12. Blank 1988, at 97–99. See also Haney 1992, at A8 ("the lion's share of research money goes to the diseases with the loudest pressure groups," citing as an example that government spends $79,000 for every American who dies of AIDS but only $600 for every death by stroke).
13. Havighurst 1977, at 313 ("This rationing function is . . . peculiarly difficult for political institutions to perform, given the public's expectations and the symbolic importance of health care."). See also Blumstein 1981; Elhauge 1996.
14. Morone 1992, at 1931.
15. Medicare has been faulted in its generosity for not employing any form of means testing for its first 30 years. Until the 1995 legislation, it charged the wealthy the same premiums as the lower middle class. During its first 20 years, Medicare used the highly inflationary indemnity model of insurance preferred by the medical establishment. More recently, its new method of hospital payment has been criticized for unduly favoring large, influential teaching hospitals. See, generally, Christensen 1992. These perceived excesses are among the primary targets in the recent Republican campaign for Medicare reform.
16. Brown 1991, at 28, 35.
17. Daniels 1991, at 2234; U.S. Congress 1992a, at 8; Nagel 1992, at 1976 (over two-thirds in focus groups were medical professionals and only 8 percent were poor); Leichter 1992, at 1961 (same).

18. Klein 1993a, at 74.

19. 388 So. 2d 470 (La. Ct. App. 1980).

20. Ibid. at 472. The couple had duplicative coverage under nine separate policies amounting to several times more than the actual cost of treatment, and they had "been hospitalized for more than four months [over the prior three years] and [had] claimed in some nine lawsuits against these companies during that time, over $15,000." Nevertheless, the court ordered coverage because the insurance policy did not explicitly require treatment to be medically necessary and because the wife had several small children at home who prevented her from resting.

21. See, e.g., Dallis v. Aetna Life Ins. Co., 768 F.2d 1303, 1304 (11th Cir. 1985) (coverage exists for "immuno-augmentative therapy" for cancer, costing $11,000 and provided in a Bahamanian clinic, even though it has "never been approved by any of the various agencies of the United States Government, nor has it ever been proven to be effective"); Shumake v. Travelers Ins. Co., 383 N.W.2d 259 (Mich. Ct. App. 1985) (insurer must pay $17,478 for laetrile and nutritional therapy for lung cancer, even though FDA disapproval meant that it was illegal to ship laetrile in interstate commerce), appeal denied, 425 Mich. 859 (1986); Tudor v. Metropolitan Life Ins. Co., 539 N.Y.S.2d 690, 692 (N.Y. Sup. Ct. 1989) (finding coverage for mercury vapor testing by a physician who "treats the whole person, with biochemical methods and emphasis on elemental deficiencies and food allergies"). But see Free v. Travelers Ins. Co., 551 F. Supp. 554 (D. Md. 1982) (finding no coverage for laetrile); Bruno v. Security Gen. Life Ins. Co., 522 So. 2d 1242 (La. Ct. App. 1988) (finding no coverage for nutritional supplements prescribed by "holistic" physician).

22. See cases collected and discussed in Hall and Anderson 1992, at 1650.

23. See, e.g., Mount Sinai Hosp. v. Zorek, 271 N.Y.S.2d 1012 (N.Y. Civ. Ct. 1966) (involving such a contract). Surprisingly, this language still persists in some contemporary contracts. See, e.g., McLaughlin v. Connecticut Gen. Life Ins. Co., 565 F. Supp. 434 (N.D. Cal. 1983); Schroeder v. Blue Cross & Blue Shield, 450 N.W.2d 470 (Wis. Ct. App. 1989).

24. See Institute of Medicine 1985, at 136–40; Mehlman 1986, at 784–94 (comparing three different concepts of "waste," the first considering only the effect of the technology on the patient, the second incorporating the cost of the technology, and the third converting patient benefits into dollars so that benefits can be compared with the cost of the treatment).

25. See Zuckerberg v. Blue Cross & Blue Shield, 487 N.Y.S.2d 595, 600 (N.Y. App. Div. 1985), aff'd, 490 N.E.2d 839 (N.Y. 1986) (approving insurer's denial of coverage for nutritional therapy treatment of cancer and stating that the denial would have "the desirable effect of affording greater protection to . . . patients who are especially vulnerable to unfounded claims of miraculous cures"). Perhaps the patronizing nature of this justification explains why courts have rejected it so consistently. Except in the most obvious cases of quackery, it stands to reason that insurers should defer to patients' and doctors' own decisions about whether a treatment is safe. Therefore, insurers might fare better in court if they used a less disingenuous justification, that is, if they defended primarily on the basis of cost effectiveness, or even granting cost effectiveness, on the basis of uninsurability.

26. For instance, the five criteria that the Blue Cross and Blue Shield Association use in making its technology assessment recommendations to its constituent plans ask only whether the technology improves net health outcomes equal to the alternatives. They contain no consideration of whether equally effective alternatives are less costly or whether the incremental increase in net health outcomes is justified by the additional costs. See Pirozzi v. Blue Cross-Blue Shield, 741 F. Supp. 586, 590–91 (E.D. Va. 1990); see also

Kalb 1989, at 1115–16 ("[P]rivate insurers virtually never consider the costs of a technology when determining whether it is reasonable or necessary. . . . Specifically, private insurers have not attempted to contain costs by systematically excluding wasteful technologies from coverage.").

27. 54 Fed. Reg. 4302–10 (1989).

28. Institute of Medicine 1989.

29. Insurers lost somewhat less often (48%) under specific exclusions than under general exclusions (57%), but this difference was not sufficient to be statistically significant. For instance, insurers in the 1980s lost dozens of cases involving "autologous bone marrow transplant" (ABMT) for breast cancer when they relied on the general "experimental" treatment exclusion. In 1990s, they redrafted their contracts to exclude this treatment specifically, but in the next round of litigation physicians had developed an alteration of the procedure referred to as "peripheral stem-cell rescue," which involves collecting the retransplanted cells from the bloodstream rather than from the bone marrow. Even though this new version was even more experimental than the older version, some courts reasoned that it was sufficiently different to preclude the application of the specific exclusion of ABMT for breast cancer, or at least to make this a debatable question which, owing to the rule that all ambiguities resolve against the insurer, resulted in an automatic win for the patients. For this and other reasons, insurers still continue to lose about half of these cases. See generally Anderson and Hall 1996; Hall et al. 1996.

30. The judicial distortion of scientific facts has received much attention across a range of legal issues. See generally Wessel 1980; Wessel 1988; Huber 1993; Developments 1995. In the context of health insurance disputes, see Costich 1991.

31. See Champagne et al. 1991, at 388.

32. Eminent jurist Judge Jack Weinstein observed that "an expert can be found to testify to the truth of almost any factual theory, no matter how frivolous, thus validating the case sufficiently to avoid summary judgment and force the matter to trial. . . . Juries and judges can be, and sometimes are, misled by the expert-for-hire." Weinstein 1986, at 482.

33. Various statements by the parties could be taken to waive contractual rights, or details of their relationship may create heightened duties. Also, patients in similar conditions may do better jobs from one case to the next in presenting evidence to support their positions.

34. Elhauge 1994, at 1464.

35. Fondacaro 1995.

36. Accordingly, courts have observed that the denial of insurance coverage does not prevent the doctor from rendering care; it merely determines that, in the insurer's judgment, the subscriber pool has chosen not to pay for the particular treatment. See Goodman v. Sullivan, 891 F.2d 449 (2d Cir. 1989) (stating that the Secretary's regulation denying payment for MRI scans does not presume to supervise or control the practice of medicine, but simply refuses subsequent Medicare reimbursement for certain kinds of services; while this may influence some medical decisions, such tangential influence is inherent in Medicare itself); Association of Am. Physicians & Surgeons v. Weinberger, 395 F. Supp. 125, 134 (N.D. Ill.) (stating that the Medicare utilization review mechanism "does not prohibit a physician from performing any surgical operations he deems necessary. . . . It merely provides that if a practitioner wishes to be compensated^sfor his services by the federal government, he is required to comply with certain guidelines and procedures enumerated in the statute"), aff'd mem. sub nom. Association of Am. Physicians & Surgeons v. Matthews, 423 U.S. 975 (1975). See also Hall 1988, at 463; Havighurst and Hackbarth 1979.

37. Pirozzi v. Blue Cross-Blue Shield, 741 F. Supp. 586, 588 (E.D. Va. 1990); Dozsa v. Crum & Forster Ins. Co., 716 F.Supp. 131, 138 (D.N.J. 1989); Bradley v. Empire Blue Cross & Blue Shield, 562 N.Y.S.2d 908 (N.Y. Sup. Ct. 1990).

38. Indeed, this appears to be the construction that a number of insurers give to their experimental exclusion, when it is said that they apply it with discretion on a "case-by-case basis."

39. There is obviously a Catch-22 at play here since the refusal to reimburse at the outset will greatly slow the dispersion of the new technology. The parties to the contract may nevertheless desire this effect. Many analysts in the health policy community believe that new technological innovations are diffused much too rapidly due to the absence of the market test that is usually imposed on innovations in other industries. If new technologies must prove themselves in an adverse reimbursement environment, only those that are cost saving or that provide a clear cost beneficial improvement in outcomes will be selected.

40. David Eddy, a leading researcher and policy analyst on medical effectiveness, discusses this point with respect to ABMT treatment for breast cancer in particular, but uses terminology that contrasts a societal perspective with an individual patient perspective: "[M]any activities in medicine that make great sense from the point of view of an individual patient might not make sense when the perspective is widened to encompass other activities for other people—what we call society." Eddy 1991d, at 1449.

41. Huber 1988, at 192.

42. See Meusberger v. Palmer, 900 F.2d 1280 (8th Cir. 1990) (holding that pancreas transplant must be covered by Medicaid even though considered experimental by Medicare); Weaver v. Reagan, 886 F.2d 194 (8th Cir. 1989) (finding it arbitrary and capricious to deny Medicaid coverage for using an expensive AIDS drug in a manner not yet approved by the FDA); Pinneke v. Preisser, 623 F.2d 546 (8th Cir. 1980) (holding that Medicaid must fund sex-change operations); cf. American Soc'y of Cataract and Refractive Surgery v. Sullivan, 772 F. Supp. 666 (D.D.C. 1991) (requiring Medicare to pay for investigational intraocular lens implants that have not yet received FDA approval).

43. See Schwartz 1991, at 235–37.

44. Fuller 1978.

45. He referred not merely to judicial litigation but to the institution of adjudication in its broadest possible sense, as contrasted with the two other fundamental forms of social ordering: contracting and voting.

46 Fuller 1978, at 403.

47. Hasty v. Central States, Southeast and Southwest Areas Health and Welfare Fund, 1994 U.S.Dist. LEXIS 6570 (N.D.Ind. 1994).

48. Bechtold v. Physicians Health Plan of Northern Indiana, 19 F.3d 322 (7th Cir. 1994). See also Wilkins v. Sullivan, 889 F.2d 135, 140 (7th Cir. 1989); Goepel v. Mail Handlers Benefit Plan, 1993 WL 384498 (D.N.J. 1993).

49. See Morone 1993, at 737.

50. U.S. Congress 1992a.

51. See also Kalb 1989, who suggests distinguishing among safe, effective, and cost-effective, and limiting basic coverage to cost-effective.

52. Havighurst 1994.

53. Our approach is specified in greater detail in Hall and Anderson 1992.

54. Hall and Anderson 1992. Anderson, Hall, and Steinberg 1993. Elsewhere, Ellman and I take a step further by outlining how patients themselves could specify different cost-

effectiveness criteria by selecting budgets for designated categories of service when they sign up for insurance. Ellman and Hall 1994.

55. See Hadorn 1991a; Hadorn 1991b, at 11; Eddy 1991c,e; U.S. Congress 1992a.

56. Thomas 1993, at 135–45. See generally Stade 1993.

57. See generally Tanenbaum 1993; Frankford 1994a.

58. Schauer 1991; Schneider 1992; Sunstein 1996, 1995b; Kennedy 1976, at 1710.

59. The term "process values" was first coined and articulated by Summers 1974. See also Mashaw 1983.

60. Emerson 1940, at 152.

61. Gilmore 1977, at 110–11.

62. Kennedy 1976, at 1710.

63. Schauer 1991, at 155–56.

64. Schneider 1992, at 61.

65. Simon 1982.

66. Diver 1983.

67. See Wright 1992; Wright 1991.

68. Mechanic 1992.

69. See Goodwin 1992.

70. Elster 1992, at 224.

71. Notably, see Havighurst 1994.

72. Rosenfeld 1994, at A23, col. 2.

73. Relman 1990a, at 912.

74. Mechanic 1992, at 1721.

75. Mechanic 1986, at 147–48, 208. See also Welch 1991.

76. Quill and Cassel 1995, at 369–70.

77. Tanenbaum 1993.

78. Morreim 1987, at 34.

79. Schwartz and Aaron 1990, at A15.

80. Steinbrook and Lo 1992, at 342.

81. Hadorn 1991a, at 2223. See also Eddy 1991c, at 2136 (diagnostic and procedure codes "cannot distinguish between a carotid artery bypass procedure done for a man with 90% occlusion and [angina] symptoms versus an asymptomatic man with 40% occlusion"); U.S. Congress 1992a, at 7 (even with 700 items, "the level of heterogeneity . . . means accepting that some patient with excellent expected outcomes with treatment must forego therapy, while other patients with patently worse treatment-specific prognoses receive it").

82. U.S. Congress 1992a, at 8.

83. Myerson 1995.

84. Certainly, many groupings among these codes are possible. On the other hand, even the multitude of existing ICD categories are far too broad and lacking in specific clinical indications to be other than crude in their present form. Eddy 1991d, at 2444. Out of frustration, the Oregon Commissioners began to refer to "the tyranny of the ICD-9 codes." Hadorn 1991a,b.

85. In other words, for only two conditions, A and B, the protocol would have to consider A alone, B alone, and AB, as well as A occurs before B, A occurs after B, and A and B occur simultaneously. Dubois and Brook 1988. See also Parmley 1994.

86. Eddy 1984, at 78–79.

87. For a summary and critique of the existing effort in the public and private sector to rigorously assess medical practice, see U.S. Congress 1994.

88. Marmor and Blustein 1992, at 1549. See generally Epstein 1990; Dubois and Brook 1988.

89. Eddy 1984, at 80. Eddy continues:

> [E]ven when the best trials are conducted, we still might not get an answer. Consider the value of mammography in women under fifty, and consider just one outcome—the effect on breast cancer mortality. Ignore for the time being the radiation hazard, false-positive test results, inconvenience, financial costs, and other issues. This is one of the best-studied problems in cancer prevention, benefiting from the largest (60,000 women) and longest (more than fifteen years) completed randomized controlled trial, and an even larger uncontrolled study involving 270,000 women screened for five years in twenty-nine centers around the country. Yet we still do not know the value of mammography in women under fifty. The first study showed a slight reduction in mortality, but it was not statistically significant. The larger study suggested that mammography has improved since the first study, and that it is now almost as good in younger women as in older women, but the study was not controlled and we do not know if "almost" is good enough. Even for women over fifty, where the first study showed a statistically significant reduction in breast cancer mortality (of about 40 percent at ten years), there is enough uncertainty about the results that no fewer than four additional trials have been initiated to confirm the results. These trials are still in progress.

90. It is thought by many that the political message being sent is aimed at those who support managed care, since this type of research is fundamental to how managed care functions. See Iglehart 1996.

91 Sun 1983, at 37 (the AMA argued that "the center should not make general statements about appropriate medical care" because this was "trying to dictate the practice of medicine"); Blumenthal 1983, at 600–01 (describing the lobbying efforts of the AMA to persuade Congress to cut off funding for the center).

92. Tanenbaum 1994, at 42.

93. Hunter 1991. See generally Schon 1983; Tanenbaum 1994.

94. Mechanic 1986, at 147–48, 209. Mechanic offers an even more forceful and cogent development of this argument in Mechanic 1992.

95. Dubos 1968. See, e.g., Nease et al. 1995 (finding a substantial chance that many patients with class II (moderate) angina will be more bothered by their symptoms and limited in their activities than the average patient with severe (class III/IV) angina).

96. La Puma and Lawlor 1990; Levinsky 1990.

97. Hadorn 1991a,b.

98. Harris 1985.

99. Taurek 1977. For further elaboration of the morality of counting and comparing lives, see Kamm 1993; Rakowski 1993; Elhauge 1994; Goold 1996.

100. Mechanic 1980, at 432. See also Freidson 1970a, at 170 ("a rather thoroughgoing particularism, a kind of ontological and epistemological individualism is characteristic of the clinician"); Goss 1961, at 40 ("professionals require . . . 'individual authority': freedom to make their own trained judgment rather than according to the dictates of superiors in a bureaucratic hierarchy"); Ku and Fisher 1990. Lipsky 1980 documents and analyzes the ability of service professionals in many other different fields to defeat bureaucratic organizational controls.

101. Jesilow, Geis, and Pontell 1991 (documenting tendency of doctors to rationalize cheating based on patient benefit when they find reimbursement rules confusing, irrational, and intrusive); Rundle 1989, at A1, A8; Rosenthal 1990a, at A1, B7 ("'Many doctors acknowledge that minor deception is commonplace . . . to squeeze money out of tight-fisted

insurers who balk at paying for . . . preventative services. "If a patient needs a mammogram to screen for cancer, you put breast lump on the form," said Dr. Robert Lawrence'"); Novack et al. 1989, 2980 (finding that the majority of physicians surveyed were willing to "misrepresent a screening test as a diagnostic test to secure an insurance payment").

102. Brody 1992; Burt 1979.

103. Schauer 1991; Tanenbaum 1994.

104. Frankford 1994a.

105. Mechanic 1986, at 148.

106. Milgram 1969, at 32–43.

107. Burt 1979, at 81–82.

108. Wilson 1993, at 52.

109. See Special Report 1987.

110. See Chassin 1988, at 441. For instance, David Hadorn proposes guidelines such as: perform a CT scan for headache of "sudden or recent onset, with abnormal neurological signs," or, do bypass surgery in cases of "unstable or persistent angina that is unresponsive to maximal medical therapy or in which side effects are incapacitating." Hadorn 1992c.

111. See Hall 1991, at 144 quoting AMA 1990, at 23. And this is precisely the disclaimer that Milliman & Robertson attaches to its widely used guidelines. Myerson 1995.

112. Freidson 1985, at 28. See also Marylander 1980, at 16. ("Very few established administrative routines in hospitals cannot be abrogated or countermanded by a physician claiming medical emergency.").

113. Fleck 1992, at 1607.

114. Callahan 1989, at 362.

115. Fleck 1994.

116. See also, Goold 1996; Eddy 1991a; Symposium 1990, at 16–23.

117. Emanuel 1991.

118. Fleck 1992, at 1624. See also Goold 1996.

119. Egan 1990; Hadorn 1991a, b; Eddy 1991c.

120. Still, the Office of Technology Assessment found that the list suffered from missing codes, duplicate and illogically placed codes, and apparently illogical relative rankings such as placing medical therapy, which is usually tried first, lower than surgical therapy, for the same condition. U.S. Congress 1992a, at 7.

121. Eddy 1991c, at 2138; Hadorn 1991b, at 16.

122. Daniels 1993, at 230. Daniels gives the following additional examples from Oregon: Having to wear eyeglasses was rated slightly worse than not being able to drive a car or being confined to bed. "Other weightings clearly reflected cultural attitudes and possibly bias: having trouble with drugs or alcohol was given the second most negative weighting of all conditions, much worse than, for example, having a bad burn over large areas of your body or being so impaired that one needs help to eat or go to the bathroom." Ibid.

123. Fox and Swazey 1974 at 231–32.

124. See Thomas 1993.

125. For instance, Northwestern National Life Insurance Company 1990 found that 50 percent of people would have the most trust in a national panel of medical professionals. A panel of consumers came in a distant second, at 18 percent.

126. Fox and Swazey 1974, at 232. See also Annas 1985.

127. Sehgal, Galbraith, Chesney et al. 1992.

128. Blakeslee 1990, at B7, col.4.

129. Calabresi and Bobbit 1978.

130. Ibid. at 19–21.

131. Hadorn 1991a, at 2219.

132. Blumstein 1981.

133. Shapiro 1987. See also Shapiro 1994; Pildes 1991.

134. Nelson 1994, at 339.

135. Calabresi and Bobbit 1978, at 21, 22, 26.

136. Fleck 1992; Fleck 1987; Fleck 1990; Nelson 1994.

137. Here, I am responding to the argument in Fleck 1987.

138. Besharov and Silver 1987.

139. For a thorough analysis of the political legitimacy of bioethics consensus panels, see Moreno 1995, especially Chapter 4. For further development of the problem of fair representation, see Goold 1996.

140. On both this next point and the prior points, David Eddy's analysis is very informative in Eddy 1990.

141. As Mary Ann Baily observes,

> The rules one would personally choose, given one's own preferences over health states, may not be the rules one considers appropriate when everyone will be forced to contribute to the cost of implementing them. For example, one woman who desperately wants children bankrupts herself for in vitro fertilization treatments, yet believes they should not be included in a societally guaranteed level of care; another woman considers the opportunity to bear a child so important that some infertility treatment, as well as care for pregnancy and delivery, belongs in the guaranteed level, even though she herself prefers to remain childless (Baily 1994, at 39–40).

142. Kahneman, Slovic, and Tversky 1992; Elster 1982, at 237.

143. In one fascinating study, physicians tended in their group-based decisions to order fewer tests with uncertain benefit, and they gave less weight to the personal concerns of patients. Redelmeier and Tversky 1990.

144. Fleck 1992, at 1625.

145. Responses were even closer between a new cancer treatment that would give 100 patients one extra year of life (44 percent) and one that would completely cure five patients (40 percent). Medica Foundation 1994.

146. E.g., AMA 1994a.

147. Moreno 1995.

148. Courts might be viewed as a notable exception since their decisions are highly case specific, but they, too, suffer from capacity constraints. Due to the costs of litigation, only the rare payment dispute ends up in litigation. Unlike other third-party authorities, however, courts are unable to issue rules in lieu of case review.

It might also be thought that insurance companies individualize their medical decisions when they process claims, but this is mostly a ministerial function based on rudimentary information rather than an extensive case review. Therefore, claim processing tends to proceed by internal rules rather than expert discretion. Where such discretion is exercised, such as in the small minority of cases that are referred to the insurer's medical director or to outside consultants for review, the review is based on a paper record rather than on direct patient contact. Therefore, that review lacks the immediacy and personal contact of the model discussed in text.

149. Veatch 1991b, at 24. See also Mehlman 1996. For a Critique, see Goldberg 1996.

150. That is, they agree to accept some or all of the financial and treatment risk in exchange for a fixed fee per enrollee.

151. This is Fred Schauer's term.

152. For additional explanation of this healing phenomenon, see the discussion and sources cited in Chapter 2.

153. Brody 1992, at 195.

154. Freidson 1970b, at 98 (arguing that as a defense to the evaluations of outsiders, physicians impute more uncertainty to their work than in fact exists); Freidson 1970b, at 164 (citing the tendency of physicians to emphasize the "primacy of firsthand clinical experience," thereby "exaggerating the acceptability of varying opinions").

4

Physician Bedside Discretion

The preceding discussion explains that fundamentally three different mechanisms are conceivable for making health care spending decisions. Cost-sensitive treatment decisions can be made by patients, by physicians, and by third parties (primarily private and governmental insurers, but also various regulatory or review organizations). Elsewhere in our economy, cost/benefit trade-offs are usually made through the purchasing decisions of individual consumers. Chapter 2 explains that this simple market mechanism is not generally available or desirable for health care because the unpredictability of illness causes us to purchase insurance, and the complexities of medical judgment cause us to delegate vast authority to our physicians. Some role for consumer rationing may be preserved to the extent that insurance is incomplete (requiring, for instance, patients to pay deductibles and coinsurance) and to the extent that informed-consent requirements place the ultimate authority in the hands of patients. But because insurance will never be entirely abandoned, and because patients will always rely to some significant degree on their physicians' recommendations, medical spending decisions are necessarily made through the agency of insurance and the agency of physicians.

Of these two alternatives, virtually all commentators agree that those who foot the bill for medical care may set some external limits on the particular items they will fund. Thus, for both patients and third parties, the debate is only over the specifics of what, where, and how medical spending decisions will occur. In contrast, bedside resource allocation by physicians remains much more controversial at a level of fundamental principle. Unlike as with other mechanisms, it is necessary to ask whether this mechanism is proper at all. Physician bedside rationing occurs when doctors, influenced by professional, administrative, or financial incentives, decide that a particular item of treatment is not worth its costs, despite its possible or probable benefits. This physician-driven mechanism for making health care spending decisions is exemplified by HMOs, which (as described in more detail in Chapter 5) reward their physicians for economizing and penalize them for going over budget. It is also embodied in practice settings described below such as government hospitals, which operate under severe budget constraints that require physicians to act parsimoniously in order to balance the competing needs of their many patients.

OPPOSITION TO PHYSICIAN BEDSIDE RATIONING

Even though it is commonplace for physicians to make resource allocation decisions in many conventional practice settings, ethical opposition to physicians playing this role is widespread and heartfelt. Victor Fuchs, an economist who champions health care rationing, expresses the common attitude of concern: "The commitment of the individual physician to the individual patient is one of the most valuable features of American medical care. It would therefore be a great mistake to turn each physician into an explicit maximizer of the social-benefit/social-cost ratio in his or her daily practice."[1] Embracing this concern, the dominant position among medical ethicists and within the medical profession is a nearly absolute[2] moral prohibition against physicians ever considering the costs of treatment to any degree. Norman Levinsky, a prominent Boston physician who publishes frequently in the nation's most prestigious medical journals, presents the standard argument for this role-based ethic by analogy to the lawyer's role:

[P]hysicians are required to do everything that they believe may benefit each patient without regard to costs or other societal considerations. In caring for an individual patient, the doctor must act solely as that patient's advocate, against the apparent interests of society as a whole, if necessary. An analogy can be drawn with the role of a lawyer defending a client against a criminal charge. The attorney is obligated to use all ethical means to defend the client, regardless of the cost of prolonged legal proceedings or even of the possibility that a guilty person may be acquitted through skillful advocacy. Similarly, in the practice of medicine, physicians are obligated to do all that they can for their patients without regard to any costs to society. . . . It is society, not the individual practitioner, that must make the decision to limit the availability of effective but expensive types of medical care.[3]

Robert Veatch, the director of the Georgetown University Kennedy Institute of Ethics, one of the world's most renowned centers for bioethics, uses the following rhetorical flourish to place his qualms about bedside rationing on a quasi-contractual footing:

Asking physicians to be cost-conscious . . . would be asking them to abandon their central commitment to their patients. In effect they would be asked to remove the Hippocratic

Oath from their waiting room walls and replace it with a sign that reads, "Warning all ye who enter here. I will generally work for your rights and welfare, but if benefits to you are marginal and costs are great, I will abandon you in order to protect society."[4]

Many other representative views from influential authorities are collected in the Appendix to this chapter.

I will refer to this ethic as the physician's ethic of absolute quality. This position advocates that, from the physician's perspective, literally any marginal medical benefit, no matter how small, is worth absolutely any price because we want doctors in their role as healers to behave as if each of our lives is priceless. Adherents believe that rationing either is not necessary or that it must be imposed from external, societal sources.

A divergent wing of less absolutist physicians and ethicists takes a view that is more accommodating to bedside rationing. They recognize the necessity of rationing and are willing to contemplate physicians' incorporating economic costs into their clinical judgment in some manner, since they see this as superior to rationing solely by market forces or by insurer or governmental fiat.[5] Still, most adherents to this minority view impose the constraint that physicians be strictly insulated from any personal stake in their economizing decisions. Physicians are allowed to mediate a conflict between the health care needs of one patient and those of a group, but they may not be financially rewarded for rationing. Thus, bedside rationing is permissible only if the savings go entirely to other patients within a closed financing system, as occurs in Great Britain or in a nonprofit, group-model HMO that pays its physicians a straight salary.[6]

Only a very few ethicists go beyond this intermediate stance and openly embrace economic incentives for physicians to limit care. The leading voice is Haavi Morreim, but she seems to accept resource allocation by physicians more out of a sense of resignation, as a matter of economic or practical necessity, than from a firm basis of moral justification.[7] No one has yet articulated a complete moral and political defense of physician rationing under the influence of financial incentives.[8]

As a consequence, federal legislative policy has been greatly influenced by the dominant ethical view. In 1986, Congress banned hospitals from knowingly making any payment, "directly or indirectly, to a physician as an inducement to reduce or limit services provided [to Medicare or Medicaid patients]."[9] This legislation was in response to the uproar from the medical profession when a chain of proprietary hospitals in California proposed to reward physicians for staying within reimbursement limits that Congress had set for Medicare payments to hospitals.[10] This ban was initially written to extend to HMOs, but after learning that this would prohibit the manner in which most HMOs pay their physicians, Congress suspended the ban on HMO incentive plans pending further study.

Realizing that an absolute prohibition on any direct or indirect incentive to withhold care would unrealistically ban all forms of payment except fee-for-service, Congress has been more ambivalent in its recent legislative policy about financial inducements for physicians to limit services. Nevertheless, it continues to express considerable concern. A 1990 law subjected Medicare HMOs to regulatory oversight of their physician incentive arrangements and prohibited "specific payment[s] . . . as an inducement to reduce or limit medically necessary services provided with respect to a specific individual."[11] States have not yet followed suit, but several have considered bills to require HMOs to disclose their financial incentive plans.

Financial incentives to minimize treatment are also proving controversial in litigation. In an increasing number of lawsuits, plaintiffs' lawyers are arguing that an HMO physician's decision to withhold treatment, such as a Pap smear or biopsy to detect cancer, was inappropriately influenced by an undisclosed financial incentive plan. The common law is still in a very tentative state because most of these cases have been settled or dismissed for procedural reasons prior to trial. In the only two reported decisions, one court ruled that an HMO incentive plan does not constitute fraud or breach of warranty because such plans are consistent with public policy and are not intended to interfere with sound medical judgment,[12] and another ruled that it was proper to exclude evidence that profit motivation might have caused an HMO physician to fail to hospitalize a patient with labor complications, observing that such evidence "was only marginally relevant [to malpractice] and potentially very prejudicial."[13] However, one trial court refused to dismiss a similar suit, ruling that triable issues of fact existed over whether an incentive plan contributed to the doctor's alleged negligence.[14] In another case,[15] a California jury charged an HMO more than $12 million in compensatory and $77 million in punitive damages for refusing to fund medically necessary cancer treatment. At trial, the plaintiff's attorney introduced evidence that the HMO medical director responsible for the decision was compensated partly on the basis of how much money he saved the company. The legality of physicians making medical spending decisions is thus very much unsettled as a matter of common law as well.

Physician rationing can also be attacked under disability laws. The Fourth Circuit has ruled that federal statutory law requires honoring the parents' wish to continue aggressive life-support for a baby born with virtually all of its brain missing and with a minimal life expectancy, even though such treatment would "exceed the prevailing standard of medical care."[16] The lower court reached the same conclusion on the grounds that withholding expensive treatment due to poor prognosis would constitute prohibited disability discrimination.[17] Disability discrimination is also the grounds on which the Bush administration at first refused Oregon permission to ration care to its Medicaid recipients.[18] There is a fundamental and unresolved tension between coherent rationing criteria, which devote more medical resources to those who have the most to gain, and the requirement in disability discrimination law that opportunities and entitlements be distributed without regard to physical condition.[19]

This summary of the law is not intended necessarily to criticize the wisdom or accuracy of these individual rulings under their particular areas of legal doctrine.

It is intended only to document the unanimity between the ethical and the legal communities in their opposition to bedside rationing. As this chapter will demonstrate, such a position is out of step with current economic and medical realities and is not supported by careful application of the principles of medical ethics. The objective is to establish only the weak thesis that physicians may balance benefits against costs in some circumstances and to some degree, not the strong thesis that this is the only or the dominant means for enforcing spending limits.

This critique proceeds from positions that are both external to and internal to traditional medical ethics. It maintains first that the individual rights and role morality bases for the absolute prohibition are inferior to the larger moral and political concerns that medical ethics tends to neglect. This chapter goes further, however, to show that the physician's ethic of absolute quality cannot be sustained even within the prevailing framework of medical ethics. Each of the competing values of beneficence and autonomy that underlie conventional medical ethics is capable of permitting physicians to serve simultaneously as medical and economic agents for their patients. Before undertaking this analysis, however, we must first look more closely at just what bedside rationing entails and how it compares with the alternatives.

THE NATURE AND EXTENT OF BEDSIDE RATIONING

An Example of Bedside Rationing

To help focus the more abstract discussion that follows, consider this concrete example of physician bedside rationing based loosely on a mishap my wife suffered:[20]

As we were playing tennis, she lunged at the net for one of my dastardly (accidental) drop shots and badly strained her knee. An orthopedist's examination based on physical symptoms produced the diagnosis that, with about 90 percent certainty, she had suffered only a ligament strain; therefore, only bed rest was needed. Our further questioning of the doctor revealed, however, a 10 percent chance of a more serious ligament tear that, if it existed, would lead to permanent, slight impairment in 10 percent of such cases unless promptly corrected by surgery. Thus, there was a one-in-100 chance that simply waiting and watching could result in a weakening of my wife's knee—no visible limp, but such that she would no longer beat me at tennis as often as she usually does. An expensive magnetic resonance imaging scan could have resolved this remaining uncertainty, but would have cost $1200. Patterns of physician practice are sufficiently variable in these circumstances that it would not constitute negligence either to perform the surgery immediately or to simply wait and not perform an MRI scan. The doctor, who worked for an HMO, declined to order this additional test. The diagnosis was nevertheless correct and my wife is still the better tennis player (although now she lets me win my drop shots).[21]

There are several critical characteristics of the form of physician resource allocation just illustrated. First, this does not constitute the crass attitude of expendability that rationing critics often attack; rather, it consists of the prudent trimming of incrementally beneficial services. Larry Churchill has observed that much of the opposition to bedside rationing can be explained by the fear that doctors will "play God" by overtly sacrificing life or health for some social agenda.[22] Thus, many of the critics of physician rationing quoted above and cited in the Appendix focus on dramatic, life-and-death decisions such as terminating all treatment for the elderly or for a severely injured child.[23] But I, too, agree that it would be too corrosive of the treatment relationship for physicians to make high-stakes, high-drama rationing decisions without consulting their patients or relying on explicit regulatory or contractual authority. I see physicians declining to order a confirming diagnostic test, an extra day in the hospital, a more expensive drug, or a referral to a specialist when the stakes are low or their confidence in diagnosis and prognosis is fairly high already.[24]

Second, this example illustrates that the form of physician decision making I envision does not allow "substandard" treatment. It permits the denial of marginally beneficial treatment only where doing so is consistent with the prevailing standard of care and thus does not constitute malpractice. However, since the legal standard of care is determined by professional custom, physician rationing may result in a less demanding malpractice standard than currently exists.[25] Therefore, tort law provides only a partial brake against physician abuse. Nevertheless, it protects against physicians whose resource allocation decisions are far more severe than the norm. As economist Lester Thurow explains, "The medical profession now has professional norms concerning what constitutes bad medical practice. Those norms have to be expanded to include cases in which high costs are not justified by minor expected benefits."[26] Bedside rationing should not allow sharp departures from prevailing norms; it should only permit gradual evolution of those norms.

In a third respect, my example is misleading. Although it cites statistical probabilities for purposes of illustration, physician authority for resource allocation, as I envision it, would not require *explicit* cost/benefit calculations to be routinely made at the bedside level (although such calculations would not be prohibited). Instead, various mechanisms—education, peer influence and financial incentives—would cause physicians to internalize cost considerations within their intuitive clinical judgment, encouraging them to adopt a more conservative, less interventionist practice style. Cost/benefit tradeoffs would be largely implicit in physicians' thought processes, just as medical risk/benefit calculations at present are more often made through heuristic judgment than with rigorous calculation.·

This style of physician rationing is exemplified in a more extreme form in Great Britain. There, despite severe financial constraints that result in the British spending only one-third per capita what we do, physicians seldom consciously engage in explicit cost/benefit calculations.[27] British health economist Alan Williams explains that physicians there have absorbed [these much more severe cost] considerations comfortably within what they would still regard as their own clinical judgment rather than as part of any wider "extraneous" economic or social responsibility. . . . "The open and direct opinion This would cost too much, is rarely expressed and, I suspect, not often consciously entertained as a discretionary factor." . . . [Resource constraints are] so deeply embedded in the clinical consciousness that they come to be thought of as wholly within the realm of clinical autonomy.[28]

Likewise, in the United States, Luft has observed that

it is extremely unlikely that HMO physicians reflect upon the impact on their bonuses each time they consider a follow-up visit or an extra test. Instead, certain routine patterns are probably developed that tend to be consistent with their economic incentives. Inconsistent patterns may be reexamined and slowly adjusted to reduce conflict with system incentives.[29]

Potential Abuse of the Authority to Ration

This style of implicit, discretionary resource allocation is subject to strong criticism on the ground that doctors are humans prone to error and bias, and so their decisions have been shown to be highly variable,[30] inconsistent,[31] and influenced by irrational and illegitimate factors. For instance, physicians show a persistent refusal to honor patients' requests for withdrawal of life support, and a troubling inability to accurately predict their patients' value choices in this regard.[32] Those who are familiar with physicians' bedside behavior as it now exists under unlimited insurance fear that "bedside rationing is likely to result in gross injustices in which like cases are not treated alike. If rationing is left to the physician's discretion, with doctors being exhorted to save society money because of the runaway costs of health care, an array of arbitrary and inconsistent decisions is likely to result."[33]

Perhaps the most troubling sign of potential abuse from physician bias is mounting evidence that doctors treat patients differently according to their race and socioeconomic status, and that these differences cannot be accounted for by the patients' health status or insurance coverage.[34] For instance, a large number of studies document that blacks receive aggressive and invasive treatment such as bypass surgery and angioplasty for heart disease significantly less often than do whites with similar conditions and insurance.[35] This clearly disturbing evidence suggests either a subtle or overt racial bias among health care providers and institutions.[36] This evidence may not be quite as disturbing as it first appears, however, considering the fact that these procedures are typically overprescribed, and therefore those who receive fewer may be better off, or at least no worse off. Few of these studies measured actual health outcomes caused by disparate treatment, and one that did found that blacks fared better in the short term and just as well in the intermediate term.[37]

Moreover, it is noteworthy that the same bias can exist under rule-based democratic rationing as under discretionary professional rationing. Therefore, we lack any clear indication that individualized physician discretion will lead to worse bias than institutionalized or bureaucratized rationing. For instance, the rules that govern allocation of scarce organ transplants result in blacks receiving these lifesaving procedures far less often than do whites because blacks are penalized by the tissue-matching criteria contained in organ allocation rules. Blacks awaiting transplants have many fewer tissue matches because blacks are much more reluctant to donate their organs for transplant than are whites.[38] Some commentators have criticized these tissue-matching criteria as being excessively harsh and unnecessary in light of recent medical advances that partially overcome tissue incompatibility problems.[39]

Regardless of how we interpret these particular pieces of empirical evidence, there is no doubt that physicians presently are flawed and biased to some degree in their clinical judgment. Asking them to incorporate costs in their treatment decisions will only increase the severity of these abuses since they would then tend even more strongly toward harmful undertreatment. Cause for concern can already be seen in the manner in which physicians allow lifestyle factors such as occupation and sexual orientation to masquerade as medical factors in allocating organ transplants[40] and in the abusive practices that have occurred in some government-sponsored HMOs treating elderly and low-income patients.[41] Physician rationers will undoubtedly tend to favor more articulate, higher-educated patients who are better equipped to voice their demands. "We all have a natural tendency, often unconscious, to favour the attractive, the verbally fluent, the intelligent and those from our own background over the inarticulate, the ugly, the stupid, and those from different cultures."[42] Doctors will also undoubtedly devote disproportionate time to high-visibility diseases or to those that command their research or intellectual interests. This speculation is confirmed to some extent by Henry Aaron and William Schwartz's study of the manner in which rationing decisions are made by British physicians.[43] They found that conditions such as cancer that the public especially dreads, or ones such as hemophilia that have a focused interest group, receive disproportionately more physician attention than other, more ordinary and diffused, conditions such as heart disease.

It is possible to rebut these assertions by observing that the little empirical evidence directly on point is more encouraging than these naysayers admit. Studies of physician behavior when intensive care units are crowded reveal that doctors implicitly respond with plausible rationing criteria. They systematically screen out the less serious cases, and there is no apparent denial of service to dying patients.[44] One intriguing study that presented physicians hypothetical resource allocation problems found that their decisions are generally consistent with ones made by nonphysicians, that physicians have a "clear preference for the efficient use of scarce resources," but that they "deviate from pure efficiency in response to concerns over equity," for instance, by attempting to equalize the end-state health status of patients who present with different conditions, and by devoting somewhat more to the care of the young than the old.[45] Similarly, physicians in England appear to consider patient age, aggregate medical costs, and costs of alternative care in deciding where to cut back on resources.[46]

Another strong piece of empirical evidence comes from studies of the quality of care in HMOs, particularly the RAND Corporation's extraordinary Health Insurance Experiment, which used a rigorous randomization protocol to compare the health of different population groups assigned to traditional insurance, HMOs, and out-of-pocket payment arrangements.[47] Virtually all of these studies have concluded that patients fare at least as well, if not better, in HMOs than under traditional fee-for-service indemnity insurance.[48] The one notable exception is that initially, sick, low-income patients assigned to HMOs in the RAND study end up somewhat worse off than their fee-for-service counterparts for some measures of general health status.[49] However, other studies have found no worsening of health resulting from the adoption of prepaid or managed care programs for Medicaid patients.[50] Another piece of potentially negative HMO evidence is that HMO patients, when questioned about factors such as physicians' technical skills, waiting time for appointments, physician courtesy, and accessibility through the telephone, appear less satisfied than fee-for-service patients. However, these differences in consumer satisfaction are not dramatic, and they are more strongly correlated with the size and type of practice setting (solo versus group) than they are with the type of insurance (fee-for-service versus prepaid).[51]

Based on this accumulation of evidence, the fear that physician bedside rationing as it is currently practiced will lead to widespread serious abuse is not presently well founded. The very fact that researchers are reporting massive amounts of this type of information in the form of physician "scorecards" and HMO "report cards"[52] suggests that the potential for abuse is diminished, since intensified oversight will help caution physicians to be more vigilant in examining their internal motivations and biases and will help weed out those whose performance is unacceptable. Implicit rationing has been criticized because it tends toward secretiveness, but this is not a necessary attribute of bedside rationing. Physician discretion can be preserved while publicizing the patterns of distribution and resulting health outcomes and encouraging improvement. By way of analogy, the fact that educators such as myself make mistakes and display bias in the classroom does not justify teaching class by computer or cancelling class altogether; instead, the appropriate corrective remedy is to expose and correct the errors as best possible. Those who espouse the renewal of virtue ethics believe that it is at least possible for doctors to "cultivate the habit of acting justly" as an "important safeguard against [unconscious] bias."[53] Even those who are more cynical might be comforted to know that HMOs are beginning to explore ways to tie physician compensation to explicit performance measures such as patient satisfaction and actual health outcomes.

Nevertheless, the possibility of undetectable and uncorrectable abuse by physician rationers is certainly not unimaginable. Therefore, a more compelling basis for moderating opposition to bedside rationing is to compare it with the flaws in the viable alternatives articulated in the prior chapters. Critics of rationing sometimes suffer from the "nirvana fallacy" of assuming that a perfect alternative is possible. In Garrett Hardin's words, they "befuddle the issue by professing a petty faith in counterfactual conditionals . . . such as a 'heroic answer must be found,' [which] implies that there *is* a 'heroic' and painlessly acceptable answer."[54] Regrettably, there is not. The alternatives to internalizing cost constraints in physicians' clinical judgment are either (1) to force patients to always make these trade-offs themselves by preventing them from purchasing insurance, an alternative that is obviously undesirable, or (2) for private insurers and employers, driven by profit-making concerns, or for the government, driven by budget-deficit concerns, to impose cost constraints explicitly through cookbook medicine.

Bedside Rationing in Practice

Resource allocation by physicians can also be defended more pragmatically by observing the many conventional settings in which doctors routinely make decisions contrary to the immediate medical interests of their individual patients. These situations are much more ordinary and commonplace than the extreme situations of battlefield and emergency room triage that rationing opponents acknowledge as allowable exceptions.[55] Indeed, the documented exceptions to the rule against bedside rationing might be thought to be so widespread that they constitute the norm. Therefore, rationing opponents have an improbable position to defend. In actual practice, society has demanded only appropriate, not total, devotion to individual patient interests. As Stephen Toulmin has observed:

In an ideal world, no doubt, all our working institutions, and the whole society, would command the loyalties of individuals unambiguously. . . . But this remains an ideal or aspiration, not a statement about the world we actually live in. . . . Life rarely allows us the luxury of standing in one-and-only-one relationship to one-and-only-one person or institution. . . . [E]ver since Socrates, clear headed moral analysts have recognized that no *single* obligation of this kind imposes on our conduct anything more than a presumptive, all-other-things-being-equal claim.[56]

Physicians routinely and properly compromise absolute medical quality for patients who lack insurance, which was the norm prior to the 1960s. Arnold Relman has remarked that, then, "the physician's economic incentives were in a sense more sharply in conflict with his professional duty to act in the patient's interest,"[57] yet this conflict posed no ethical obstacle to physicians considering the costs of treatment. Indeed, it might be thought unethical not to do so. The same holds true today for the 40 million Americans without health insurance and, to some extent, for the vast majority of the rest of us who pay for part of the costs of treatment out-of-pocket.

Bedside rationing is also commonplace in government institutions operated under fixed budgets by salaried physicians. Municipal hospitals, Veterans Administration hospitals, military medical institutions, and the Indian Health Service constitute a significant portion of the medical establishment and serve as training institutions for a large percentage of medical students.[58] In each, physicians practice daily in resource-constrained environments that require them to be vigilant about costs and prioritize among patients to an extent that clearly sacrifices some degree of optimal patient benefit. Similar facility shortages plague many private hospitals as well in the form of restricted intensive care beds, which makes resource allocation by physicians an "everyday occurrence" in some hospitals and "likely to occur at least some of the time in many hospitals."[59] In rural areas with fewer medical resources and shortages of personnel, doctors are forced to take a less-than-optimal approach that considers how best to allocate resources within the community.[60]

In various public health arenas, physicians' duties to the state or to the public good routinely override their obligations to individual patients. Psychiatrists are under an ever-present tort-law and regulatory duty to prevent their patients from causing harm to themselves or others, a social concern that is contrary to their patients' expressed wishes.[61] Physicians also act as society's agent and sometimes against their patients' interests when they accurately certify their patients' health status to various government agencies and private institutions from which their patients seek benefits or special dispensation. Examples include patients applying for disability and worker's compensation benefits, seeking exclusion from jury duty and military service, claiming insanity to avoid criminal responsibility, or seeking to qualify for high-risk jobs such as an airline pilot. [62] Similarly, all physicians must report gunshot wounds, infectious diseases, and child abuse to the proper authorities, contrary to their patients' individual interests.[63] Surveying all these many "intrusions" led one set of authors to observe: "Those halcyon days of an unhindered, dyadic doctor-patient relationship never really existed. . . . Our society has long recognized that . . . in [some] instances, physicians are obligated to serve as agents of the government."[64]

Physicians advance other public health goals such as childhood immunizations and prudent use of antibiotics in a manner that can compromise a margin of individual patient safety. Where immunizations are widespread enough to create a "herd immunity," no individual patient is exposed to significant risk by foregoing immunizations, but if a large number of patients refuse immunizations due to the risks of side effects, the herd immunity is lost. Thus, for individual patients, an immunization can sacrifice a margin of safety more for the benefit of society than for their individual benefit (depending on the relative magnitude of the competing individual risks of contagion versus side effects).[65] Physicians seldom disclose this fact when they recommend, or insist upon, vaccinations. Similarly, some physicians discourage overuse of antibiotics in order to avoid strains of bacteria becoming resistant.[66] Contrary to common understanding, this is much more of a threat to the public generally than it is to individual patients, since aggressive use of antibiotics usually does not create antibiotic resistance in the patient's immune system but instead in the bacteria's genetics. Therefore, when doctors are taught to use antibiotics conservatively, they are sacrificing a slight margin of individual patient safety for the benefit of the public at large.

Conflicted medical practice reaches even the pinnacle of the medical establishment in the form of medical research. The randomized clinical trial, the gold standard of experimental methodology, "routinely asks physicians to sacrifice the interests of their particular patients for the . . . benefit of society."[67] When physicians ask patients to participate in such trials, they assign them randomly to a treatment group, either standard or experimental. Often, the physician believes one of these groups is not optimal; therefore, the requirement of perfect "equipoise" in the expected success of each treatment option under study is rarely met. At best, the physician can claim uncertainty as to which is best.[68] The nation's most preeminent physicians are willing to undertake this slightly conflicted role (with their patients' consent) in order to pursue society's and their own personal interest in the advancement of medical science.

Physicians also regularly engage in a mild form of rationing at a more mundane level of everyday primary medicine. They allocate their own time and attention according to a rough sense of triage among daily demands, to the slight (and sometimes considerable) inconvenience of some of their patients.[69] They also adopt prudent clinical heuristics that avoid extravagant expenditures merely to pursue tiny increments of medical benefit, such as by taking a wait-and-see approach to an apparently minor illness rather than investing enormous time and money into ruling out any possibility of a more serious ailment. As a British physician ethicist explains, "If one were to take thoroughly to heart the idea that as curative doctors we should *never* allow concern for cost to others to deflect us from doing whatever we could to benefit our patients, then diagnostic services would be overwhelmed as we tested for rare but possible problems."[70] For instance, it is not possible to say purely on grounds of individual patient benefit that monthly Pap smears are not warranted to rule out all possible risk of cervical cancer, that physicians should not prescribe antibiotics purely for placebo effects, or that patients should be refused routine, whole-body MRI scans to find undetected imperfections of all kinds, yet the failure to pursue such treatment is considered to be perfectly sound professional practice.

This is physician bedside rationing at an almost imperceptible level. The accepted rationale is that, while physicians may not force unwanted treatment on their patients, they are not required to offer treatment they considered nonstandard, unethical, or unprofessional.[71] In some cases, the objection may be a moral or religious one, but in most of these cases it is clear that economics and general prudence play a part. In either event, the physician is trading off a strict sense of the patient's individual medical benefit for a personal or societal concern.

Physician rationing has surfaced recently in a more dramatic and ethically controversial fashion, but one that nevertheless illuminates the inconsistencies within mainstream clinical ethics. Several articles in leading medical journals over the past few years have invoked the concept of medical "futility" to argue that physicians may withhold cardiopulmonary resuscitation (CPR) efforts from debilitated patients unlikely to survive to leave the hospital. Astonishingly, some of these articles argue that physicians may do so despite the patient's and family's objection and perhaps without even consulting them.[72] These proposals are not radical alterations of traditional practices but reflect a growing consensus that existing practice should receive explicit ethical rationalization. One experienced physician openly admits that "many of those who die in nursing homes are tacitly allowed to die without further attempt at salvation"; "doctors and nurses frequently decide quietly to approach nursing home residents with benign neglect of medical problems."[73] Similar unilateral decisions have been reported for severely deformed or brain-damaged newborns.[74]

Although the appropriate limits of this newly visible concept of medical futility are still being debated,[75] what is significant for us here is that the concept implicitly incorporates a cost/benefit calculation.[76] For CPR denial, the data do not show that resuscitation is absolutely futile in the sense that no patients are successfully resuscitated; they show only that these patients do not live very long or have a very meaningful existence.[77] For example, one study advocated withholding CPR from patients who come to the emergency room in cardiac arrest, observing that in 185 successive such patients given CPR at one hospital, none survived long enough to be discharged from the hospital. However, 9 percent of the patients were successfully resuscitated and lived for an average of 12 days, and in other studies, 1–2 percent survived to leave the hospital, albeit in a debilitated or comatose state.[78] Likewise, for the comatose patient, the argument is that there is little, not zero, medical benefit to continuing costly treatment that merely preserves primitive biological processes but does nothing to restore functional or mental capacity.[79] Futility is invoked as a euphemism to limit this cost/benefit analysis of life-sustaining treatment to only the most extreme categories of terminally ill and comatose patients.

While these applications of the futility characterization are at best controversial and at worst dead wrong, analogous judgments of prudential balance go into determining accepted medical practice in a much more routine and legitimate fashion whenever physicians decline to pursue extreme long-shot possibilities to the nth degree. As one physician has observed, there would hardly be an outcry if an artificial valve implant operation were withheld from a permanently comatose patient.[80] A second example comes from the report of physicians who refused to continue administering extracorporeal membrane oxygenation (ECMO) to a terminally ill and comatose child severely injured in a two-story fall. ECMO is an extremely expensive technology developed to temporarily replace heart and lung functions for only a short period, such as during surgery or while waiting for a transplantable organ to arrive. The doctors reasoned that it would exceed the standard of care to devote this extraordinary expense for a patient who would never recover and who was likely to die in any event, even though it would extend the child's life somewhat.[81] Perhaps vegetative state is a distinctive, limiting category that keeps it from being generalized to all medical care, but the point still holds that, in at least some cases, many people consider it to be legally and ethically acceptable for physicians to set resource-sensitive limits at the bedside.

Physicians have conflicted obligations in other, more specialized settings that nevertheless are considered socially acceptable and ethically tolerable.[82] Military doctors are obliged to get their patients back into battle as quickly as possible and to call attention to those they think are unfit to serve.[83] Similarly, doctors for sports teams have a duty to their employers to prevent player malingering and to report accurately the condition of players too eager to return to the game.[84] Doctors who treat workers at industrial clinics have analogous conflicting obligations to company and patient.[85] Of a different stripe altogether, but still quite significant and commonplace, is the conflict that an obstetrician must mediate whenever opposing interests arise in treating a mother and fetus, or the dilemma that a family physician faces when the treatment preferences of a minor differ from those of the parents, or when the parents themselves disagree and the physician must side with one or the other. Finally, doctors who assist in live organ donations, for instance, by operating to remove a kidney, agree to compromise a margin of safety for the donor patient to benefit another patient.

In view of these many examples, one could well conclude that the legendary allegiance of American physicians solely to each patient's absolute best medical interests is the stuff of myth, not rigorous ethical analysis. One physician summed up the credulity of those who hold this position: The opinion . . . that physicians must not be put in the position of judging between the interests of an individual patient and the limitations of society as a whole is astonishing, because their statements contradict the daily experience of nearly every practicing physician I know.[86]

In the blunt but astute words of Emily Friedman, "to muddy the waters by saying that physicians have never rationed care is hypocrisy."[87] Still, it is necessary to examine the analytical framework of medical ethics to determine whether somehow these many instances can be reconciled with a general prohibition on physicians considering costs or, perhaps, whether these instances are themselves unethical and should be prohibited. If, indeed, resource allocation by physicians is ethically appropriate in some instances, it is important to understand on what basis in order to know the proper forms and limits. The problem is that, in order to even broach this subject in a constructive manner, we must overcome the ethical and legal taboo that has been placed on physician bedside rationing.

THE MORAL AND POLITICAL STATUS
OF MAINSTREAM MEDICAL ETHICS

The clear majority voice among medical ethicists and within the medical profession against bedside rationing carries considerable moral weight, simply by virtue of the respect we are inclined to give to this community of opinion. Most leading medical ethicists are trained in philosophy, often from a religious perspective, and medicine is one of the most revered professions in society. Doctors have devoted careful thought to this problem, and we in the legal, agnostic, and profane world should hesitate to question their considered conclusions.

However, their conclusions deserve weight only to the extent that the framework of mainstream medical ethics has intellectual and public policy legitimacy. If the framework is defective or limited, medical ethics is laying claim to more authority than it is entitled to. This section demonstrates that the prohibition of physician rationing should not be uncritically accepted as governing dogma because it suffers from limitations of three sorts: (1) It is focused too narrowly on the concerns of individual physicians and patients and not enough on the broader perspective of distributive justice; (2) it is contingent on the particular financing schemes that prevailed over past decades and therefore is subservient to a societal decision to alter the basic form of insurance; and (3) role morality arguments that refer by analogy to lawyers are unconvincing unless adversarialism is in fact uniformly embraced as a desirable way to practice medicine.

The Hyperindividualism of Contemporary Clinical Ethics

The modern field of bioethics emerged in two distinct eras: the foundational and the contemporary. Prior to about 1970, medical ethics was the province of practicing clinicians, who used ethical concepts to frame codes of professional conduct. The first modern work of medical ethics was Thomas Percival's *Medical Ethics: Or a Code of Institutes and Precepts Adopted to the Professional Conduct of Physicians and Surgeons*, written in 1803 to settle the professional squabbling and turf battles that were causing a decline in the public's confidence in the profession. Percival's work became the model for each of the succeeding versions of the AMA's code of medical ethics. Consistent with the ancient Hippocratic tradition of Greek medicine, the resulting ethical principles were primarily concerned with maintaining order among members of the profession and fostering public respect for professional authority.

David Rothman's history of bioethics critiques this early phase for "elevating medical etiquette over medical ethics, for moving ever so nimbly from high-minded intuitions—do no harm—to professionally self-serving propositions—do not slander a fellow doctor or . . . contradict him in front of his patients."[88] This was a physician-centered, professional code approach to ethics written by doctors, about doctors, and principally for the professional benefit of doctors.[89]

Single-minded devotion to a patient's best medical interests, without concern for costs, emerges as one of the central tenets of this physician-centered, Hippocratic code tradition. The pledge of devotion fosters public confidence, the exclusion of competing social concerns simplifies and focuses the doctor's task solely on the craft of medicine, and the "spare-no-expense" mentality obviously enhances income potential. Lacking any broader social consensus, however, the professional code framework that supports these injunctions does not generate compelling ethical force.[90] All that can be said of its edicts is that they represent the collective views of physicians on the best way to conduct their profession. Whether this manner of regulating professional affairs is desirable from the patient's or society's perspective is still an open question.[91]

The contemporary phase of medical ethics, which is differentiated by the new-age label "bioethics," developed directly in reaction to the physician-centeredness of professional ethics. Motivated by the 1960s civil rights movement and the Watergate-era skepticism of status quo authority, the bioethics movement adopted a patient-centered framework that defined medical ethics in terms of individual rights. Bioethics was led by academic philosophers and theologians rather than practicing physicians, and it adopted as its foremost guiding principle respect for patient autonomy, as best exemplified by the legal innovation of informed consent doctrine.

This fundamental shift in perspective only reinforced the antirationing dictate.[92] Total devotion to patient interests and the exclusion of social cost considerations are fully consistent with the principle of patient autonomy. Physicians are required by virtue of their fiduciary responsibility to act solely as agents for their individual patients and to abjure any personal conflict of interest, even if this frustrates efficient distribution of societal resources.[93]

While modern bioethics has brought about much valued reform, its patient-oriented focus has been criticized for being excessively individualistic and suffering from an insular quality that segregates it from broader currents of political and moral thought.[94] This myopic quality may result in part from the occupational setting in which much bioethics work is done. Many leading medical ethicists hold jobs on, or are associated with, the faculties of medical schools for the purpose of providing clinically oriented ethical training to student doctors. As a consequence, their focus tends to be more on the clinical aspects of discrete patient–physician encounters than on the broader social concerns of reimbursement and coverage.[95]

Because many scholars in mainstream bioethics are primarily concerned with the issues that traditionally have confronted doctors in their daily clinical practice, until recently they have not attacked as vigorously the broader problems of distributive justice that legislatures, insurance companies, and private employers now face.

Critics have also observed that professional bioethicists are charged with the difficult role of shifting from dispassionate theoretical analysis in their analytical scholarship to practical, reform-oriented advocacy in their training of physicians. Too often, the roles become intertwined such that practical training is sometimes accused of being too theoretical, while the analytical writing in the field can sometimes assume a pedantic quality. In the view of one critic, certain foundational positions are taken as articles of faith that seem to require acceptance as a condition of entry to the field.[96]

Thus, although contemporary bioethics has rectified the distortion in perspective that came from viewing the treatment relationship only through the eyes of the physician, the new, patient-oriented perspective still suffers from myopic attention to the individual treatment relationship. I do not mean to say that mainstream bioethics has ignored broader concerns of social justice altogether, only that this has not been its principal focus. This clinical orientation causes many bioethicists to ask what forms of resource allocation are proper only from the perspective of a presently sick patient seeking treatment and discourages them from examining the perspective of healthy potential patients contemplating how to structure an insurance arrangement. Consequently, mainstream medical ethics has yet to fully address questions of resource allocation within medicine and across other sectors of the economy.[97]

A broader moral and political perspective undermines the physician ethic of absolute quality by noting the larger social harms that accrue if physicians are insulated from considering costs. Demanding that cost be no object in treatment decisions is one reason that health insurance is now priced out of the reach of 15 percent of the population. Therefore, to allow patient-oriented medical ethics to drive questions of distributive justice would be to "succumb to precisely the sort of individualistic morality that has sustained the inequities in health care for so long."[98] As British economist Alan Williams aptly puts it, "not to seek to become more efficient is what is unethical, because inefficiency means needlessly worsening the health of the people that doctors are there to serve. . . . [I]n my vocabulary the term to be applied to someone who acts without regard to costs is not 'ethical,' but 'fanatical.'"[99]

Under the competing view of medical ethics, the individualistic principles of beneficence and autonomy must operate within the constraints of distributive justice. Individualist principles can only instruct us how best to spend the money that society has made available; medical ethics cannot redefine the ultimate ends of social justice. Thus, "the beneficence principle, where applicable, simply requires that whatever resource the individual is entitled to . . . be employed for the maximal benefit of this individual."[100] It does not require that a particular level of benefit be funded. Similarly, the autonomy principle does not create a right to limitless resources; it only gives the patient control over how his available resources are spent. In short, an individual-rights orientation cannot force patients to purchase a more expensive brand of ethics than they can in fact afford.[101]

The physician ethic of absolute quality is also rejected under the communitarian perspective that is in vogue in other areas of moral and political theory. Communitarianism dismisses a rigid individual-rights orientation in favor of a perspective that stresses collective rights and individual responsibilities.[102] This perspective is more prevalent in Europe, where social insurance systems predominate, facilitating a much more successful reconciliation than we presently enjoy between the collective view of economic thought and the individualism of medical ethics. Communitarianism undermines the prohibition of bedside rationing because it allows for some compromise of individual rights to achieve broader social objectives. For instance, communitarianism would support the notion that an insured patient owes an obligation to others in the insurance pool to constrain her use of marginally beneficial health care resources.[103]

A prominent example of how communitarianism supports a multiplicity of rationing mechanisms is found in the recent work of physician ethicist Ezekiel Emanuel.[104] He applies a theory of liberal communitarianism to problems of medical resource allocation by arguing that insurance subscribers select among divergent communities of ethical principles when they choose a particular insurance plan. Among those principles are the mechanism and criteria for resource allocation. Emanuel sees this individual choice among competing communities of thought as the only feasible method for constructing coherent moral principles in a political state that adheres to the foundational principles of liberal democracy. Liberalism's commitment to strict neutrality on individual values precludes state enforcement of moral dictates where unanimity of opinion is in fact absent. The ban on bedside rationing would be one such illicit normative proscription.

The Economic Contingency of Fee-for-Service Ethics

The absolute prohibition on physicians making medical spending decisions is also undermined at its foundation by the moral pluralism advanced in the work of philospher Alasdair MacIntyre. He argues in his seminal book *After Virtue*[105] that moral principles are culturally contingent, not universal in their truth. There is no sure foundation from which to choose between rival moral arguments because their different premises are conceptually incommensurate. Morality is dependent on cultural cohesiveness; therefore, a moral scheme has no more force than its defining context. Remove that context and the scheme becomes arbitrary or meaningless. In MacIntyre's view, this is why our pluralistic society has been in a continuous state of moral decay ever since the unsuccessful attempt of the Enlightenment to replace an authoritarian religious moral framework with ethics based on individual rationality. He sees the inability to defend moral absolutes in a climate of moral pluralism as accounting for the "shrill tone" that characterizes much moral argument, which often exaggerates the certainty and universality of moral positions almost in inverse proportion to the strength of support for the position.

In bioethics, the leading exponent of this brand of moral contingency and moral pluralism is Tristram Engelhardt. Rather than attempting to derive a single moral view from religious authority or from the brute force of human rationality, Engelhardt advances a "secular pluralistic ethic" that "establishes the possibility of a multiplicity of concrete moral views."[106] He warns that those who are "accustomed to the sure answers of a religiously grounded ethics"[107] will fail to grasp the inherent limitations of secular reasoning. In his view, "it is hopeless to suppose that a general moral consensus will develop regarding any of the major issues in bioethics."[108] While each of us may subscribe to a concrete moral code, it is fallacious to believe that particular moral judgments are subject to categorical resolution. In Engelhardt's view, bioethics is restricted to the minimal, procedural role of overseeing the "geography" of ethical debate, not providing absolutist answers to particular problems.

Both MacIntyre and Engelhardt warn against the temptation to elevate individual beliefs to the grand scale of universal moral principle that ethics enjoyed when it was dominated by religious fervor prior to the Enlightenment. Thus, the fact that a number of thoughtful physicians and patients feel strongly and sincerely about the moral degeneracy of HMOs provides no basis for framing those personal beliefs in absolutist or categorical ethical terms. Doing so is an example of what MacIntyre describes as the "vulgarized facility of modern moral utterance" to give "moral countenance . . . to far too many causes."[109]

Moral contingency is nicely demonstrated by viewing the physician ethic of absolutist quality against the backdrop of changing health insurance systems. Seen in this light, this ethic is an idiosyncratic artifact of the culture of attitudes and behavior generated by outmoded forms of insurance.[110] Demanding that doctors provide all treatment of any medical benefit, despite its cost, assumes that a world of unlimited resources is available for medical treatment. Therefore, it fits all too conveniently the form of open-ended, unregulated, fee-for-service payment that predominated prior to 1980. Patients can easily afford such an absolutist ethic if they are fully insured and have to share in little or none of the costs of treatment themselves, and doctors can eagerly respond since to do so only magnifies their income and professional standing. Insisting that cost is no object when it comes to health frees physicians from any constraints on their ability to practice their profession to the highest degree of their training and technical skill. One must question, then, whether this ethic has any greater foundation than providers' self-interested glorification of a particularly generous method of payment.

From the perspective of a patient *without* insurance, a money-is-no-object ethic is hardly compelling. This ethic did not prevail in the period prior to World War II when insurance was not commonplace, and it surely does not prevail for the tens of millions of patients who presently lack insurance. For those who still have insurance, their insulated status is increasingly jeopardized precisely because the medical profession continues to insist on an unaffordable ethic. The ethic is suspect, then, not only because of its historical and economic contingency, but because it paradoxically is causing the very economic collapse that is undermining its raison d'êntre. Absent first-dollar, fee-for-service insurance, there is no ethical basis for insisting that physicians provide absolute quality, yet it is this ethic that is making such insurance increasingly unaffordable. In short, the ethic is self-destructing.

To respond that high-minded ethical concerns prevail over baser economic ones misses the point; in this arena, the two are intertwined. "It is not just the demands of efficiency that lead us to 'put a price on life' in conditions of moderate scarcity; it is the demands of justice itself."[111] Some timeless ethical principles—fundamental liberty and due process, for instance—are held by society to be of such foundational importance that they may not be easily compromised or entirely sacrificed for merely instrumental reasons of economic efficiency. The demand that physicians remain oblivious to costs is not of this intrinsic moral stature.

There was an earlier stage in the historical evolution of health care financing when ethics and economics were thought to be in fundamental conflict, and it was ethics that was forced to yield. When Medicare and Medicaid were enacted as part of Lyndon Johnson's "Great Society" social reforms, medical professional societies raised the radically different ethical objection that insurance in *any* form is corrupting. Herman Somers and Anne Somers report that the ethical argument used then shared remarkably in the same tones of absolutism that characterize the opposition to physician rationing now:

Leading medical societies have repeatedly asserted that good doctor-patient relations and good quality care depend on a particular form of medical economics: the patient or his family must personally choose and directly pay the physician. Some medical spokesmen extend the argument to condemn every kind of third party arrangement designed to help in the financing of medical care. A former president of the Association of American Physicians and Surgeons asserts flatly that all third party programs—private or public—"historically result in less satisfactory and inferior medical care."[112]

It is now clear to us that this opposition to all forms of insurance was an inferior brand of ethics. Today, when the debate is between different *forms* of insurance—unrestricted fee-for-service (traditional indemnity), heavily regulated fee-for-service ("utilization review" and preferred provider organizations), or group-based prepayment (HMOs)—we should be equally suspicious of arguments going to the preservation of a particular payment arrangement. Just as the greater demands of social justice forced the ethic of individual reliance to give way to the ethic of absolute quality, now, the disintegration of insurance requires us to relinquish absolute quality.

Seen in this light, the anachronistic prohibition of bedside rationing acts somewhat like an ancient taboo in a primitive culture that survives long past the destruction of the context that initially gave it intelligibility.[113] To continue to hold fast to the rule that physicians must ignore costs, after the era of unconstrained reimbursement has disappeared, is to arrogate to it an artificial ethical stature it does not deserve. Because this ethic is historically and economically contingent, we must discard it when larger social, political, and economic forces require the surrounding payment culture to change. In short, we stand in need of a new ethic that recognizes the existence of variable levels of funding and that is sensitive to the possibility that greater injustice is done if insurance is not affordable at all.

The Limits of Role-Based Adversarialism

The extremism of an absolutist ethic can sometimes be reconciled with the pragmatism of the real world by invoking concepts of role morality. Role morality recognizes the instrumental status of professional ethics yet is often able to maintain an extremist ethic by arguing that an abnormal ethical stance is necessary for the profession to adequately serve its social function. Thus, while it is generally not permissible to kill, the role morality of the military allows, even requires, soldiers to kill in order to serve the social function of national defense.[114]

Legal ethics is the model of role morality on which the prohibition of bedside rationing is based. A foundational principle of legal ethics is that lawyers are to pursue their clients' interests zealously, setting aside any concern for social justice such as the client's guilt or undeservedness.[115] One widely quoted statement of this principle occurred in Lord Brougham's 1820 defense of Queen Caroline against King George IV's charge of adultery: "An advocate, in the discharge of his duty, knows but one person in all the world, and that person is his client. To save that client by all means and expedients, . . . he must not regard the alarm, the torments, the destruction which he may bring upon others. Separating the duty of a patriot from that of an advocate, he must go on reckless of consequences."[116] This edict of client devotion is so strong that prominent judges and academics have argued (albeit subject to some dissent) that lawyers must put perjurious clients on the stand in some circumstances and may discredit and humiliate opposing witnesses known to be truthful.[117] For instance, a lawyer defending an accused rapist is expected to brutally expose the victim's private sexual practices even if the lawyer privately suspects his client's guilt.

Doctors argue that the ends of medicine demand the same extreme devotion to their patients' immediate treatment interests, even to the obvious severe detriment of society's ability to care for other patients. This analogy between doctoring and lawyering cannot be drawn so easily, though. The mere fact that both are learned professions does not automatically establish that they are governed by the same role morality.[118] Role morality justification depends narrowly on the precise instrumental connection between the particular behavior and the relevant social objective.[119] For legal ethics, strict client devotion is demanded by the adversarial system of adjudication, which is designed to arrive at the optimal determination of justice via a contest of competing extremes. In such a system, the lawyer's single-minded pursuit is counterbalanced by the opposing lawyer's equally zealous advocacy, with a neutral judge and jury serving as the ultimate arbiter of the merits of the competing arguments.

To justify by analogy an equivalent role morality for doctors would require showing that an adversarial system of medicine is equally (1) present *and* (2) desirable *and* (3) that physician oblivion to costs is equally essential to this system of medicine. An adversarial system of medicine in fact is evolving as private and public payers increasingly impose rigorous review standards for medical appropriateness. Thus, one might argue that extreme adversarialism by doctors counteracts the insurer's or hospital's tendency to spend too little.[120] However, to posit this possible justification is not to establish its desirability in theory or its uniform acceptance in practice.

In fact, adversarial medicine has not been uniformly adopted. Adversarialism characterizes primarily the indemnity form of insurance, which separates the financial risk-bearing function from the treatment function. The HMO model of insurance, which combines these two functions, obviates the adversarial nature of third-party reimbursement by internalizing financial incentives within the primary-treatment decision maker. Thus, the role that society in fact places on physicians practicing in an HMO environment is a nonadversarial one that justifies a nonabsolutist role morality.

Paradoxically, adversarial medicine is loudly denounced by the same medical establishment that advances the absolutist physician ethic. Doctors consider themselves the ultimate arbiters of medical appropriateness, and they vigorously oppose the establishment of any counterbalancing role representing the purchaser's or insurer's interest. Echoes of this vicious denunciation of adversarial medicine can be heard at virtually any social or professional gathering of doctors. Therefore, the conception that doctors in fact hold of a properly structured medical system is inconsistent with the single-minded role morality they assert for themselves. Doctors cannot have it both ways. If medicine is to avoid the adversarial qualities that most people oppose, physicians will have to assume a different role, one with an ethic that allows them to internalize the constraining forces that they argue should not be imposed from external sources.

In sum, we reach the same conclusion via yet another route: Medical ethics is subservient to the financing system within which society asks physicians to practice. Role morality is more of an argument by description than by normative prescription, that is, it calls on doctors to adapt to the role they are in fact asked to serve; it does not define what the role should be. Therefore, role morality carries no ethical bite at the larger level of political and social decision making that is presently reshaping the role physicians should play in health care rationing. At most, it is able to counsel physicians on how best to carry out their function as health care rationers; it does not allow them to refuse this role outright.

This relentless critique of the existing framework of ethical analysis seems to leave no room for physicians to refuse to make medical spending decisions. To the contrary, I mean only to argue that an absolute ban on any such role cannot be taken as an article of faith simply because this appears to be an established ethic within medicine. There may, however, be other grounds for limiting physician discretion to allocate resources. Some aspects of medical practice may create a stronger foundation for ethical objection than this critique suggests so far. The physician's role ethic may be supported by the unalterable attributes of sickness and the possession of superior technical knowledge, not just the happenstance of a particular type of insurance. Therefore, I will next turn to the ethical analysis that derives from these more permanent features of medicine to assess the strength of the restriction on physicians ever considering the costs of treatment.

BENEFICENCE AND AUTONOMY

The branch of medical ethics that is focused on the treatment relationship is dominated by two distinct moral principles: beneficence and autonomy.[121] In starkest (and somewhat oversimplified) relief,[122] beneficence looks to medical benefit as the primary ethical criterion whereas autonomy looks to patient self-determination. Beneficence tends toward a consequentialist and physician-determined ethic. It encourages physicians to act according to their judgment of what is best for the patient's health. Autonomy, in contrast, fosters an intrinsic (sometimes labeled "Kantian" or "deontological") value and is more patient centered. It professes (again, in its most extreme form) that doctors should take orders from their fully informed patients. It is remarkable that principles as divergent as these two each are thought to generate, in such an absolute form, a prohibition of physician rationing. The remainder of this chapter explores how this consequence is thought to obtain and why it is wrong, first examining beneficence and then autonomy.

The Principle of Beneficence

Kinder and Gentler Paternalism

Patient benefit as the guiding principle originates in the Hippocrates's admonition *primum non nocere* (first, do no harm). Technically, this Hippocratic maxim states only the passive nonmalfeasance principle, possibly because, at the time, there was little affirmative good that medicine was capable of. In the modern context, in which the power of medicine has been vastly increased, the maxim has been reinterpreted to operate in a more activist vein. In its most extreme form, beneficence is seen as supporting an intensely paternalistic role for doctors. Beneficence traditionally was invoked to justify physicians dictating all aspects of medical treatment without regard to the possibility of differing patient values about such matters as what constitutes tolerable medical risk and which form of medical benefit is preferable. Contemporary versions of beneficence moderate this paternalistic strain, however, by requiring that doctors define medical benefit in terms of each patient's own value system and by limiting paternalistic intervention to situations where fully competent decision making is not possible.[123]

The leading exponent of this contemporary brand of beneficence is Edmund Pellegrino,[124] who has done much of his work with David C. Thomasma.[125] These two ethicists ground their philosophical basis for beneficence on the brute physical and psychological facts of illness, which constitute "nothing less than an ontological assault."[126] Because serious illness creates intense anxiety, vulnerability, and an altered sense of self, it inherently undermines the unity of mind and body; a seriously ill person is, at a very profound level, not truly herself. She is fundamentally compromised in both her physical and mental capacities in a manner that exceeds other severely debilitating conditions such as impoverishment or imprisonment. This state of "wounded humanity,"[127] coupled with the power that physicians possess through their vastly superior knowledge and skill to diagnosis and treat illness, necessitates patients placing ultimate trust in their doctors' decisions. This trust, in turn, demands the physician's utmost fidelity to the patient's best medical interests so that this intense need for trust is honored and not abused.

These elements of trust and vulnerability are classic incidents of a fiduciary status. A prohibition on cost considerations for fully insured patients therefore would seem to flow automatically from these potent and permanent aspects of the treatment relationship. Physicians who compromised quality of care out of a concern for costs to society would be violating a patient's trust by trading the patient's interests off for the (medical or nonmedical) interests of others. Moreover, a physician who compromised on medical quality out of a concern for her own (or her employer's) financial well being would be engaged in a blatant conflict of interest, in contravention of universally held requirements of fiduciary responsibility.[128]

Consequently, Pellegrino and Thomasma offer unmitigated criticism of the "gatekeeping" role that HMO physicians play in constraining patients from seeking expensive testing, specialist consultation, or hospital admission. They see the argument for gatekeeping as "an ethically perilous line of reasoning" that is "morally unsound and factually suspect," and which they liken to the morality of "the Soviet physician, which makes the good of the polity and society the prime principle of medical ethics."[129] In the words of another staunch critic, gatekeeping

is an untenable and hopelessly conflicted role that undermines the voluntarism and earned trust which lie at the heart of the family physician's effectiveness. . . . [It] transforms an intimate, covenantal relationship into a hard-edged contract between strangers . . . [and it] involves family physicians in structures of power, secrecy, and risk that are foreign to their traditions and ideals, and reduces their role to that of a corporate watchdog.[130]

Yet, despite this apparent solidity of thought between beneficence and barring physicians from any resource allocation role, this prohibition cannot withstand more careful analysis of the foundations of the beneficence principle. The basis for giving physicians a prominent role in determining patient benefit is ultimately instrumental: Patients' welfare will best be advanced if their care is determined, or at least carefully counseled, by their physicians rather than by relegating doctors to the ministerial role of, say, a barber whose only function is to strictly follow client instructions of where and how much to cut. Focusing on the instrumental aspect of this justification reveals the absence of any intrinsic command that *medical* benefit be the ultimate criterion of patient welfare. Surely a sensible account of patient benefit must include a mix of economic as well as medical welfare.

Ex Post versus Ex Ante Views of Beneficence
At least for uninsured patients, the beneficence principle must allow physicians to factor costs into their treatment recommendations. It is only for fully insured patients that the beneficence principle requires physician oblivion to costs. Not all *forms* of insurance, however, support this conclusion. This is so only for insurance that is chosen because of its comprehensive and unlimited characteristics. A patient who chooses a more limited form of insurance, or one that explicitly asks the physician to consider costs, has expressed a value preference for less than optimal medical benefit. To fail to honor this choice would be to contradict the patient's own view of his or her best interests and therefore to return to the intensely paternalistic version of beneficence that reigned before the advent of contemporary bioethics.

The flaw in using beneficence to prohibit physician rationing for all insured patients is the application of the principle only at the time of treatment, not at the time insurance is purchased. This skewed perspective leads to the erroneous thinking that when doctors consider costs for an insured patient, they are necessarily trading off the patient's welfare for the welfare of others in society. This is true only from the ex post (after the fact) perspective of an already fully insured patient who is presently sick; only then is it in the patient's best interest to demand extravagant care. From the ex ante (before the fact) perspective of a presently healthy patient who is purchasing insurance, however, asking the doctor to assume a role that considers costs is asking him to trade off one aspect of the patient's interest for another: short-term medical for long-run economic.[131]

David Eddy illustrates this ex post/ex ante distinction by asking whether it is worth it to pay $10,000 per dose for a hypothetical new drug that improves by 1 percent the chance of surviving one year after a heart attack. He observes that "[e]very one of us has two minds when we make a decision about whether a health care activity is worth its cost. We have one mind when we are well, sitting in our living rooms, paying taxes, or writing out a check for health insurance. We have another mind when we have a health problem and are sitting in a physician's office."[132] Thus, the conflict in perspectives is not between the patient and society but between two equally rational preferences of a single individual, only in different circumstances.[133]

If the beneficence principle is applied at the point where the potential patient is deciding how much health care coverage she can afford, it is quite capable of allowing physicians to assume the role of both an economic and a medical treatment agent, if this is consistent with a patient's ex ante view of her own best interests. Because costs saved on one medical use can purchase other medical benefits, a rationing role viewed from the ex ante perspective can fairly be viewed as maximizing the patient's overall medical welfare. Balancing the patient's economic welfare with her medical welfare can benefit the patient's medical interests by allowing the purchase of more comprehensive insurance, by making insurance minimally affordable, or by freeing the money for use in arenas that might prevent health problems from arising, such as better food, shelter, exercise, etc. As Alan Williams explains, because costs are the same as foregone benefits, physician rationers are not cost/benefit maximizers, they are benefit/benefit maximizers.[134]

Beneficence-based opponents to physician rationing fail to see this basic point because they consider patient benefit only in the ex post position of one who has already purchased insurance and therefore has no (or little) cost at stake. But nothing in the beneficence principle requires this myopia. If, indeed, the nature of an insurance arrangement freely chosen calls on the doctor to be oblivious to costs, then beneficence demands absolute quality. But, if patients freely choose a different form of insurance, all that beneficence should require is that physicians best implement the actual value choice the patient has made. Nonpaternalistic beneficence does not justify imposing a richer brand of medicine or ethics than the patient can afford, so long as patients have reasonable opportunities to choose their insurance (which many do not) and the decision they make lies within the range that society in general finds minimally decent.[135]

Pellegrino and Thomasma, two of the strongest beneficence-oriented critics of physician rationing, themselves offer an account of beneficence that legitimates this extension of the principle. They carefully delineate a hierarchy of four levels at which patient benefit should be defined: (1) The Good of Last Resort, (2) The Good of the Patient, (3) The Particular Good, and (4) The Biomedical Good. The last of these refers to technical medical proficiency; this is preceded by the patient's own perception of what medical outcome is best for him in the circumstances; this medical objective should be consistent with the patient's general value system; and foremost is the patient's broadest conception of his ultimate objectives in life.[136] This ordering demands that the patient's nonmedical values be consulted first before striving for absolute medical proficiency. Pellegrino and Thomasma acknowledge, then, that "one could choose to reject the good of the body in favor of other goods—saving one's own or one's family's money."[137] Since beneficence in their view requires physicians to honor this choice,[138] bedside rationing is affirmatively embraced by the internal logic of Pellegrino and Thomasma's own framework. Hence, the beneficence principle offers no support for their resolute rejection of the gatekeeping role.

Beneficence might create more opposition if doctors had rights superior to the patient's to refuse a medical spending role the patient desires. However, physicians' rights as a professional are strictly derivative of patients' interests. This is precisely why medical ethics is said to be role-based. Individual physicians do have intrinsic, personal rights to refuse to enter a particular treatment relationship and to assert fundamental ethical objections to particular procedures such as abortion, but physicians *as a group* have no higher claim that would trump patients' desires in the strong fashion that would bar any form of bedside rationing. Thus, a particular physician cannot be forced to work for an HMO, but he also may not prevent other physicians from deciding they wish to do so.

The Rule-Deterrent Argument

Shifting now to a different tack, it is possible to construct a beneficence defense for the physician's ethic of absolute quality by invoking concepts of role morality that are founded on rule instrumentalism. Beneficence ethicists might respond that, although particular bedside rationing decisions may be desirable in some individual cases, on a larger scale, the moral foundations of professional ethics would be undermined if physicians were to abandon the manifesto of absolute fidelity to patient health. This rule-deterrent view of ethics sees moral injunctions serving the instrumental purpose of improving the human condition. It uses ethical rules to set ideal end points toward which imperfect humans strive but which they are never expected to reach.[139] It finds its most powerful modern statement in the resurgence of "virtue ethics," which attempts to improve moral character by focusing on desirable psychological traits and attitudes rather than on concrete rules of behavior.[140]

This view of ethics contemplates an innate tension between the inevitable imperfection of human nature and the absolutism of moral injunctions. Therefore, moral absolutes that exert a desirable influence need not be rejected simply because they are ultimately unachievable or even counterproductive. Whether ethical rules should be stated in absolute or qualified terms is determined more by the pragmatics of maximizing their psychological impact than by principled analysis of ideal settings.

For instance, this rule-instrumentalism is perhaps the best justification for continuing to prohibit physician-assisted suicide at the same time that we allow passive killing of patients when they (or their families) request the withdrawal of life support. A doctor's healing role requires a clear injunction against killing patients.

Using euphemistic and spurious causation arguments, society has allowed *passive* euthanasia (the withdrawal of life-support) despite this injunction, but *active* euthanasia would be too blatant to reconcile with the absolute ethic of life preservation. Consequently, even though a strong case might be made for assisting voluntary rational suicide in cases such as a terminally ill cancer patient racked with uncontrollable pain, we maintain the prohibition nevertheless because of the deterrent effect this clear rule has in other medical situations.

Likewise, the beneficence-oriented ethicist might argue that the ethic of absolute medical quality must be maintained at the individual patient level despite strong arguments against it at a societal level. An exaggerated expectation of physician loyalty serves the hortatory function of inspiring an ethos of patient devotion that motivates better physician behavior than would otherwise exist. Marc Rodwin adopts this view:

Even if financial incentives promote desirable clinical choices they may encourage the wrong kind of attitude in physicians . . . [by] compromis[ing] the commitment and ethos that prompt physicians to act in the interests of patients. . . . Herein lies the irony: law and rules are sometimes needed to promote attitudes and an ethos that is deeper and stronger and more important than the rules themselves.[141]

But for the very reasons that support this rule-instrumentalism argument, it is possible to preserve an ethos of absolute quality in theory at the same time that we countenance its contradiction in practice. The teleologic character of ethical maxims, their always striving toward but never reaching an ideal end point, contemplates inherent tensions and outright contradictions between what doctors profess and how they act. For instance, with respect to physician-assisted suicide, we presently tolerate a contradiction between the Law on the Books that declares this to be homicide and the Law in Action which, through prosecutorial discretion or judicial leniency, had never actually imprisoned any physician for actively assisting in a patient's death until Dr. Kevorkian's open defiance gave the legal system no other choice.[142]

This view of ethics can tolerate an environment in which physicians are allowed to make cost-constrained treatment decisions at the same time that we urge them never to lose sight of each patient's absolute medical benefit, so long as the contradiction is not so blatant or severe that cynicism is widespread and the ethos is destroyed. At present, we tolerate a stark dichotomy between medical ethics' professed adherence to a rule of absolute patient loyalty and the reality documented above of myriad routine violations of this rule.[143] An even greater tension between ethic and practice is successfully maintained in Great Britain where, despite severe physician rationing caused by a funding level that is one-third our per capita annual expenditure, British doctors still profess just as strong an ethic of absolute quality.[144]

This lip-service respect can be attacked as a gross hypocrisy,[145] but it also illustrates that, to the extent ethical maxims are justified primarily by their rule-deterrent function, that function is not destroyed by bedside rationing. Indeed, a greater contradiction between ethics and practice may, like a stretched rubber band, serve only to strengthen the pull of ethical rules. As the potentially corrupting influences become stronger, a beneficence ethic might only become more resolute even though actual compliance may be diminished. This explains why the absolute-quality manifesto thrives in the relatively barren soil of the British National Health Service and why it persists in America in the face of the numerous contradictions that exist in actual medical practice. Paradoxically, then, bedside rationing might further reinforce the vigilance of a beneficence orientation.

I must admit that I find this to be a weak and somewhat distasteful defense of bedside rationing, but I remind the reader that it is intended to respond to the precise objection posited (rule-deterrent beneficence) rather than to build a positive case for rationing. Thus, to those who would view this argument as relegating medical ethics to superficial, hypocritical, or fraudulent status, the challenge must be put to them: How has medical ethics avoided this denigration in more conventional treatment settings, where resources are limited? If we need not abandon the pretense of absolute fidelity in those settings, we need not do so in the HMO setting. If we must for HMOs, so must we elsewhere. It is untenable to demand that the ethic of perfection be literally enforced in only innovative practice settings.

Respect for Patient Autonomy

The prohibition against physician rationing is also viewed as fundamental to an ethic that emphasizes the preeminence of patient autonomy. The rationale is much the same as under beneficence, although grounded in intrinsic rather than instrumental values. Libertarian thought supports a negative autonomy explanation that prohibits physician-initiated, cost/benefit trade-offs because patients cannot be coerced to sacrifice even a small margin of benefit for the welfare of others in society. A positive autonomy rationale is that physicians have affirmatively agreed with their patients to play a cost-insulated role. The positive autonomy position is frequently supported with the social compact style of reasoning popularized by John Rawls.[146] This position argues that bedside rationing would contradict patients' expectation of undivided loyalty and absolute quality, an expectation created by physicians' pledge to the Hippocratic oath. A third line of argument, harkening to Kant and Mill, advances the most extreme position: that bedside rationing is impermissible even with patient consent since it sacrifices an unallowable degree of inalienable autonomy.

Each of these justifications for the absolute prohibition is flawed, either in its abstract conception of what constitutes autonomy and whether it is alienable, or in its conviction about what preferences people actually have. The argument in this section, simply put, is that individuals may or may not agree to their physicians making cost/benefit trade-offs on their behalf, but we should not presume their desires when it is possible to ask them. When people authorize their physicians to ration, respect for autonomy demands that we honor this wish.

The Social Compact Against Bedside Rationing
Robert Veatch is the leading proponent of the hypothetical contract branch of autonomy-based medical ethics. He advances a "triple-contract theory" for resolving bioethical dilemmas that asks what agreement has been reached (1) by society, (2) between society and the medical profession, and (3) between individual physicians and patients.[147] Veatch posits that, at the second level, society has assigned a special ethical role to physicians that commits them to ignore cost considerations except in the most dire circumstances of temporary shortage, leaving ordinary resource allocation issues to external control through other social mechanisms.[148] I say "posits" because Veatch equivocates on the derivation of this social compact. He offers no satisfactory explanation as to whether this agreement in fact exists, whether it does not exist but should, or whether it is only one of several plausible arrangements for resource allocation that society might choose. Nevertheless, his personal view is quite absolute: "[I]t should not be the physician's responsibility to eliminate [treatment] on cost grounds if that physician believes on balance that the procedure is even infinitesimally beneficial to the patient." [149]

The social compact model offers a useful heuristic device for solving certain moral problems. It can be misapplied, however, if it is used to invoke norms of consent to justify what are in fact paternalistic impositions. "[T]here is a profound moral gulf between the actual consent of an individual and that individual's presumed consent."[150] Actual agreements have moral force because the promisor undertakes a commitment of the will.[151] The mere fact that a hypothetical transaction is indisputably thought to be highly desirable to me in no way creates a personal moral obligation under this will theory to submit. The same applies to my individual commitment to a social compact.[152]

Hypothetical contracts gain their moral force in an entirely different way than the will theory that applies to individual agreements. Properly employed, social compact theory uses contract only as a metaphor to invoke an idealized reasoning process to generate social rules for distributive justice. Hypothetical contracts have such transcendent moral force that they render actual consent irrelevant. To this extent, hypothetical contract analysis is, in some manner, opposed to individual autonomy since it can limit the allowable range of actual agreements. Stated in a more positive manner, hypothetical contracts promote the rationality component of autonomy at the expense of the individual preference and consent components.

Accordingly, social compact theory is carefully limited to situations where no actual choice can be exercised or where the choice exercised is illegitimate. Even then, the hypothetical contract heuristic requires such a high degree of confidence in order to adopt its universally applied conclusions that it is incapable of yielding concrete substantive solutions for very many real-world problems. The following discussion will elaborate why, on both of these counts, social compact theory fails to prohibit bedside rationing: (1) An actual, properly conducted, insurance enrollment process is not so inherently defective that market decisions should be overruled by hypothetical, ideal agreements. (2) Moreover, even if actual contracts were absent or fatally defective, it is a misapplication of the highly abstract Rawlsian framework to think that it can generate universal and unqualified agreement to something as concrete as a particular treatment relationship or professional role.

The Content and Validity of Actual Agreements to Ration

An ethic founded on patient autonomy must honor bedside rationing where patients in fact choose this role for their physicians. Philosopher David Gauthier explains that, in any moral scheme, the analysis starts with actual agreements. Ethical constraints are imposed only when self-interested transactions are insufficient to produce a social optimum. "Morality arises from market failure. . . . [T]he perfect market, were it realized, would constitute a morally free zone, a zone within which the constraints of morality would have no place."[153] Actual agreements may be suboptimal either because they do not exist—perhaps transaction costs prevent agreements from being reached—or because actual agreements are flawed in some manner. Flaws might exist because of imperfections in information or rationality, or because larger interests ("externalities") are at stake than those of the immediate parties. A hypothetical contract analysis remedies these flaws by supposing what agreements would be reached under ideal, unbiased conditions for deliberation.

A properly run HMO enrollment process is capable of producing unbiased agreements, subject to satisfying the informed-consent requirements of sufficient information and lack of coercion that are discussed in Chapters 6 and 7. Subscribers will have affirmatively consented to physician rationing if told that the insurance plan they choose authorizes their doctors to exercise cost-sensitive clinical judgment in order to lower premiums or expand benefits.[154] Externalities are not generally present, since the primary interests are those of the immediate parties. Therefore, positing ideal deliberators is not needed to remove biasing self-interest. The only possible flaw is that subscribers might make poor judgments about the desirability of physician rationing, which is hardly an autonomy-based foundation for an absolute prohibition.

Veatch bases his argument on the many defects of physician rationing noted earlier in this section, principally, the inability of physicians to accurately replicate the values of their patients. "I am convinced that reasonable laypeople . . . would not want to transfer the allocational decisions, even the microallocational decisions, to others who ought to reach different decisions than they themselves would reach."[155] In doing so, however, he commits the classic nirvana fallacy of supposing that perfect replication is available in some other manner. Since patients of necessity must transfer their spending decisions to someone else if they desire to preserve any form of affordable insurance, the question becomes: Which, among several imperfect proxies, is least bad? It is implausible to assert that, on the whole, treating-physicians' views are less aligned with patient preferences than those of insurance companies, government regulators, or supervising physicians.

At most, a hypothetical contract analysis might set the outer bounds of rational agreement. It is reasonable to prohibit forms of physician decision making to which only a tiny minority of subscribers would submit, since extreme aberrations are likely to be mistaken decisions or too difficult for society to implement through pooled-insurance arrangements. But a hypothetical contract could not preclude physician authority to consider costs altogether unless it were reasonable to assume that virtually no patient would agree to any version of this role. Although the question has seldom been presented squarely, the little survey evidence that exists (discussed on page 64) suggests significant support for physician rationing, compared with the alternatives.

Autonomy-based ethicists sometimes simply assert that patients' and society's expectations are to the contrary, but this begs the question. Supposed patient desire for what is presently the norm is too easily invoked as a cover for paternalistic imposition of a physician-dominated code of ethics. For instance, precisely the same form of reasoning was used by a lower court in the *Quinlan* case[156] to justify imposing life-support against the father's wishes in order to uphold the traditional vitalism ethic that is now considered defunct:

A patient is placed, or places himself, in the care of a physician with the expectation that he (the physician) will do everything in his power, everything that is known to modern medicine, to protect the patient's life. . . . Society has come to request and expect this higher duty. . . . The nature, extent and duration of care by societal standards is the responsibility of a physician.

The New Jersey Supreme Court, with the strong support of both beneficence- and autonomy-based ethicists, saw that the patient's and family's actual wishes superseded the ethic the medical profession presumed that society wanted. For the same reasons, Veatch's contract-based arguments are unconvincing. Although the social compact might once have prohibited physician rationing, this notion is subject to defeat simply by observing that the social and economic circumstances that gave rise to past understandings—such as the affordability of comprehensive and unregulated fee-for-service insurance—have radically changed.

The Indeterminacy of Rawlsian Analysis

Moral and political theorists have warned that one must guard against the tendency of hypothetical contract analysis to arrogate personal opinion to universal rule. This tendency to elevate individual beliefs to the grand scale of universal moral principle is inherited from religious-based ethics and is carried into modern times by Kant's "categorical imperative."[157] Robert Veatch himself explains that the nature of ethical analysis is to generate universal or absolutist positions. "If we consider the judgment one of ethics we believe that others ought to reach the same judgment about the rightness of the action that we have reached. . . . To the extent this is possible, we can be said to be rendering an ethical judgment rather than merely expressing a preference."[158] Thus, to resolve an issue from an ethical perspective, especially from a social compact perspective, biases the analysis against a pluralistic solution by assuming that a universal answer is not only possible but inevitable. To the contrary, very few specific social problems can be resolved with the level of generality and unanimity required of the Rawlsian "original position." Rawls makes this very point in his most recent book.[159]

The particular configuration of an insurance plan and the structure of individual physician–patient relationships are not the kinds of high-level abstractions capable of generating the degree of confidence required by the hypothetical contract heuristic. The idealized deliberators in Rawls's "original position" do not have individual characteristics and so cannot specify their preference for particular social rules and practices. Thus, the primary substantive propositions produced by Rawlsian analysis are extremely general statements such as, "each person is to have an equal right to the most extensive basic liberty compatible with a similar liberty for others."[160] Lower-order applications of these very abstract principles must be resolved by actual consensual processes, such as contract and voting, to fill in the vast complexities of legal and social order. A constitutional convention adopts a general sociopolitical framework consistent with the original principles, a properly elected legislature promulgates subsidiary laws, and the courts apply those laws to particular cases.[161] At these lower levels, the pure hypothetical contract usually is capable of specifying only decision mechanisms and decision rules, not the substance of the decision.

The propriety of physician bedside rationing is one of the countless social problems that must be left to these lower-level decision processes, either through market transactions or legislative regulation. This substantive neutrality does not deny individual physicians and ethicists their freedom to argue for the adoption of a particular rule, but their views must be taken as no more than the expression of personal opinion. To give them more public policy weight than this would be tantamount, in Robert Clark's words, to using hypothetical contracting as an imaginative device for "elites" to impose their views paternalistically while declaring false allegiance to individual will.[162]

The Inalienability of Autonomy

A more straightforward but equally unavailing philosophical basis for disallowing all forms of bedside rationing is that patient autonomy is inalienable. An informed election of an insurance arrangement under which physicians make cost-sensitive treatment decisions might be thought to limit autonomy in two ways: one decisional and the other physical. First, the patient is foreclosed from subsequently overruling a physician's decision to deny a marginally beneficial test or procedure.[163] Second, the slight possibility that the treatment in question might save the patient's life or markedly improve her physical or mental functioning means that election of a physician rationing role may lead to impairment of the patient's freedom of physical action.

Some ethicists, influenced by the writings of Kant and Mill among others, hold the value of autonomy in such ultimate regard that they view it as inalienable. In Arthur Kuflik's account, "Philosophers otherwise as divergent in their views as Locke, Spinoza, Rousseau and Kant, all subscribed, in one form or another, to the following thesis: . . . nobody can reasonably obligate himself not to function as a morally autonomous agent."[164] Imanuel Kant and John Stuart Mill represent the two extremes of the intrinsic versus instrumental spectrum of reasons given in support of the value of personal autonomy. Kant places intrinsic moral value on autonomy because it is the human condition necessary to "function as a critically reflective moral agent."[165] We are morally responsible agents only to the extent that we are free to make our own decisions. The primary function of individual rights is to preserve this freedom. Personal autonomy is particularly central to medical decision making because one's body is so fundamental to one's ability to function and to one's fundamental sense of self.[166]

Mill places equal stress on autonomy but approaches the issue from the utilitarian perspective that an individual's assessment of his own welfare is far more likely to be accurate than an assessment by a third party.[167] In order to preserve this cornerstone of utilitarianism, Mill argues that autonomy-defeating choices should be prohibited.[168] "The principle of freedom cannot require that [one] should be free not to be free. It is not freedom, to be allowed to alienate [one's] freedom."[169] Thus, he argues in a widely quoted passage that voluntary slavery should be prohibited.[170] Kant and Hegel have extended these sentiments much further by arguing, on a similar basis, that it is not permissible to alienate any aspect of personal sovereignty. In essence, one may unalterably dispose only of one's property but not of one's time, services, or other personal attributes.[171]

Society presently accepts the validity of these arguments by declaring certain autonomy-limiting decisions to be off-limits. Consent is not a defense to maiming or killing, and agreements to submit to slavery or to waive rights to bankruptcy, divorce, or voting are not enforceable. Likewise, in the medical context, agreement to dangerous or mutilating experimentation is forbidden.[172] Some commentators go further and argue that patients may not consent to an unnecessarily risky medical experiment because their rights "cannot be waived or abrogated. They are inalienable. The right to be treated as an individual deserving the physician's best judgment and care . . . is inherent in every person. This right, based on the concept of dignity, cannot be waived."[173]

These arguments, particularly as extended to the present problem, seriously misconstrue both the nature of autonomy and the concept of inalienability. The first mistake is to collapse into a single concept the two distinct notions of freedom of will and freedom of physical action. Philosopher of law Joel Feinberg distinguishes between de facto and de jure autonomy, the former being merely the ability to act and the latter being the more essential sovereign control over the former.[174] Robert Nozick makes a similar point by observing that debates over autonomy are frequently clouded by confusing two distinct concepts: (1) autonomy as an end-state goal that should be affirmatively pursued, and (2) the correct view, that autonomy is a side constraint, one that cannot be violated as we pursue differing normative ends.[175] Finally, Gerald Dworkin reaches the same conclusion under a split-level view of autonomy that distinguishes between the primitive instinct for self-gratification—the motivation of a mere "wanton"[176] who acts impulsively on any first-order preference—and a person's more critical reflection about his primary desires.[177] One is autonomous, not to the extent that one has the freedom to pursue first-order desires, but rather to the extent that one endorses those desires and the restrictions imposed on them. For instance, it would make sense to speak of an autonomous addict as one who chooses not to fight an addiction. From this perspective, to foreclose on autonomy grounds the ability to constrain one's base preferences is to exalt subhuman wantonness to a revered moral status.

It is a favorite argument of physician-oriented medical ethics to mask paternalism as autonomy by conflating simple freedom of action and the more complex values that underlie reflective autonomy.[178] For example, one sees early in the debate over the right to die the specious argument that informed refusals of life-sustaining care are not enforceable because allowing a patient to die would be autonomy-defeating. Autonomy arguments such as these are now readily seen as disguised forms of paternalism[179] in that they allow doctors to argue that they must control medical decision making because they know best what will preserve the patient's health and hence the patient's autonomy-enhancing freedom of action. Arguing, as some have done, that patients cannot refuse beneficial treatment because autonomy is inalienable confuses the *relinquishment* of autonomy with the *exercise* of autonomy[180] and converts autonomy from a right to a duty.

Properly conceived, freedom-constraining decisions can be autonomy-enhancing. We strengthen, or at least exercise, our autonomy by constraining some of the options available to us in order to create a different, more valued, range of opportunities. As law professor Michael Shapiro has observed, "[i]nterfering with or discouraging such choices may thus impair autonomy, though done in its name."[181] This irony is fundamental to our basic conception of freedom of contract. The entire body of contract law, and hence all private markets, is founded on the insight that making promises binding can be freedom-enhancing, to the extent that most people consider it immoral not to carry out self-constraining promises. Charles Fried makes this basic point: "In order that I be as free as possible, that my will have the greatest possible range consistent with the similar will of others, it is necessary that there be a way in which I may commit myself. It is necessary that I be able to make nonoptional a course of conduct that would otherwise be optional for me."[182] Because it is clearly specious to argue that autonomy defeats every materially constraining decision, something more than physical harm must be shown before patients can be denied the right to authorize physicians to make medical spending decisions.

A second line of argument, one that relies on the intrinsic justification for holding autonomy inalienable, is equally flawed. The intrinsic importance of autonomy is thought to make it inalienable because mere instrumental gains cannot justify autonomy's sacrifice. This argument, however, fundamentally misconceives the nature of inalienability that philosophers working in the Kantian tradition would ascribe to autonomy. Margaret Radin explains that the inalienability concept has been used too freely to commingle a disparate collection of meanings.[183] Rights may be inalienable in a number of widely varying senses. Inalienability is rarely used to say that a decision is strictly forbidden; this prohibitory meaning is reserved for fundamental, constitutive actions such as giving away a right to vote or to marry. In most circumstances, rights are said to be inalienable only to mean, as in The Declaration of Independence, that they cannot be taken away against one's will, not that one cannot give them away. Alternatively, it is meant that they cannot be transferred in a certain fashion, such as through market transactions (organ donation and adoption are examples). In yet another plane of meaning, other rights are said to be inalienable in the more profound, metaphysical sense that any attempt to rid oneself of the right is simply futile or conceptually nonsensical. For example, we might say that one's personhood is inalienable.[184] It would be an empty gesture to say that alienation in this sense is prohibited under penalty of law.

Which meaning of inalienability applies to personal autonomy over medical decision making? In the Kantian tradition, autonomy is an irreducible element of moral humanity.[185] It is inalienable in the conceptual incoherence or futility sense, not in the prohibitory sense. Whether humans are autonomous in the Kantian sense does not depend on their wealth, freedom of movement, or other tangible attributes. Autonomy is an ontological given. It exists simply and utterly by virtue of one's humanity.[186] The Kantian vein of bioethics postulates autonomy as an a priori attribute of humanity that accounts for the possession of moral and political rights. Because we are potentially autonomous individuals, each of our persons and preferences must be intrinsically valued as ends in themselves which cannot be sacrificed unwillingly as means to achieve larger social objectives. These universal moral and political conditions are not subject to change; they simply exist. "[O]ne simply is autonomous, inescapably, and efforts to escape one's autonomous status are foredoomed to conceptual failure. Being autonomous is, in this sense, *mandatory*."[187] Thus, restrictions of freedom can be said to violate rights or interests, but it is incoherent to say that they diminish autonomy in this deontological sense.

Properly conceived, freely chosen decisions to restrict one's range of opportunities serve to promote autonomy if freely and knowingly entered into. Accordingly, society endorses many autonomy-constraining decisions, even those that can lead to cataclysmic results. The law enforces contractual obligations to the brink of bankruptcy, and it erects elaborate protections in support of the right to terminate life-sustaining treatment. Research subjects may consent to sacrifice some margin of comfort or safety in the pursuit of scientific experimentation.[188] Through plea bargaining, criminal defendants may waive constitutional rights and voluntarily assume long-term punishment. Some states even permit psychiatric patients to commit themselves to a limited period of mandatory treatment.[189] The plethora of these laws is such that the contrary rules listed above are clearly the exception, based on prudential grounds rather than on any absolute requirement that autonomy be preserved.

For instance, many commentators believe that Mill and others, while correct in arguing against voluntary slavery, were wrong to base these arguments on personal autonomy. According to these commentators, the strongest basis for prohibiting voluntary, permanent servitude lies in the prudential argument that history has shown that the institution of slavery leads to great social injustice.[190] Moreover, in most instances, slavery is not voluntary in origin. Even if voluntary slavery were real, one can easily question the rationality and appropriate level of the disclosure required to exercise a truly autonomous choice of this magnitude. Therefore, society has concluded that the costs of policing the propriety of totally freedom-abdicating agreements outweigh the very slight potential benefits that might come from allowing such agreements.

Naturally, one might attempt to replicate this style of argument for any self-constraining form of agreement, but to do so requires convincing and detailed empirical support. This is not the form of argument that lends itself readily to an absolute prohibition of marginal sacrifices in medical benefit, nor is it an argument that anyone has advanced. Perhaps this is because of the dearth of evidence, discussed above, that bedside rationing leads to harmful results.

Still, one can object that, while it is permissible to constrain one's range of activity, the principle of autonomy prohibits relinquishing the very right to make this decision. Thus, the right to die does not infringe personal autonomy if a patient or guardian makes the decision, but no euthanasia advocate would argue that a patient may delegate to a doctor the very decision of whether or not he should die. It is this unalterable abdication of responsibility that most rankles autonomy-based ethicists about bedside rationing. The concern is not that cost-constrained refusals of potentially beneficial treatment will be made, but that the decisions will not be made by the patient himself. This more demanding objection requires further search for a more convincing response.

Ulysses and the Sirens

Two fundamental aspects of medical treatment under insurance overcome the objection that a patient's appointment of his physician as a rationing agent entails an impermissible relinquishing of decisional autonomy: (1) the distortion in perspective that results from the purchase of insurance and (2) the differing preferences a patient may have at two points in time. The assertion that a patient may exercise but may not delegate the decision to die does not hold if the patient anticipates that the decision must be made when she will be incompetent. Such is the case of a comatose patient dependent on life-support. In these situations, society strongly endorses the patient's appointment of a friend or family member to make the decision for them. At least in theory, nothing precludes the appointment of the physician. It is true that, usually, this appointment carries with it rather specific instructions on what actual decision to make, but such instructions necessarily leave some measure of discretion. For example, a patient might instruct the appointee to let her die only if she becomes terminally ill, meaning that she is expected to live less than a year, and only if treatment withdrawal can be done without pain or severe discomfort.

In the present inquiry, the purchase of insurance creates another form of incapacity—insensitivity to costs—that warrants, and indeed necessitates, delegating cost/benefit trade-off decisions to someone else. Autonomy is honored by empowering this delegation of rationing authority, just as it is honored by allowing named surrogates to refuse care for comatose patients. Whether doctors should be appointed, and how detailed their instructions should be, are not, under this objection, matters or fundamental principle but merely go to the practicalities of how best to replicate and carry out the patient's wishes.

Honoring an autonomous decision to delegate authority to a surrogate does not avoid, however, a second dilemma for autonomy. Unlike conventional medical surrogacy, which can be revoked at any time and particularly as death approaches, the delegation of rationing authority is made irrevocably—at least for the duration of the insurance contract. An irrevocable insurance election, unlike a living will, places in conflict two equally autonomous decisions. At the time of purchase, a subscriber to a limited-option insurance plan desires to sacrifice some marginal medical benefit for the sake of lower premiums. In contrast, at the time of dire but potentially curable illness, an insured patient wishes full-blown, state-of-the-art treatment without regard to expense. Neither position is inherently more legitimate from an autonomy-promoting perspective. The value of autonomy provides a meaningful critique only when applied to a single decision at one point in time. It cannot easily resolve the dilemma created when two autonomous decisions, separated in time, contradict each other. A constraint on autonomy will necessarily occur regardless of which preference is honored. Honoring the second preference will deny the earlier self the economic savings, while honoring the first preference will deny some margin of beneficial treatment to the later self. We simply cannot ask in the abstract which the patient prefers because she has contradictory preferences over time.

Philosophers and public policy theorists have invoked the Homeric myth of Ulysses and the Sirens to probe similar dilemmas.[191] Ulysses was told that in one portion of his journey he would pass the island of the Sirens, whose enchanting song was so seductive that no man could withstand the temptation of trying to swim ashore in the rough waters, causing his inevitable demise. Being forewarned, Ulysses had his crew plug their ears with wax. He, however, wanted to hear the alluring song while simultaneously protecting himself from the danger, so he instructed his crew to tie him firmly to the mast and ignore any later commands to set him loose.

This story has been used repeatedly to demonstrate the rationality and moral legitimacy of strictly enforcing some self-constricting decisions that are at least temporarily irrevocable. Precommitment, also referred to as "auto-paternalism" or "anticipatory self-command," is commonplace in everyday life, on both small and large scales. People set alarm clocks and discard cigarettes and alcohol to protect themselves from the less rational impulses that may overtake them later, and they expect those around them to honor the earlier, clear-headed decisions. People also take marriage vows, enlist in the army, and invest in pension funds in a manner that, while not strictly foreclosing a modified course, knowingly attaches significant penalties to a change of mind. That people may later regret these decisions which cannot easily be undone does not lead society to declare them immoral, illegal, or impermissibly autonomy-defeating. Rather, society views most of these examples as highly rational exercises of personal autonomy for the very reason that they constrain other preferences.

Nevertheless, some self-binding decisions do impair autonomy impermissibly. The possibility of severe regret causes the law to limit the degree of future deprivation that may be caused by irrevocable precommitments. The examples of waiving rights to divorce and to bankruptcy have already been mentioned. Similarly, a mother cannot give irrevocable consent before birth to give a child up for adoption.[192] Taking a medical example, courts would not be inclined to honor the prior instructions of a former Jehovah's Witness to refuse blood transfusions, however irrevocably made at the outset, if she should later renounce the religious faith that gave rise to the earlier pronouncement.[193]

In sum, this analysis produces the indeterminate insight that the validity of precommitment turns on the strength of a variety of factors. The first is the possible degree of deprivation that advance irrevocable consent can cause. Whereas Ulysses suffered only a minor inconvenience, voluntary slavery agreements are unenforceable, consent is not a defense to maiming or killing, and money can be prematurely withdrawn from pension accounts under special circumstances such as permanent disability or early death. We are also more inclined to honor precommitment commands if they are designed to protect against anticipated periods of irrationality or extreme temptation and if they govern events that are not too distant in the future.[194] Thus, a number of states allow mental patients to commit themselves voluntarily to a fixed period of psychiatric hospitalization without the possibility of changing their minds, although not for too long.[195]

How are these general guidelines applicable to the situation of potential insurance enrollees who bind themselves to their doctors' future decisions to deny potentially beneficial treatment because of cost? First, observe that insurance enrollment might be viewed as entailing no future restriction at all; it could be seen as only a present-consumption decision to purchase a less expensive, comprehensive insurance plan. An analogy can be drawn to purchasing a car without an airbag. This usually is not viewed in these complex moral terms as a constraint on one's choice to be more protected in the event of a future accident. Rather, it is viewed simply as purchasing a cheaper car, with its attendant safety risks. Similarly, the purchaser of less expensive insurance has the benefit of all that she has purchased, and so this decision may be viewed as not restraining autonomy to any extent.

It is also worth noting that the validity of a choice-constraining insurance agreement is less controversial than the Ulysses problem since Ulysses did not create contract rights or vested property interests in others that might be used to reinforce his self-constraining decision. The Ulysses paradigm poses only the enforcement of a purely personal vow. The self-constraint of agreeing to physician rationing is contained in an insurance agreement, which entails reciprocal promises between two contracting parties as well as obligations to the pool of other subscribers. The objection that one contracting party later may feel "buyer's remorse" is no more relevant here than in any other binding contractual relation. The obligations that attach to promissory actions, by virtue of the expectations or property interests they create in others, impose overriding moral and legal considerations that differ from the purely isolated self, constraint in the Ulysses paradigm.[196]

Viewing insurance enrollment nevertheless as a pure form of prior self-constraint, the precommitment to implicit or marginal bedside rationing results in only a modest degree of deprivation. While it may be argued that precommitment is impermissible for health care generally since life and death decisions are risked, only a very small portion of health care decision making clearly involves such high stakes. Most decisions are at the margin, either incrementally improving an already-ample safety margin, or futilely grasping at straws to avoid a near certain demise. On the other hand, physicians should not be given unfettered authority to consign their patients to a premature death or a clearly avoidable disability. As discussed in Chapter 5, the degree of allowable risk and the range of allowable decisions will be set by contractual limits, by the strength of the rationing incentive, by counterbalancing professional and legal norms of appropriateness, and by other forms of collective judgment.

It is also important to recognize that the time frame of precommitment via insurance enrollment is limited. Arguments have been advanced that the Ulysses paradigm should not permit the young to determine irrevocably the level of health care they will receive when they are old because most people are unable to form an abstract appreciation of such a remote and radically different form of themselves. The concern is that the young would tend to excessively discount their distant needs and therefore make "foolhardy, precipitous, or uninformed" decisions about their welfare in old age.[197] Recognizing these traits, society employs tax policy—in the form of social security taxes and Individual Retirement Accounts (IRAs)—to mandate or encourage retirement savings. The form of physician rationing I envision is markedly different, however, since the election is made through the insurance enrollment process, and health insurance agreements are typically subject to annual change either through contract renewal by employers or through open enrollment for workers at large firms.

Finally, as noted above, the precommitment entailed in HMO enrollment is properly viewed as protection against an anticipated period of irrational influence caused by the distorting incentives of insurance. Economists call this insurance-induced form of irrationality "moral hazard." They are not referring to the type of moral problems under examination here but to those entailed in, for instance, setting fire to a fully insured but bankrupt business. It is perhaps unfortunate that this pejorative label has been extended generically to all forms of distorting incentives created by insurance, since most examples, such as demanding all beneficial medical care, are perfectly legal and morally respectable. Nevertheless, the moral hazard label reminds us of the central point of this analysis, that this respectable behavior certainly is not morally compelled. For many people, modifying this distorting effect of insurance may be necessary in order to make insurance affordable at all. In other words, the decision for many subscribers will not be whether to allow any form of precommitment; rather, the decision will be which of the two is the more rational form: forgoing insurance altogether or choosing insurance that entails rationing. This is equivalent to the contrast between Ulysses's sailors plugging their ears and his tying himself to the mast. The deafened sailors were denied any pleasure from the Sirens' song while Ulysses enjoyed the privileged position of hearing their music while protecting himself from catastrophe.

Still, one can correctly observe that it is impossible to know one's own true preferences until confronted with the brute reality of bypassing a small but distinct possibility for cure at a time of dire distress. The terminally ill patient's last-gasp desire to receive any and all possible treatment may be so overwhelming that a healthy individual could not truly appreciate it through mere psychological projection. One of autonomy's greatest defenders, John Stuart Mill, observed that the utilitarian ground for honoring individual choice erodes where the person has no basis in experience to make the judgment: "The presumption in favour of individual judgment is only legitimate where the judgment is grounded on actual,

and especially on present, personal experience; not where it is formed anteced-
ently to experience, and not suffered to be reversed even after experience has
condemned it."[198] There is no resolute response to this heartfelt attack on bedside
rationing.[199] That is why the Ulysses situation is a true dilemma. No perfect solution can be found.

It is possible, however, to offer the following observations about the psychological reality of preference formation. Jon Elster has invoked a second piece of
folklore known as the sour grapes fable as a metaphor for what he calls "adaptive
preference formation."[200] In the classic fable, a wolf repeatedly jumps for a bunch
of tempting grapes that dangle just out of its reach. The frustrated wolf mutters to
itself as it stalks away that they were probably sour anyway. What this fable teaches
us is that preferences and expectations tend to shape themselves to people's realistic opportunities. In forward movement, what is possible is desired, and our wants
become our needs. But in reverse direction, once firmly convinced that something
is truly unattainable, we are quite capable of the easy rationalization that it was
not of any real import to begin with.

In the present context, one imagines great frustration for the patient denied full-
blown, state-of-the-art treatment because our expectations have been conditioned
by the previous availability of unlimited medical resources. If we rationally and
consciously choose to allow physicians or others to set limits, however, our psychological expectations are likely to adapt themselves accordingly as our attitudes
and beliefs are changed by the resource allocation mechanism we select.[201] Empowering physicians to set limits may reduce, not enlarge, the cognitive disso-
nance between our medical wants and the care that a limited funding scheme makes
available. Thus, bedside rationing may tend to dissipate the very autonomy-based
dilemmas that objectors conjure up.

CONCLUSION AND FURTHER INQUIRIES

It is a deviant view of morality that seeks to prohibit all forms of physician discretion to allocate health care resources at the bedside, a view that too conveniently
supports the self-interested political and economic aims of those with a stake in
traditional reimbursement methods. Some form of bedside rationing is permissible under each leading ethical framework—utilitarian, libertarian, and communitarian. The strongest attack is based on a Kantian sense of autonomy, but
autonomy is too often invoked as a philosophical glorification of liberty in an
attempt to infuse a social argument with an incontestible quality.[202] This does not
succeed for the very reason that the reflective dimension of autonomy is a higher-
order concept than the simple expansion of material opportunities. Therefore,
bedside rationing easily survives even the staunchest autonomy-based attack.

Discarding the conventional physician's ethic of total devotion to each individual patient's maximum health benefit only begins the discussion, however. We

still have substantial ethical and analytical work to do in constructing the new ethic to take its place. Doctors cannot be expected to plunge into the brave new world of rationing with no ethical guidance whatsoever. Fortunately, many insightful ethicists and physicians have turned their attention to forging this new ethic.[203] Although this work is still highly formative, the gist of the new ethic is that each physician should allocate available resources impartially among his own patients.[204] Physicians are not required to achieve universal social justice or perfect economic efficiency; their aim is to do the best they can with the resources at hand for their own patients and others within the same group. The incentives that affect their behavior should influence them in their professional, not their personal or private, lives,[205] and they should be guided by concepts of honesty, stewardship, virtue, and professionalism.

The shift from individual patient welfare to patient group welfare is not as radical, then, as turning physicians into welfare maximizers for society at large. The group focus still honors a sense of commitment to the individual patient by respecting the patient's own choice of insurance and practice setting. It also fosters a practice style conducive to fair and equitable treatment. Within the individual physician's horizon, all patients should be treated equally, without regard to ability to pay. In the words of noted physician ethicist John La Puma, "the underlying framework is no longer patient autonomy, it's fairness."[206] Each physician adapts his clinical judgment to form a practice style that fits within the resource constraints of his practice setting. In doing so, she considers the fairest methods for allocating among competing needs within the group. This does not require every physician to act uniformly. Resource differentials and practice patterns can still vary among practice settings. But uniformity within a setting allows physicians to maintain an attitude of fidelity to each patient's best medical welfare.

This brief sketch of a new medical ethic only scratches the surface of the concepts that must be articulated in order for the ethic to be implemented. The range of unanswered questions raised by these emerging concepts tells us that rejecting the absolute prohibition has not carried us very far down the path of understanding the proper conduct of physician rationing. Nevertheless, we have accomplished at least this much: Validating incentives for physicians to make cost/benefit tradeoffs at the bedside under some idealized circumstances removes the ethical, political, and legal taboo that presently attaches to any acknowledgement that physicians may ever consider the costs of treatment, and so allows open inquiry into these important questions. Yet we still have not fully answered certain fundamental questions that affect the legitimacy of this entire enterprise. If the moral legitimacy of bedside rationing depends on autonomous choice, then constraints in the range of insurance options may render illegitimate the choices made during insurance enrollment. Even where adequate choice is offered, the choice cannot be considered informed without some disclosure of the incentives and mechanisms that produce discrete resource allocation. Moreover, we have yet to clearly articulate the allowable range of rationing choices. At some point, the incentives for physicians to abuse their patients' best medical interests may become too strong, and the resulting treatment refusals may be too severe. These are the topics examined in Chapters 5–7.

APPENDIX

The following are representative views of those medical ethicists and physicians or physician organizations that appear to oppose any role for physicians making resource allocation decisions at the bedside.[207] For contrasting views, see sources cited in notes 5–8 of this chapter. See generally John M. Eisenberg, Doctors' Decisions and the Cost of Medical Care 81 (1986) (discussing traditional opposition to considering social costs); Susan Wolf, Health Care Reform and the Future of Physician Ethics, Hastings Cent. Rep., March–April 1994, at 28, 32 (documenting AMA's opposition to rationing); E. Haavi Morreim, Balancing Act: The New Medical Ethics of Medicine's New Economics 45 (1991b) (collecting traditional ethical positions opposing physician rationing); E. Haavi Morreim, Fiscal Scarcity and the Inevitability of Bedside Budget Balancing, 149 Arch. Intern. Med. 1012 (1989) (same).

Ethicists and Other Theorists

Ruth Macklin, Enemies of Patients 160 (1993):

[E]ven if expenditures for health care need to be cut, rationing at the bedside is an unethical way to go about that task.

Frank H. Marsh and Mark Yarborough, Medicine and Money: A Study of the Role of Beneficence in Health Care Cost Containment 90 (1990):

It is inconceivable morally that a physician can act in the patient's best interests, while . . . promoting the economic welfare of the institution he represents.

Edmund D. Pellegrino and David C. Thomasma, For the Patient's Good: The Restoration of Beneficence in Health Care 172–73, 187 (1988):

arguing that physician gatekeeping is "ethically perilous," "morally unsound," and "moving in the direction of the code of the Soviet physician."

Robert M. Veatch, A Theory of Medical Ethics 285 (1981):

[I]t should not be the physician's responsibility to eliminate [treatment] on cost grounds if that physician believes on balance that the procedure is even infinitesimally beneficial to the patient.

Charles Fried, Rights and Health Care—Beyond Equity and Efficiency, 293 New Engl. J. Med. 241, 243 (1975):

The physician who withholds care that it is in his power to give because he judges it is wasteful to provide it to a particular person breaks faith with his patient.

Andrew Griffin and David C. Thomasma, Pediatric Critical Care, 143 Arch. Intern. Med. 325, 327 (1983):

[T]he physician-provider must continue all treatment efforts without regard to society's just demands for conservation of scarce resources.

Robert P. Rhodes, Health Care Politics, Policy, and Distributive Justice: The Ironic Triumph 105 (State University of New York Press, 1992):

Forcing physicians to do violence to their oath of healing the sick threatens the moral foundations of the profession. Rationing must be done at the level of policy, not at the point of delivery.

Mark A. Yarborough and Andrew M. Kramer, The Physician and Resource Allocation, 2 Clin. Geriatr. Med. 465, 471 (1986):

arguing that physician gatekeeping creates a "morally unacceptable conflict of interest"

The same view is shared by most of the legal academics that have written on the subject:

Barry R. Furrow, The Ethics of Cost-Containment: Bureaucratic Medicine and the Doctor as Patient-Advocate, 3 Notre Dame J. L. Ethics Public Pol. 187 (1988); Maxwell J. Mehlman, Rationing Expensive Lifesaving Medical Treatments, 1985 Wis. L. Rev. 239 (1985); Maxwell J. Mehlman, Health Care Cost Containment and Medical Technology: A Critique of Waste Theory, 36 Case West. Res. L. Rev. 778 (1986). See also Edward B. Hirshfeld, Should Ethical and Legal Standards for Physicians be Changed to Accommodate New Models for Rationing Health Care?, 140 U. Penn. L. Rev. 1809 (1992) (representing the AMA).

The single most influential book on medical ethics takes a surprisingly ambivalent position. In their first edition, Beauchamp and Childress adopted the standard absolutist position: "Physicians are to do all they can for their patients without counting society's resources and without taking into account the range of factors . . . that policymakers rightly should consider." Tom L. Beauchamp and James F. Childress, Principles of Biomedical Ethics 195 (1st ed. 1979). Their latest edition does not contain this statement, nor does it appear to discuss directly who should be the rationing decision maker for incremental, cost-saving treatment. Instead, Beauchamp and Childress focus on the substantive criteria to be used in the form of overt rationing required by severe shortages and dramatic, life-or-death decisions. See Tom L. Beauchamp and James F. Childress, Principles of Biomedical Ethics 378, 382–86 (4th ed. 1994) (acknowledging importance of decision-making question but not discussing it in any detail). They do, however, acknowledge the ubiquity of HMOs using financial incentives to encourage physicians to conserve resources, which they say creates a "worrisome conflict of interest," but which they do not state is categorically unethical. Ibid. at 438–39.

Physicians and Medical Organizations

American Medical Association Council on Ethical and Judicial Affairs, Code of Medical Ethics: Current Opinions with Annotations 4–5 (1994b):

A physician has a duty to do all that he or she can for the benefit of the individual patient. . . . The treating physician must remain a patient advocate and therefore should not make allocation decisions.

American Medical Association Council on Ethical and Judicial Affairs, Ethical Issues in Managed Care, 273 JAMA 330, 332 (1995b):

The physician is obligated to provide or recommend treatment . . . [that] will materially benefit the patient. . . . Physicians should not engage in bedside rationing.

Marcia Angell, Cost Containment and the Physician, 254 JAMA 1203, 1206–07 (1985):

As individual physicians, we must do the very best we can for each patient . . . spending whatever is necessary for effective medical care.

See also Marcia Angell, Medicine: The Endangered Patient-Centered Ethic, Hastings Cent. Rep., February 1987, at 12 (Suppl.); Marcia Angell, The Doctor as Double Agent, 3 Kennedy Institute of Ethics J., 279–286 (1993):

As long as we are spending enormous resources on an inherently inefficient and inflationary system we cannot justify asking doctors to withhold beneficial care to save money for third-party payors. Doing so serves a largely political agenda and endangers the patient-centered ethic that is central to medicine.

Allen R. Dyer, Patients, Not Costs, Come First, Hastings Cent. Rep., February 1986, at 5, 6:

answering "emphatic 'No'" to physician rationing.

Howard H. Hiatt, Protecting the Medical Commons: Who Is Responsible?, 293 New Engl. J. Med. 235, 239 (1975)

A physician . . . must do all that is permitted on behalf of his patient. . . . [S]ociety should settle for no less.

Edward B. Hirshfeld, Should Third Party Payors of Health Care Services Disclose Cost Control Mechanisms to Potential Beneficiaries?, 14 Seton Hall Legis. J. 115, 130–31, 147 (1990):

describing AMA's recognition that cost-consciousness creates conflict of interest between patient and physician.

John L. Puma et al., Ethics, Economics, and Endocarditis: The Physician's Role in Resource Allocation, 148 Arch. Intern. Med. 1809, 1819 (1988):

Resource allocation decisions must be made as social policy choices . . . not in medical offices [or] hospital rooms.

G. Gayle Stephens, An Opposing View, 28 J. Fam. Pract. 698, 701 (1989):

arguing that "the gatekeeper role is hopelessly conflicted, ethically unmanageable, clinically naive, professionally ungratifying, and historically unnatural."

Daniel P. Sulmasy, Physicians, Cost Control, and Ethics, 116 Ann. Intern. Med. 920, 920 (1992):

[R]ationing decisions by individual physicians at the bedside are morally unacceptable.

See also, Erich H. Lowey, Cost Should Not Be a Factor in Medical Care, 302 New Engl. J. Med. 697, 697 (1980) (letter to editor) (citing Nazi Germany in attack on cost-benefit analysis); Joseph F. Boyle, Should We Learn to Say No?, 252 JAMA 782 (1984) (opposing physician rationing); B. Zawacki, ICU Physician's Ethical Role in Distributing Scarce Resources, 13 Crit. Care Med. 57–60 (1985) (same).

Notes

1. Fuchs 1984, at 1573.
2. The only exception is for temporary situations of dire constraints such as natural disaster, battlefield triage, or emergency-room trauma cases.
3. Levinsky 1984.
4. Veatch 1986, at 38.
5. Churchill 1987, at 106–112 (ethicist); Menzel 1990, at 12–13 (ethicist); Brody 1987b, at 5–17 (ethicist); Welch 1991, at 223–226 (physician); Cassel 1985, at 550, 563 (physician); Ellsbury 1989 (physician); Glover and Povar 1991 (physician and policy analyst); Goold and Brody 1995, at 135 (physician ethicists); Jecker 1990 (ethicist); Orentlicher 1996 (physician ethicist); Ubel and Arnold 1995 (physician and ethicist).
6. The leading exponent of this compromise position is philosopher Norman Daniels. See Daniels 1987, at 75–78; Daniels 1986. See also Rodwin 1993, at 156–62; Cassel 1985, at 550, 558; Reitemeier and Brody 1988, at 284, 290; Wolf 1994, at 28, 37–38.
7. See Morreim 1991b , at 65–66 (conflicts of interest are now "inescapable for physicians"; "it is no longer plausible to demand that physicians literally always place patients' interests above their own"). Albert R. Jonsen and colleagues also recognize that physician rationing makes good economic sense. See Jonsen et al. 1986, at 149–50, 154. However, their style of analysis is, for the most part, to outline relevant ethical considerations without taking a definitive stance.
8. The best works I have encountered so far are the brief developments in Glover and Povar 1991, at 13–24; Friedman 1986; Orentlicher 1996; and Ubel and Arnold 1995.
9. 42 U.S.C. § 1320a-7a(b).
10. For a critique of this legislation, see Hall 1988, at 499–504.
11. 42 U.S.C. § 1395mm(i). Implementing and interpretative regulations have been proposed at 57 Fed. Reg. 59024 (Dec. 14, 1992), to be codified at 42 C.F.R. § 417.479. See Chapter 5 for further explanation of this law.
12. Pulvers v. Kaiser Foundation Health Plan, 160 Cal. Rptr. 392, 394 (Cal. App. 1979). The court observed that the jury found that no negligence was committed.
13. Madsen v. Park Nicollet Medical Center, 419 N.W. 2d 511, 515 (Minn. Ct. App. 1988).
14. On the other hand, the court also ruled that financial incentive plans are not per se in violation of public policy. Bush v. Dake, No. 86–25767, Mich. Cir. Ct., Saginaw County,

April 27, 1989, summarized in 17 Health Law Digest, No. 8, at 16. The case was subsequently settled. See Rodwin 1993, at 168–73.

15. See Pollock 1993, at B5 (discussing Fox v. HN Management Holdings).

16. In re Baby K, 16 F.3d 590, 596 (4th Cir. 1994). This ruling is based on the Emergency Medical Treatment and Active Labor Act (EMTALA), 42 U.S.C. §1395dd (1988), which requires hospitals to examine and, as appropriate, treat or transfer anyone seeking emergency care regardless of the patient's insurance or financial status.

17. In re Baby K, 832 F. Supp. 1022, 1028–29 (E.D. Va. 1993) [relying on the Americans with Disabilities Act of 1990, 42 U.S.C. §§12101–12213 (Supp. V 1993)], aff'd on other grounds, 16 F.3d 590 (4th Cir. 1994).

18. Oregon's rationing list was subsequently approved by the Clinton administration, however, following substantial revision in its methodology and content. See Chapter 3 for further discussion.

19. The following sources examine this fundamental conflict in a variety of contexts: Crossley 1993; Hadorn 1992b; Orentlicher 1994; Peters 1995; Stade 1993.

20. Some of these facts are made up, and others are my imprecise and untutored understanding of medical facts as I recall them being explained to me several years ago. However, whether accurate or not for the precise conditions I describe, this hypothetical is representative of the type of decisions physicians make all the time.

21. Obviously, if the outcome of omitting the test had not been this sanguine, the tone of my story would not be so flippant. However, given the low odds of maloccurrence and the fact that I am purposefully avoiding any imputation of tort liability in the present discussion, this is a fair basis for evaluating the type of physician rationing I advocate. A contrasting example can be found in the emotionally gripping first-hand account by a physician who failed to diagnose a pregnancy by declining (on grounds of cost and inconvenience to the patient) to perform an ultrasound, resulting in the mistaken abortion of a live fetus. Hilfiker 1985, at 72–77.

22. Churchill 1987, at 106.

23. For example, Levinsky 1984 focuses on heart and liver transplants; Puma et al. 1988 address the denial of a heart valve replacement for an alcohol and drug abuser in severe cardiac distress; Griffin and Thomasma 1983 use the case of a five-year-old hit by a car who recovers from a deep coma and multiple serious injuries after months of intensive care; and Yarborough and Kramer 1986 use the extreme example of terminating all care for the elderly.

24. As a consequence, the opposition to physician rationing (as I define it) may not be as severe as I portray at the outset. See, e.g., Brennan 1991, at 177, 183, 186–87 (physician rationing is permissible except for dramatic, life-and-death decisions). Nevertheless, as I document earlier and in the Appendix to this chapter, several prominent authorities in medical ethics oppose physician rationing in any form, and most medical ethicists oppose physician rationing induced by financial incentives.

25. See Hall 1989.

26. Thurow 1984.

27. "Whenever possible, British doctors recast a problem of resource scarcity into medical terms. They have developed standards of care that incorporate economic reality into medical judgments." Aaron and Schwartz 1984b.

28. Williams 1988, at 1183–85 (quoting Sir Raymond Hoffenberg, then president of the Royal College of Physicians).

29. Luft 1982, at 275.

30. See Wennberg and Gittelsohn 1982, at 123; Wennberg and Gittelsohn 1973, at 1104; Paul-Shaheen, Clark, and Williams 1987.

31. Pearlman et al. 1982.

32. Orentlicher 1992; SUPPORT 1995.

33. Macklin 1993, at 161.

34. See Randall 1993, at 160–62; AMA Council 1990, at 2344–46. See also AMA Council 1991, at 559–562.

35. Ford and Cooper 1995.

36. The inference of racism is inconclusive because the studies employ only crude measures of health status, and they do not control for other, more innocuous possible causes. For instance, they do not fully account for counterindications for the measured procedures, or for the possibility that blacks on average prefer less interventionist medicine. See Ford and Cooper 1995.

37. Another study found that, although blacks received less treatment than whites at the same hospitals, because blacks on average were treated at better hospitals, there were no overall differences in the quality of care. See Ayanian 1994.

38. Ozminkowski, Friedman, and Taylor 1993.

39. Ayres, Dooley, and Gaston 1993.

40. Gianelli 1992, at 1; Developments 1990, at 1636; Pearlman et al. 1982; Halper 1985, at 73–78.

41. Chavkin and Treseder 1977.

42. Toon 1994, at 587. See also Katz 1985. Lipsky 1980, at 107–111 documents and discusses the ubiquity of this phenomenon in many other service professions.

43. Aaron and Schwartz 1984a.

44. Strauss, LoGerfo, Yeltatzie et al. 1986 ("we conclude that physicians can effectively ration intensive care beds on a regular basis"); Singer, Carr, Mulley et al. 1983, at 1156 ("Although physicians systematically chose the more severely ill patients for admission to the ICU . . . , there was no apparent age discrimination"); Selker, Griffith, Dorey et al. 1987 ("for no group [admitted or excluded] did mortality increase when the CCU was full. These data suggest that physicians can safely adapt to substantial reductions in the availability of CCU beds"). But see Kalb and Miller 1989 ("There is evidence that rationing as it is now practiced is biased and inequitable"); Crane 1975 (finding that doctors use a mix of patient/family wishes, medical prognosis, and social factors to ration ICU beds). See generally Anspach and Renee 1993 (extensive, nonjudgmental ethnographic description of decision making process affecting life-and-death decisions).

45. Homan 1993.

46. Aaron and Schwartz 1984a.

47. The extraordinary rigor of the study comes from the fact that it was a designed and controlled social experiment, one of the largest in history, rather than simply a study of existing natural patterns. This allowed the researchers to control for numerous confounding variables, such as healthier patients preferring one form of insurance over another. For additional discussion, see Chapter 2, and Newhouse and The Insurance Experiment Group 1993.

48. See Bates and Connors 1987, at 57 (reviewing literature which concludes that for Medicare beneficiaries quality of care in HMOs is at least equal to that of fee-for-service insurance); Cunningham and Williamson 1980 (reviewing 27 studies of HMO quality, of which 19 found HMOs superior to other settings; remaining eight studies found HMOs either to be equivalent to other settings or else study findings were inconclusive); Franks and Clancy 1992, at 426–27 (summarizing literature on risks of undertreatment in HMOs); Miller and Luft 1994 (same); Weiner 1986 (same).

49. Newhouse and The Insurance Experiment Group 1993, at 346.

50. See, e.g., U.S. General Accounting Office 1993.

51. See Rubin et al. 1993.

52. See Physician Payment Review Commission 1995, at 339; Lasker et al. 1992.

53. Toon 1994, at 587.

54. Hardin 1980, at 61–62. See also Callahan 1989, at 356–57 ("we need to pit the methods of rationing against each other, not against the ideal world in which we all wish we lived").

55. See Winslow 1982; Childress 1983.

56. Toulmin 1986, at 783–85. Accord Churchill 1987, at 110–11. ("None of us have the luxury of loyalty to only one principle or the simplicity of unambiguous devotion to one and only one person or set of persons. . . . Unalloyed allegiance is an impossible standard of purity of motive, and anyone who believe themselves capable of it may be subject to other overestimates of their virtue and ability as well.") See generally Erde 1996.

57. Relman 1985b, at 103, 105.

58. Welch 1991, at 225.

59. Kalb and Miller 1989; Otten 1989.

60. Jecker and Berg 1992.

61. Symposium 1978.

62. Stone 1979, at 244.

63. Hall 1985, at 159–60; Developments 1985, at 1542–48.

64. Holleman, Edwards, and Matson 1994.

65. James 1988; Anderson and May 1990. This is referred to as the "prevention paradox." Brock and Wartman 1990, at 1599. See also Mansfield 1991, at A11. ("The media and the health-care industry act together to perpetuate the myth that vaccination solves problems without necessarily making new ones.")

66. See Welch 1984, at 63.

67. Hellman and Hellman 1991, at 1586.

68. Freedman 1987; Schafer 1982; Gifford 1986.

69. Gillon 1988, at 116–18.

70. Ibid. at 128. See also Williams 1988, at 1184 ("despite their protestations to the contrary doctors never have behaved without regard to the costs of their actions").

71. Brett and McCullough 1986.

72. For leading examples in this literature, see generally Gray et al. 1991; Marsh and Staver 1991; Murphy 1988. For a broad survey of this debate, see generally Boozang 1993; Schneiderman et al. 1990.

73. Gillick 1988, at 749. See also Lo et al. 1985 (documenting that doctors regularly withhold cardiopulmonary resuscitation (CPR), sometimes without consent or over the patient's and family's objection); Rosenthal 1990b (reporting that medical teams frequently just go through the motions by performing half-hearted resuscitation efforts behind drawn curtains, charades known as "Hollywood codes"); Orentlicher 1992 (surveying the range of situations in which patient choice is suppressed by medical norms).

74. Paris, Crone, and Reardon 1990, at 1013 (reporting such a case); In re Baby K, 16 F.3d 590 (4th Cir. 1994) (finding such action illegal under federal statutes governing hospital emergency services). Even the otherwise heavily "pro-life"-oriented "Baby Doe" regulations that issued from the Reagan administration allowed the cessation of treatment for severely brain-damaged newborns where treatment is judged "virtually futile in terms of survival." 50 Fed. Reg. 14887 (1985). However, these regulations do not address the question of disclosure or consent.

75. Symposium 1995a.

76. See Murphy and Finucane 1993; Schneiderman et al. 1990, at 953 (advocating definition of futility that allows cessation even though treatment is effective in up to

1 percent of cases); see also Gray et al. 1991 (observing that huge commitment of resources is made to largely unsuccessful resuscitation attempts); Rosenthal 1990b (reporting that doctors "question whether futile resuscitations, which can cost thousands of dollars and tie up precious intensive care beds, make sense in an era of rising health costs").

77. Wolf 1988, at 199; Tomlinson and Brody 1990; Lantos, Singer, Walker et al. 1987; Youngner 1988; Veatch and Spicer 1992; Truog, Brett, and Frader 1992.

78. Gray, Capone, and Most 1991.

79. Paris, Crone, and Reardon 1990, at 1013 (arguing that even successful efforts to maintain long-term physical functioning of a severely brain-damaged infant are "futile . . . unless a reversal or amelioration of the underlying condition could be expected"); Schneiderman, Jecker, and Jonsen 1990 (defining treatment as "ineffective" if it merely preserves unconscious bodily functioning or leaves a conscious patient in a highly dependent state of intensive care).

80. Miles 1991.

81. Paris et al. 1993.

82. Useful surveys are contained in Rodwin 1993, at 256; and in Murray 1986; and in Erde 1996.

83. Howe 1986.

84. Murray 1984.

85. Walsh 1986.

86. Peterson 1985. Accord Elkowitz 1986, at 123 ("medical resource allocation enters the day-to-day practice of every physician at any level").

87. Friedman 1986, at 351.

88. Rothman 1991, at 102–03.

89. Veatch 1981, at 24–26. See also Fox 1979, at 83. ("Most physicians, philosophers, and historians have assumed the major questions in the field to be who shall practice medicine, in what relationships with other practitioners, and with what obligations to patients, institutions, and public authority.")

90. Sociologist Eliot Freidson characterizes the medical profession as harboring an "imperialistic ideology . . . a self-deceiving view of the objectivity and reliability of its knowledge and of the virtues of its members. . . . Its very autonomy has led to insularity and a mistaken arrogance about its mission in the world." Freidson 1970a, at 370.

91. Veatch 1981 at 97, 106 ("a professional ethics grounded in nothing more than agreement, custom, or vote by a group's members can have no ethical bite. . . . It is doubtful such a standard can be called an ethic at all").

92. The paradoxical congruence of historical and contemporary medical ethics against physician rationing is best exemplified by the fact that Robert Veatch, one of bioethics' harshest critics of the professional code basis for medical ethics, and who first declared that the "Hippocratic ethic is dead," Veatch 1981, at 154–59, 170, has explicitly resurrected Hippocratic individualism in his attack on physician rationing, claiming that this practice renders the Hippocratic oath a fraud.

93. One statement of this individualism theme that has been particularly influential in medical ethics is Fried 1975, at 244.

94. Rothman 1991, at 241–46; Emanuel and Emanuel 1992, at 2226; Schneider 1994. A useful summary and annotation of the literature tracing the history of bioethics and critiquing its isolation from larger bodies of political and economic thought can be found in Rodwin 1993, at Appendix C.

95. This individualism may also result from the religious orientation of the philosophical training that many of the early leaders in the field received. Religious doctrine, and the tradition of church/state separation, reinforce a neglect of matters relating to political

economy. ("Render unto Caesar what is Caesar's. . . .") In contrast, more secularly trained philosophers, such as Norman Daniels and Allen Buchanan, demonstrate a richer appreciation for the distributive justice framework in which these issues arise.

96. Wikler 1991, at 236. Wikler attacks the brand of "clinically oriented bioethics . . . that brandishes 'Principles' of all sorts on an as-needed basis," idem at 248, and he characterizes much of the work in bioethics as "mantra-driven ethical analysis . . . [in which] novel insights and turns of argument are virtually ruled out . . . [and] masses of naively faithful repeatedly inton[e] a small set of magical words in hopes of achieving a short cut to enlightenment." Ibid. at 240.

97. For further elaboration of this critique, see Fox 1979, at 82, 90; Fox and Swazey 1984; Clouser and Gert 1990; Green 1990. For a response to these and other attacks on bioethics, see Gorvitz 1986; Lustig 1992.

98. Churchill 1987.

99. Williams 1985, at 2, 5. In Norman Daniels' words, "a rationing system based on ability to pay violates fundamental requirements of justice. . . . It thus constitutes a greater moral evil than either the need to place a price on life or the need to restrict the autonomy of the physician in the pursuit of absolute quality." Daniels 1985, at 138.

100. Buchanan and Brock 1989, at 192.

101. See Schwartz and Grubb 1985, at 19.

102. See generally Gardbaum 1992; Gutman 1985; Walzer 1983; Sandel 1982.

103. See Chapter 7 for further development of this analysis.

104. Emanuel 1991.

105. MacIntyre 1981.

106. Engelhardt 1986, at 385.

107. Ibid. at 12.

108. Ibid. at 40.

109. MacIntyre 1981, at 104.

110. See Daniels 1987, at 71–74 (contrasting the "Unrestricted Ideal Advocate" model of ethics that depends on the luxury of retrospective, fee-for-service reimbursement, with the "Ideal Advocate" model, which operates within the constraints of limited resources).

111. Daniels 1985, at 138.

112. Somers and Somers 1961, at 413–14, quoting Doenges 1959, at 28.

113. MacIntyre 1981, at 105.

114. See Gewirth 1986.

115. Luban 1988; Schwartz 1978.

116. Quoted in Luban 1988, at 54.

117. Freedmen 1966.

118. For instance, lawyers are under a stricter duty of confidentiality than are physicians. See Hall 1985, at 176–77.

119. Luban 1988, at 104–47.

120. See Hadorn 1992a, at 80–81 (developing the analogy between medical review systems and legal adversarialism).

121. Owing to the influence of bioethicists at Georgetown University's Kennedy Institute of Ethics in establishing this widely dominant analytical framework, the beneficence/autonomy recitation has come to be known as the "Georgetown mantra." Wikler 1991, at 239. The classic work is Beauchamp and Childress 1979. The mantra also includes "nonmalfeasance," but for the present purposes, this can be treated as a version of beneficence. The fourth element, justice, as noted above, has received much less development to date and therefore is treated as less central to mainstream bioethics.

122. What follows is an overgeneralization that exaggerates the actual differences in the operationalization of these principles. As implemented, these principles tend to be more moderated and nuanced than described here.

123. See generally Childress 1982.

124. The seminal essay is Pellegrino 1979.

125. Their most comprehensive account is Pellegrino and Thomasma 1988. See also ibid. 1981. A recent, exemplary addition to this approach is Emanuel and Emanuel 1992, who advocate a "deliberative" model under which physicians attempt to persuade patients which value choices they should make, rather than mechanically implementing the intervention a patient chooses from a neutrally presented list of options.

126. Pellegrino 1979, at 44.

127. Ibid. at 45.

128. Chapter 5 pursues the latter point in considerably more detail.

129. Pellegrino and Thomasma 1988, at 172, 173, 187.

130. Stephens 1989, at 704.

131. This fundamental point, which has been made previously and at greater length by Menzel 1990, and Havighurst 1992, has systemic importance across a broad range of health care problems. See Chapter 3 for additional discussion, in connection with the role of the courts in resource allocation.

132. Eddy 1990. Donabedian makes the same point by explaining that patients are "optimalists" at the time of insurance purchase but "extreme maximalists" when they are sick. Donabedian 1983.

133. Eddy 1991d, at 1449. Norman Daniels uses the same distinction to solve the anti-utilitarian objections that otherwise would apply to redistribution of health care resources from the elderly to the young. He develops a "prudential lifespan account" of the proper *longitudinal* allocation of health care resources *within* a person's lifetime in order to avoid interpersonal welfare problems that arise if the allocation is viewed as one across persons at a point in time. Daniels 1988, at 41–46. See also Gibbard 1983, at 153, 156–58; Menzel 1990, at 10.

134. Williams 1988, at 1185.

135. The crucial qualifications introduced in this sentence are explored in Chapters 6 and 7.

136. Pellegrino and Thomasma 1988, at 87–91.

137. Ibid. at 47.

138. Pellegrino himself argues elsewhere that it would constitute "moral abandonment" for a doctor not to "make every effort to learn as much as he or she can about the many dimensions of what constitute the patient's best interests." Pellegrino 1991, at 82.

139. See MacIntyre 1981, at 50–51 (analyzing morality in terms of the disjunction between human nature in its untouched state and human nature as it could be if it realized its full potential); Shapiro 1994 (demonstrating how legal rules have symbolic value apart from their principled justification or their actual effect); Shapiro 1988b, at 1559–61 (observing usefulness of "clumsy institutions" that superficially support one value system but simultaneously perpetuate opposed values by constantly holding open opportunity for disfavored values to gain preeminence); Mackie 1977, at 107–08, 134–35 (discussing distinction between the narrow sense of morality, which is a guide to specific conduct that counteracts natural inclinations, and the broader sense of morality, which is universal and contemplative); Emmet 1994 (analyzing how moral ideals can affect behavior and attitudes without being meant to serve as a precise guide to conduct).

140. See Pellegrino and Thomasma 1993, at 11–12, 18–22 (describing revival of virtue ethics and the distinction between virtues and moral rules).

141. Rodwin 1993, at 245.

142. Glantz 1988.

143. See also Elkowitz 1986, at 124 (reporting on survey of 15 physicians and medical students, and finding sharp dichotomy between how they characterize their treatment decisions and how they actually behave).

144. See Aaron and Schwartz 1984b ("Confronted with the need to allocate scarce services . . . , many doctors alleviate their own discomfort by persuading themselves that some treatable patients would not benefit at all"); Williams 1988 (British doctors ration "despite their protestations to the contrary"); Gillon 1988 (exposing contradiction of the ethic of absolute quality held by British physicians); Menzel 1990, at 8 (British physicians go to great lengths to preserve patient-centered ethic in the face of obvious rationing).

145. Leonard Fleck 1992 views this form of implicit, unacknowledged rationing as a "convenient device for societal self-deception" that "insulates the consciences of societal decisionmakers from critical moral self-reflection."

146. See generally Rawls 1971.

147. See Veatch 1981, at 134–38.

148. Ibid. at 283–86.

149. Ibid. at 285.

150. Dougherty 1990, at 36. See generally Elhauge 1994 (explaining moral distinction between actual and presumed consent).

151. See Fried 1981, at 3 (discussing the moral basis for contract enforcement).

152. See Hume 1953, at 43, 48–50.

153. Gauthier 1986, at 84.

154. Menzel 1990, at 14. Menzel does not carry this argument as far as he might, however, because he addresses consent to particular treatment decisions rather than to a generic resource allocation mechanism. Under the latter view, the enrollment decision validates a whole range of rationing decisions, thereby avoiding the need to adopt the more controversial "presumed consent" argument that Menzel does. See generally Elhauge 1994 (advocating informed insurance selection as means of choosing generic rationing criteria). Additional analysis of Menzel's position can be found in Chapter 6.

155. Veatch 1990, at 472.

156. 348 A.2d 801, 818 (N.J. Super. Ct. Ch. Div. 1975), modified and remanded, 355 A.2d 647 (N.J.), cert. denied, 429 U.S. 922 (1976).

157. See Engelhardt 1986, at 12–14; MacIntyre 1981, at 48.

158. Veatch 1991a, at 114.

159. Rawls 1993, at 336–40.

160. Rawls 1971, at 60.

161. Ibid. at 196–201, 358.

162. See Clark 1989, at 1721–22.

163. In actuality, the physician may not be denying the procedure per se but only insurance coverage. However, without insurance the patient may not be able to afford the treatment. Moreover, depending on how the legal doctrine of informed consent applies, the patient may not even know that potentially beneficial treatment is being withheld.

164. Kuflik 1984, at 271.

165. Ibid. at 287.

166. In Gerald Dworkin's terms, human beings are "embodied creatures," meaning not just that people are creatures that inhabit bodies, but that people *are* their bodies. Dworkin 1988, at 113.

167. Mill 1975, at 102–03. It may be, though, that Mill thought that the psychological experience of autonomy itself is so welfare-enhancing that its preservation is required by immediate—not merely consequential—utilitarian grounds. If so, then Mill also reasons in the same intrinsic vein as Kant, only for hedonistic rather than moral reasons. See Feinberg 1983, at 473.

168. Other welfare-based arguments for inalienability are developed in Calabresi and Melamed 1972, at 1113–14; Kuflik 1986, at 84–87; Rose-Ackerman 1985, at 937–41. Economists argue that inalienability rules can be justified as a second-best governmental response to various forms of market failure caused by externalities and transaction costs, or as a means to achieve certain nonefficient, distributional goals.

169. Mill 1975, at 126.

170. Mill writes: "[B]y selling himself for a slave, [man] abdicates his liberty; he forgoes any future use of it beyond that single act. He therefore defeats, in his own case, the very purpose which is the justification of allowing him to dispose of himself. . . . The principle of freedom cannot require that he should be free not to be free." Ibid.

171. See Radin 1987, at 1891–98 (describing but disagreeing with this position of Kant and Hegel).

172. Kidd 1953, at 212.

173. Hellman and Hellman 1991, at 1587.

174. See Feinberg 1983, at 462–63.

175. See Nozick 1974, at 28–35.

176. This term originated with Harry Frankfurt, who uses this split-level conception to explain free will. See Frankfurt 1971, at 11.

177. Dworkin 1988, at 108 (defining autonomy as "a second-order capacity to reflect critically upon one's first-order preferences and desires").

178. See, e.g., Komrad 1983, at 40–43 (advocating limited paternalism as desirable in that it can be used to increase the patient's autonomy).

179. E.g., Strasser 1988, at 111–16.

180. See Feinberg 1978, at 123 (arguing that the right to die is not inconsistent with the inalienability of life).

181. Shapiro 1988a, at 355. Shapiro adds that using "autonomy police" to guard against even excessively self-constricting choices "may harm autonomy more than [help] it." Ibid. at 354; see also Dworkin 1988, at 65–78 (arguing that more choice is not always preferable where there are costs of increased choice).

182. Fried 1981, at 13.

183. See Radin 1987, at 1852–54 (reviewing various meanings); see also Barnett 1986, at 186–91 (same); McConnell 1984, at 27–33, 53–56 (same).

184. More prosaically, I am reminded here of a George Carlin joke about the futility of trying to throw out a trash can.

185. This characterization does not fully reflect Kant's actual view of autonomy. Rather, it reflects what some modern bioethicists have made of his sometimes-conflicting positions. Thus, this summary attempts to describe only the modern Kantian tradition, not to be an accurate historical account of Kant's own treatment of these subjects. For discussion of the details of Kant's actual views, see generally Murphy 1970; Sullivan 1989.

186. See Hill 1989, at 91, 93, 96–97.

187. Ost 1984, at 309.

188. See Kidd 1953, at 211. However, their decisions are closely supervised by external review of the research proposal, and the decision to participate cannot be made irrevocable. See 45 C.F.R. §§46.101–.124 (1993).

189. The primary legal objection to minimum stay agreements is not disagreement with the principle of advance commitment but the lack of adequate disclosure and informed consent. Thus, courts have struck down voluntary commitment statutes for defects in the patient's competency and the process for obtaining consent. See, e.g., Ex parte Romero, 181 P.2d 811 (N.M. 1947). In contrast, where a patient was fully appraised at time of admission, a federal court allowed enforcement of a six-month stay for narcotics addiction. Ortega v. Rasor, 291 F. Supp. 748, 752 (S.D. Fla. 1968) ("[t]he Court will not permit the petitioner to terminate his treatment simply because the road to recovery is bumpy"). Only one court has squarely held that specifically enforcing an agreement to remain in treatment constitutes "involuntary servitude," amounting to a substantive due process violation. Ex parte Lloyd, 13 F. Supp. 1005, 1007 (E.D. Ky. 1936). See generally Dresser 1982 (surveying but opposing the law allowing voluntary commitment contracts); Note 1993 (analyzing ability of mental patient to given irrevocable advance consent to a course of treatment).

190. See, e.g., Dworkin 1988, at 128–29.

191. For the most frequently cited source, see Elster 1979. For another insightful discussion, see Schelling 1984.

192. See In re Baby M, 537 A.2d 1227 (N.J. 1988); Robertson 1990, at 421.

193. This example is borrowed from Childress 1982, at 92.

194. Sometimes it is posited that holding precommitment agreements irrevocable is only permissible where the person would later ratify the refusal to honor her change of heart. Thus, Ulysses surely was thankful that his crew held him to his word, and I am grateful when my wife rousts me out of bed to go to work, despite my grouchy protests at the time. However, limiting the scope of legitimate precommitment agreements in this manner does not so much resolve the dilemma we face as define it away. This solution views the problem as one where different preferences are expressed at three points in time. If the critical point for preference testing is the third stage, then the decision made at the first stage is neither necessary nor sufficient; it is simply irrelevant. In other words, under this resolution Ulysses's crew would have been justified in binding him to the mast even if he had given no such command; the justification would lie in his later ratification, even if it were expressed in the fiction of presuming his prior consent. This resolution is inapposite to our inquiry, which is what moral force attaches to the earlier pronouncement. This problem can be seen clearly only if no ratification is assumed subsequent to the regret.

195. Most states allow the detention of a voluntary patient for three to five days after requesting release to ensure the continuity of outpatient care or to consider whether to institute involuntary commitment proceedings. See Brakel 1985, at 185–88 (collecting and analyzing all relevant statutes).

196. See Schelling 1984, at 99 (distinguishing between vows and contracts).

197. Wikler 1988, at 67; see also Buchanan and Brock 1989, at 107 (surveying but rejecting arguments against honoring advance directives to withdraw life-support); Cantor 1992, at 13–22 (same).

198. Mill 1929, at 960.

199. It is noteworthy, though, that this issue is subject to empirical testing, which, limited though it is, so far provides some support for holding patients to their earlier-expressed preferences. Llewellyn-Thomas, Sutherland, and Thiel 1993 (finding that patients' evaluations of the burdens of radiation treatment for cancer are consistent before and after treatment); Danis et al. 1994 (elderly patients who expressed preference to decline life-support were much more likely two years later to make the same decision than those who initially wanted life support, but black, low income, and less educated patients were more likely to

change their minds, as were patients who had been hospitalized in the interim); Boyd, Sutherland, Heasman, et al. 1990 (patients who have experienced a disabling condition view it more positively than those who have not).

200. Elster 1982, at 219, 219–38. Cass Sunstein refers to this phenomenon as "endogenous" preference formation. Sunstein 1986, at 1143.

201. For an example of this phenomenon at work in medical care, see Deyoet et al. 1987, at 141–45 (describing how patients with uncorrectable lower back pain found education just as reassuring as X-rays).

202. Jeffrie Murphy, who is a Kantian, observes that "the person who claims duress or coercion every time he simply finds life's choices hard is doing nothing more than wrongly trying to get other people to feel obligations where they really have no obligations. The currency of moral discourse is thereby cheapened." Murphy 1981, at 88.

203. For initial movements in this direction, see generally Brennan 1991; Brody 1987b; Daniels 1987; Emanuel 1991; Emanuel and Emanuel 1992; Goold and Brody 1995; Jecker 1990; Ozar 1987; Wolf 1994.

204. See Eddy 1993; Elhauge 1994.

205. That is, they should think about their patients and their reputations, not their income and debts.

206. Oberman 1994, at 3, 35.

207. In distinguishing between ethicists and physicians, I do not ignore the fact that many prominent ethicists are physicians. I am only using a convenient shorthand to refer to each group's primary occupation.

5

Motivating Physicians With Financial Incentives

So far, we have determined that it is permissible to induce physicians in some manner to consider the costs of treatment, whether this inducement occurs through education, peer supervision, practice guidelines, or other behavioral influences. A more difficult question is whether to condone the particular form of physician rationing that occurs when doctors are influenced to perform this function through various financial incentive arrangements. The problem with more acceptable, nonfinancial means for changing physicians' behavior is that they are notoriously ineffective. They either do not accurately address the way in which physicians approach clinical problems, or they fail to alter physicians' fundamental motivations and therefore are too easily ignored or circumvented. For instance, various education efforts have been shown to be somewhat successful while they are being conducted, but when they cease, physicians' behavior lapses back to its original pattern. Even practice guidelines and recommendations issued by prestigious organizations such as the NIH have little demonstrable effect on doctors.[1]

In contrast, there is no dispute about whether financial incentives will work; indeed, the controversy is over whether they are too potent. Financial incentives clearly affect physicians' behavior, as they do everyone else in society. Unlike categorical clinical rules, incentives are well suited to the judgmental and individualized discretion that characterizes much of clinical practice.[2] Various studies show that when sudden changes are made in the manner in which doctors are paid, they are capable of quite dramatic increases or decreases in the frequency with which they perform or order various procedures. In one widely reported instance, a chain of urgent care clinics switched from paying its doctors a flat hourly rate to paying them a percentage of their billings. Within six months, the doctors were ordering 16 percent more X-rays and 23 percent more lab tests per patient visit.[3]

HMOs are the setting in which we presently see the most explicit and creative use of financial incentives to induce physicians to trim out expensive care that is of slight or no benefit. HMOs motivate their primary care physicians (those who are a patient's first point of contact within the HMO) to economize in two ways. First, they pay them a fixed amount, either per annum (salary) or per enrollee (capitation), regardless of how much effort they devote to each patient's case.[4] These base pay methods place primary care physicians at risk mainly for their own time. Second, these physicians also play a "gatekeeping" role in approving expensive testing, specialist referral, and hospitalization services performed by others. Various bonus and penalty devices place these primary care physicians at financial risk for the costs entailed in their gatekeeping decisions. For example, an HMO might withhold 20 percent of a general practitioner's base pay until the end of the year to offset any excess beyond the amounts budgeted for hospitalization and specialist referral services attributable to that physician's patients. Alternatively, the HMO might augmont the physician's base pay by distributing a portion of the savings that accrue from keeping his patients' referral and hospitalization costs under budget. Some HMOs employ both bonus and penalty methods, and these incentives are often pooled among a group of physicians.

These cost-containment incentives are subject to a serious ethical objection: By rewarding physicians for withholding potentially beneficial care, they create an economic conflict of interest between the doctor and the patient. Many medical ethicists have argued that while it may be permissible to ask doctors to save money on one patient in order to better treat others, it would defile physician rationing to allow doctors to keep the savings themselves. Most ethicists draw the line on physician rationing at this point. A growing number would allow physicians to consider costs to some degree, but very few support using financial incentives as the means for prompting this behavioral change.

Just as the prior chapter rejected the notion that physicians may never trade off potential medical benefits out of a concern for costs, this chapter will analyze whether it is possible to maintain the absolute prohibition against motivating physicians to do so through financial incentives. The essence of my rebuttal is again based on patient consent. While undisclosed or extremely corrupting incentives may be prohibited outright, properly informed insurance subscribers may rationally agree to a set of strategically crafted incentives that induce doctors to act as both their medical treatment and their economic purchasing agents. This line of analysis will be developed first by summarizing the law of fiduciary responsibility and then by exploring the "agency cost" branch of economic theory. The chapter concludes by applying this analytical framework to the regulations governing physician incentive plans in Medicare HMOs.

FIDUCIARY LAW

Several commentators have argued in recent years that financial conflicts of interest in medical treatment contravene the law of fiduciary responsibility.[5] Fiduciary law is a body of principles that impose a special measure of loyalty and devotion on several classes of professionals—primarily lawyers, trustees, corporate directors, and general business agents—by virtue of their control over vital decision making and the vulnerability of their clients.[6] To protect against the resulting potential for abuse, the law holds those who are in a fiduciary status to heightened duties of loyalty, candor, and effort that exceed those imposed by ordinary legal norms.

Considering the classic attributes of fiduciary status, it is difficult to imagine stronger grounds for imposing fiduciary obligations than those that apply to physicians. As one court stated: "The relationship of patient and physician is a fiduciary one of the highest degree. It involves every element of trust, confidence and good faith."[7] Doctors have vastly superior experience in a complex body of skills and knowledge that is critical to preserving the life and restoring the health of their patients. Doctors control their patients' welfare in the most vital aspects conceivable. Sick patients, by virtue of their debilitated and vulnerable state, are abjectly dependent on their physicians' decisions. Accurate diagnosis requires patients to reveal the most personal details of their lives, and effective treatment entails a physical invasion of the most private aspects of bodily integrity. For these reasons, many courts and commentators have affirmed the fiduciary status of doctors. The Supreme Court of North Carolina expresses the standard reasoning:

The relationship of patient and physician is generally considered a fiduciary one, imposing upon the physician the duty of good faith and fair dealing. This special relationship envisions an expectation by both parties that the patient will rely upon the judgment and expertise of the doctor. Furthermore, this relation is predicated on the fundamental proposition that the physician possesses "special knowledge and skill in diagnosing and treating diseases and injuries, which the patient lacks, and that the patient has sought and obtained the services of the physician because of such special knowledge and skill."[8]

While it is easy to classify physicians as fiduciaries, it is much more difficult to specify exactly what obligations this classification entails. Fiduciary law is far from the archetypal seamless web of the law. There is no integrated body of general principles or precise doctrine that applies consistently to all forms of fiduciary relationships. Each fiduciary relationship is treated in such a situation-specific fashion that an invocation of the fiduciary concept is frequently a conclusory labeling device for positions reached for reasons independent of the formal requirements of the law. As Harvard Law Dean Robert Clark observes, "commentators have spilt many gallons of ink writing sharp observations about particular lines of cases and fuzzy banalities about the general concept, [but] . . . because the subject matter is so sprawling and elusive, there has been little legal analysis of the fiduciary concept that is simultaneously general, sustained, and astute."[9]

Nonetheless, there are basic principles of fiduciary obligation that share broad, familial resemblance across many categories of relationships.[10] One of these common elements is the prohibition of financial or other personal conflicts of interest.

"[I]t is a rule of universal application that no one, having [fiduciary duties] . . . shall be allowed to enter into engagements . . . in which he has, or can have, a personal interest conflicting, or which possibly may conflict, with the interests of those whom he is bound to protect. So strictly is this principle adhered to, that no question is allowed to be raised as to the fairness or unfairness of a contract so entered into."[11]

This principle applies directly to HMO financial incentive plans: "A physician having a financial interest in decreasing utilization of premium dollars would have the appearance, if not the reality, of being a self-serving denial-of-care agent."[12]

Consentable Conflicts

Prohibiting all conflicting financial interests would naturally preclude any form of economic incentive for physicians to engage in health care resource allocation. But fiduciary law does not erect such a prophylactic barrier to financial conflicts, either inflationary or deflationary in nature. Instead, such conflicts are usually subject only to heightened scrutiny for fairness. Indeed, this is true for almost the entire array of fiduciary principles. For the most part, they constitute a body of presumptions that influence the rigor with which independently imposed legal obligations are interpreted and enforced, rather than impose direct substantive legal obligations of their own. The primary sources of law, contract and tort, are not supplanted by fiduciary law; by and large, they are only augmented by heightened standards of enforcement, proof, and disclosure.[13]

For instance, under contract law, fiduciary status does not render agreements between principals and agents unenforceable; it only lowers the threshold of unfairness required for striking contracts down, and it reverses the ordinary maxim of "buyer beware" by requiring the fiduciary to disclose all material information. Under tort law, the fiduciary status of physicians does not radically alter their standard of care compared with other service professionals such as architects and engineers; it only restricts the ability to require their clients to waive malpractice rights, and it elevates the ordinary disclosure requirements from those of simple consent to those of informed consent.

Accordingly, fiduciary law does not mandate any particular fee arrangement. Fiduciaries can be paid by the hour, by the job, or by a percentage of the proceeds, whether or not this arrangement is contrary to the client's interest. For instance, stockbrokers are typically paid a percentage of the purchase price of the stocks they buy and sell, and a defense lawyer is paid by the hour. As a result, the broker may have a financial incentive to trade stock more frequently than is in the client's best interest, and the defense lawyer is rewarded for protracted litigation regardless of the outcome of the case. Nevertheless, these and other sufficiently clear, voluntary, and fair financial incentives are held to be consistent with fiduciary status in other arenas.[14]

In each of the major categories of fiduciary status, beneficiaries may consent to at least some degree of conflicting interest.[15] In general, a lawyer may not represent differing interests in litigation or hold a stake in the outcome that is adverse to the interests of his client, but it would infringe a client's right to select her own attorney if the law were to preclude such representation entirely. Therefore, a lawyer may undertake conflicted representation with client consent after full disclosure, if it is "obvious" that her ability to provide "adequate" service will not be compromised.[16] In other fiduciary contexts, "[o]ne employed as a [business] agent violates no duty to the principal by acting for his own benefit if he makes a full disclosure of the facts to an acquiescent principal and takes no unfair advantage of him."[17] Similarly, corporations law generally permits corporate managers to engage in conflicted dealings if their actions are ratified by a fully informed and disinterested majority of board members or shareholders.[18] Consent to some financial conflict is available even for trustees, who are subject to the most demanding of fiduciary duties. Trustees who conserve financial assets may enter into competition with beneficiaries if such actions are authorized by the terms of the trust or if a competent beneficiary consents.[19]

In the medical arena, disclosure and consent is the primary mechanism for resolving conflicts that arise in the research setting. There, the scientific goals of the experiment may compromise the participant's optimal treatment in order to benefit society and the researcher's career.[20] An even stronger application of these fiduciary precedents in the medical arena is illustrated by the "durable medical power of attorney" laws that allow patients to nominate anyone they want as their agent for making life-and-death medical decisions on their behalf. Most medical ethicists view family members as the preferred decision makers for terminating life-support[21] even though family members may have financial and emotional interests in sharp conflict with the health interests of patients. For example, family members may stand to reap financial benefits under a will, be obligated to pay for some or all of the costs of care that is not declined, or suffer greatly from the emotional effects of a prolonged period of treatment. Far from being viewed with suspicion, this authorization of an intensely conflicted agent for even the ultimate medical decision is held to be a privileged election, in part because of the intrinsic value we attach to autonomous choice over deeply personal matters like health care.

The Psychological Basis for Patient Trust

Still, these precedents are not dispositive because fiduciary law is so acutely situation specific. Special attributes of the physician–patient relationship may dictate, in this context alone, that fiduciary status imposes a total prohibition on service-minimizing financial conflicts. If one recalls the strength of the reasons for imposing fiduciary duties, it becomes clear that this possibility is not frivolous. A very strict fiduciary ethic may be needed to preserve the essential therapeutic role that trust plays in the treatment relationship. If patients were not able to trust their doctors, their anxieties and feelings of vulnerability at the prospect of exposing the innermost aspects of mind and body either would deter their seeking treatment, or would hamper the therapeutic effect of treatment, or would violate a fundamental sense of safety and integrity. Patient trust, in addition to facilitating treatment, has also been championed as intrinsically valuable. Even short-term medical relationships, such as the one created by the delivery of a baby, can generate feelings of intimacy and bonds of loyalty that are akin to close friendship or familial attachment. As summarized by Herman and Anne Somers, "[I]llness, *per se*, tends to create—even in the most intellectual of patients—an attitude of dependence, of 'regression' to helplessness, and perhaps to childlike behavior. . . . In this state, confidence in the authority and benevolence of the doctor . . . —the now familiar 'father-image'—is generally desired."[22]

Financial conflicts of interest might undermine these strong bonds of patient trust in one of two intermingled ways. First, the presence of a conflict might directly destroy trust by causing patients, justifiably or not, to mistrust their doctors. Second, even if trust were to persist despite financial conflicts, conflicts may cause physicians to violate this trust by mistreating patients for personal financial gain. In short, we must be concerned about both the appearance and the actuality of abuse. It is this concern that led Congress in 1986 to ban all treatment-minimizing incentives within hospitals for Medicare and Medicaid patients.[23] This concern has also produced carefully argued scholarly works calling for a heightened fiduciary ethic and strict legal curtailment of deflationary financial conflicts in all treatment settings.[24] Closer examination of the trust rationale reveals, however, that these concerns do not support a strict prohibition of all financial conflicts to which patients might give consent. Rather, these concerns advocate setting broad, outer limits on the range and intensity of incentives for bedside rationing.

The opponents of financial incentives overstate their case because they assume a psychological basis for trust that is far too fragile. They seem to adopt the one-dimensional view that faith in our doctors increases in proportion to the constraints placed on their authority. It is difficult to know with any assurance, however, how trust is affected by various forms of conflict. This is especially true given the elusive nature of trust and the attendant absence of empirical testing. It appears possible, however, that trust in physicians is capable of withstanding many assaults. Physician ethicist Edmund Pellegrino views a patient's trust as "ineradicable," given the intensity of the need for trust when suffering from a serious illness and faced with the highly technical, invasive, and uncertain nature of medical science.[25] To quote Herman and Anne Somers once again, "'Honor thy physician because of the need thou hast of him.' So said Ecclesiastes to the Hebrews thousands of years ago. And still, today, patients yearn to have confidence in their doctors, to idealize them, to endow them with superhuman powers."[26]

Paradoxically, trust may be most indefatigable in precisely those cases where patients are the most vulnerable, for it is the physician's very power that gives rise to trust. Contrary to the superficial assumption that we confer power only on those whom we trust, we often confer trust in proportion to the power that others have over us. In the extreme case, children have near-total trust in their parents because of the near-absolute power parents possess, regardless of the extent to which parents may or do abuse that power.[27] This human trait produces the pathetic but real possibility that increasing opportunity for abuse may only fortify the intensity of trust. This is certainly not true for all, or even most, types of power, but it is likely true for many aspects of medical power. Because patients have no choice but to trust their physicians, they may be willing to trust them regardless of how much power physicians wield, perhaps even more so as that power increases.

Another paradox of the resiliency of trust is that trust in the system of medicine can survive even when individual professionals violate that trust.[28] Patients' faith is based not only on their knowledge of the personal characteristics of their individual physicians but also on their preexisting concepts of the archetypal physician. That is why we are able to trust a doctor the first time she treats us. Without this systemic trust, modern medicine with its team approach and emphasis on specialization would not be possible. This more diffuse trust is fostered by institutional and social mechanisms such as licensure and peer review that are not necessarily undermined by isolated acts of misbehavior. Once this system trust is established, individual professionals do not have to earn their trust in each instance. People are willing to trust those whom they have no personal basis for trusting because of society's shared experience with the institution of medicine. This broader foundation for medical trust renders it more resilient than opponents of financial incentives often represent.

Violating Medical Trust

Based on the foregoing, there is reason to believe that not all financial incentives to ration care will destroy system-wide trust in medicine. A greater concern, though, is whether financial conflicts of interest will create strong temptations for individual physicians to violate this trust. Even if trust would nevertheless persist, a prophylactic prohibition of financial conflicts may be desirable to protect against any potential for abuse.

The potential for abuse is not the only side to the equation, however. If discretionary authority were conferred only where there is no potential for abuse, authority would be allowed only where the stakes are so low that the authority is irrelevant. Of equal importance, therefore, is whether banning financial incentives would diminish potential benefits. Doctors who are made completely trustworthy may be so denuded of authority that they are unable to fulfill their core professional function. Therefore, restrictions on authority must be tailored with the fundamental purpose of the relationship also in mind.

Consider as an extreme example the parent–child relationship, which is sometimes used as a metaphor for the physician–patient relationship. Parents have nearly absolute authority over the most fundamental aspects of their children's lives (food, shelter, education, medication, religious values, personality development, etc.), yet parents are subject to only minimal legal supervision of how they execute this awesome power. Far from imposing fiduciary restrictions, the law encourages the exercise of these powers, to the extent of giving them constitutional protection. Parental authority is limited only in the most extreme instances of proven abuse, and then often by simply terminating the relationship altogether by removing custody over the child. This is because parental authority is considered fundamental to the nature of the parent–child relationship. One is not a parent unless one possesses this authority. The law does not think to limit this power in order to avoid potential abuse because to do so would destroy the very substance of the relationship.

In contrast, a lawyer, who also has vast power over the fate of her client, is carefully limited by fiduciary law. A lawyer cannot enter pleas, defenses, and settlements on her client's behalf without the client's express permission, and lawyers are prohibited from a range of conflicting roles and interests. A lawyer's power is subject to these restrictions because representation and counseling, not authority or interpersonal bonding, is the fundamental attribute of the lawyer–client relationship. This core benefit of the relationship can be preserved at the same time that a lawyer is strictly limited in her judgmental prerogative with respect to certain matters.

The core of the physician–patient relationship is healing. The healing power requires the physician to wield a degree of authority over the patient's fate that is intermediate between a parent and a lawyer. This power is inherent because of the vulnerability that illness entails. It is also beneficial because of the psychodynamic aspects of the healing phenomenon discussed in Chapter 2 that create in patients the strong urge to turn their medical fate over to a professional they trust.[29] This healing role does not require absolute power over patients, but it also cannot be fully achieved without some substantial exercise of discretionary authority. Therefore, legal or ethical rules that seek to eliminate physicians' power out of concern for abuse may undermine the very basis for the healing relationship. Consider the views of these respected physician ethicists:

The goal of medical ethics is seen as defanging the powerful physician, even if he then is not the sort of person from whom we wish to seek help when we are ill. But in that case we are allowing a view of medical ethics to undermine the fundamental ends of medicine itself.[30]

No professional can function properly without discretionary latitude. The more discretionary latitude we permit our professionals, the more vulnerable we become. Yet to limit that latitude is to limit the capacity for good as much as it may limit the capacity for harm.[31]

The law is sensitive to these concerns. It modulates the fiduciary limits placed on parents, lawyers, and doctors in response not just to the potential for abuse but also according to the importance of maintaining discretionary authority. For parents, power is central to the essence of the relationship, and so it is strongly encouraged and constitutionally protected. For lawyers, power is a collateral effect of the relationship but not its purpose, and so it is discouraged and frequently disallowed. For physicians, power is both the object and an incident of the treatment relationship. Therefore, the law achieves a balanced symmetry by treating the doctor–patient relationship as an intermediate case in the range of potentially corrupting powers. The law neither encourages a large measure of physician authority nor discourages it. Patients may choose for themselves how much discretion to confer on their doctors. To deny them this right would be potentially to negate the beneficial therapeutic aspects of a physician's power out of an excessive concern for potential abuse.

These observations do not compel acceptance of financial conflicts of interest, for it is certainly possible to give physicians the power to ration without using financial influence. However, they do counsel a degree of caution in weeding out all such influence solely out of fear of abuse. Marc Rodwin is one commentator who vocalizes this excessive fear. He launches a vigorous attack on the adequacy of disclosing financial conflicts as a means for protecting against the possibility for abuse. Rodwin observes that, in other contexts where consent is allowed to validate conflicts, there are additional protective mechanisms that ensure that the conflict does not lead to abuse, mechanisms that are lacking in the physician–patient relationship.[32] For example, he argues that conflicts are consentable in the attorney–client relationship because the adversary system polices the resulting arrangement. Opponents in litigation have an incentive to ferret out undisclosed conflicts in order to disqualify opposing counsel, and judges directly supervise the adequacy of representation that occurs under those conflicts that are revealed. In corporate situations and in other principal-agent relations in the business world, the protected beneficiaries are usually on a more equal footing with their fiduciaries in terms of knowledge and sophistication than are patients under the distress of illness.

This account disregards, however, the cumulative effect of the many oversight mechanisms that protect patients' interests in the treatment relationship. Direct regulation of financial conflicts occurs through both statutory and judicial avenues. As discussed below, various federal and state statutes and their implementing regulations either prohibit particular financial incentives, require their disclosure, or regulate their terms when such incentives reward those who withhold services.

In court, a number of cases have broached the legitimacy of various incentive plans, and it is generally recognized that tort theories are available to compensate patients injured by improperly designed or administered incentive arrangements.[33] Other oversight mechanisms police more indirectly by examining the competency of treatment that results from incentive plans. These include peer review committees and subscriber grievance proceedings. Finally, physicians' own internalized ethic of patient beneficence guards against corrupting influences.

The cumulative effectiveness of these safeguards is suggested by the virtual absence, despite considerable study, of empirical support for the concern that economizing incentives as they are presently used in the HMO industry lead to patient abuse. Nearly all studies of the quality of care in HMOs conclude that HMOs are equal if not superior to traditional settings for most categories of patients.[34] "Evidence linking types of financial incentives to changes in quality of care is nonexistent."[35] The one notable exception is for sick and poor subscribers who, in the leading study, fared somewhat worse in an HMO than in a full-coverage, fee-for-service plan. This was true for some measures of health status, but these disadvantaged HMO patients actually fared somewhat better on other measures. Other studies have shown that Medicaid recipients do not suffer in states that have switched from fee-for-service systems to HMOs.[36]

Granted, these dated studies are not definitive and they do not address the precise arrangements that are now in use. But their presence demonstrates that it is possible to monitor the effects of financial incentives on an ongoing basis by observing the ultimate outcomes of patient health and satisfaction. With these safeguards in place, especially for vulnerable populations, there is no solid evidence that deflationary incentives as presently used lead to systematic abuse. In the words of one astute commentator, "Honest doctors do not knowingly and willingly place their own financial self interest above the patient's best medical interests, and those who actively decide to cheat the system can easily find ways to do so, regardless of financial arrangements."[37] In the words of another, "Ethical objections can be raised against almost any economic system. . . . If physicians can be trusted to maintain some integrity in the face of ubiquitous competing influences, it follows that physicians should also be able to cope with the potential conflict of interest in gatekeeping based insurance plans."[38]

The more critical error in arguing against financial inducement is the idealistic notion that a conflict-free environment is desirable, even if not achievable. Marc Rodwin is the leading exponent of this view. He argues that mere disclosure is preordained to fail since many patients are too weak or confused to object. This assumes, however, that no sensible patient would consent to economizing incentives because they offer no advantages to patients. The sole purpose of disclosure, then, is to police or weed out financial incentives wherever they occur. This account fails to see that disclosure also serves to identify potentially beneficial incentives and subject them to acceptance by the patient.

Patients might affirmatively desire some forms of financial conflict in order to offset other forms that also corrupt patient trust. Banning all economizing incentives in an effort to create an incentive-neutral environment assumes that such an environment is possible and that corrupting sources can be unambiguously eliminated through other means. To the contrary, potentially corrupting incentives permeate medical practice. All forms of payment create some distorting influence, as does not paying at all. Even a straight salary is not beyond reproach since it creates incentives for physicians to cut back on time and attention in favor of their own leisure, and it creates a distorting incentive to make excessive referrals to specialists.

Traditional fee-for-service reimbursement suffers from the severely distorting effect of doing too many procedures, which causes not only vast economic waste but also leads to patient injury and death from overly aggressive medication and invasive surgery.[39] Incentive opponents claim to recognize this reality, yet they rarely complain as loudly about these distortions. Indeed, they sometimes praise the ethical virtue of fee-for-service incentives for aligning physicians' and patients' interests in doing the absolute best. The usual defense of this accommodating attitude is that the distortions in rationing incentives are worse because they encourage insufficient treatment and therefore are opposed to patients' medical interests. But, as former AMA ethicist David Orentlicher observes, to the extent this is true, physicians are less likely to be influenced by rationing incentives. "With incentives to limit care, physician concerns with patient welfare will be a stronger countervailing force. . . . Accordingly, physicians and patients are likely to be very sensitive to the potential harm from incentives to limit care."[40]

Conventional medical ethics also takes a more favorable view of inflationary incentives because they "are clearly visible to all concerned" and therefore easily guarded against.[41] This fact, however, only underscores the point that explicit disclosure of financial conflicts is generally considered sufficient protection. Some insurance subscribers might desire even stronger medicine, though, in the form of counterbalancing financial incentives designed to keep the distortions of fee-for-service reimbursement in check. Yet it is only at this point that incentive opponents argue for an absolute prohibition of financial conflicts of interest. Objecting to deflationary incentives when they are intended to counteract inflationary ones is not unlike a patient racked with pain suddenly becoming fastidious about the prick of the needle that injects the morphine.

Banning particular forms of payment will never produce a pristine, incentive-free state of affairs. Therefore, banning only economizing incentives, while glorifying or tolerating fee-for-service reimbursement may perversely undermine the very basis for trust that Rodwin and others seek to preserve, preventing us from concocting the least-distorting mix of incentives. This could cause an even greater affront to fiduciary principles. Fiduciary status does not impose a single, transcendent form of payment, and neither high-minded aspirations for trust nor naive assumptions about the perfectibility of human motivation should convince us to ban all conflicts of interest. Opening the possibility for the strategic use of some conflicts of interest only begins the discussion, however. Still to be resolved are the formidable problems of what forms of financial inducement are desirable in particular settings and where to draw the outer boundary of permissibility.

AGENCY COST THEORY

An alternative perspective to fiduciary law from which to view conflict-of-interest problems is offered by the branch of economic analysis known as *agency cost theory*. Agency cost theory is a generic framework for analyzing the ubiquitous problems that occur in all economic relationships that delegate authority over significant decisions. It explores the variety of ways in which agency powers are conferred and analyzes the array of techniques that are used to prevent agents from abusing their power. The name "agency cost" reflects the focus of this theory on the variable costs and benefits of different agency control techniques. The theory sees no single or small set of agency rules as universally optimal. Instead, agency relationships require a sensitive and complex balance among oversight mechanisms, incentive structures, and limits on the scope of agency power.

Agency cost theory operates on a scale that integrates ethical, legal, and practical policy analysis, and it offers a perspective more appropriate to the role-based ethic that governs physicians. This theory recognizes that professional ethics and law serve primarily instrumental goals that shape behavior in complex ways. Therefore, it avoids the categorical generalizations and unrealistic injunctions that can hamper constructive solutions to complex problems. Agency cost theory is also superior to the fiduciary framework because it is more attuned to the multidimensional conflicts that arise among groups of insured patients and across the tiers of relationships among physicians, patients, employers, and insurers. Fiduciary law has developed primarily in the streamlined setting of individual trustees administering funds for, or providing services to, one or only a few designated clients or beneficiaries. Agency cost theory, in contrast, has succeeded in explaining how these basic fiduciary concepts should apply to the large, complex group relationships that characterize the interactions among corporations, shareholders, employees, and directors.

Before exploring how agency cost theory applies to the particular problems that confront us, it is necessary to summarize its major tenets and analytical concepts.[42] An *agent* is one who is authorized to act or decide on behalf of a *principal*. Agency relations are created because principals recognize they are incapable of choosing or executing the correct course of action as successfully as are their designated agents, owing to some special expertise of the agent or some disability of the principal. However, any such delegation of authority creates an *agency risk* in that the agent's incentives and knowledge base never perfectly reflect those of the principal. Thus, every agency relationship entails the dual handicaps that the (1) agent may not fully understand the principal's objectives, or (2) the agent may seize on opportunities to pursue his own benefit over the principal's, either by slacking in effort or by appropriating some of the value of the activity for himself. Agency relationships and these attendant risks permeate all aspects of economic, social, and political life. *Agency cost theory* categorizes and analyzes the various mechanisms that have been crafted for reducing this agency risk and enhancing the potential benefits of an agency relationship.

Earlier economic theory was deficient because it considered that these imperfections either did not exist or that they were unavoidable. Agency cost theory represents an important advance because it attempts to identify and analyze ways in which these agency risks can be minimized without unduly sacrificing the benefits that gave rise to the agency relationship in the first place. An *agency cost* is the cost (measured either by direct expenditure or by sacrifice in benefit) of either reducing or bearing these risks. Agency cost theory recognizes that there is no perfect set of agency incentives and structures: the extent to which these endemic risks can be reduced depends on the size of the risk and the costs imposed by the various techniques for its reduction.

The plethora of techniques for reducing agency risk can be lumped into two basic groups: *external monitoring* of the agent's performance and *internalizing incentives* for improving performance. Diminished effort, cheating, or other forms of poor performance can be detected through external monitoring, either by the principal or by some other agent the principal retains for the purpose. This occurs, for instance, through quality assurance techniques in manufacturing. Alternatively, the agent's compensation can be structured in a manner that internalizes self-monitoring incentives, by rewarding superior performance or penalizing poor effort. This happens, for instance, when sales agents are paid on commission. Each of these techniques involves a cost that compromises the benefit of the agency relationship. Monitoring is expensive and is never fail-safe. Incentives divert the profits that would otherwise go to the principal and may create a different set of counterproductive incentives, which themselves must be monitored. The objective is to minimize the combination of losses that result from overprotecting and underprotecting. Overprotecting is costly and deters beneficial authority; underprotecting allows opportunistic abuse to go uncorrected.

A particular technique for agency risk reduction can be imposed through one or a combination of three mechanisms: (1) voluntary assumption by the agent, (2) individual contracting by the principal, or (3) legal imposition by society. *Bonding* is the term applied to efforts by agents to craft their own trust-enhancing devices in order to make their services more attractive to principals. Bonding explains, for instance, the adoption of codes of ethics by professional groups in order to convince the public of their trustworthiness. The most common mechanism for reducing agency costs is *individual contracting*. This appears in numerous guises, such as hiring employees and agents and setting their range of authority, or structuring compensation packages to reward or punish performance. Less obvious is the role society plays in reducing agency costs through *legal rules*. The most relevant body of law is that relating to fiduciary responsibility, which shares precisely the same concerns about abuse of trust and dependency.[43] Thus, agency cost theorists view the law's imposition of fiduciary duties as a collective solution to a common set of problems that transcend a variety of agency relationships.[44]

A further branch of agency cost theory known as *relational contract theory* takes this analysis a step further by exploring the transaction costs involved in employing these various techniques and mechanisms. Relational contract theory explains that collective rules can be preferable to individually contracted rules because they reduce the time and effort involved in providing particularized specifications for complex and long-term relationships.[45] For example, parties to a commercial contract frequently agree to arbitrate disputes simply by referring to the uniform procedures specified by the American Arbitration Association rather than crafting their own complex procedural code. By reducing agency costs in this manner, the law facilitates beneficial agency relationships that otherwise would not arise.

Fiduciary law offers just such an "off-the-rack" set of rules that apply generically to many agency relationships without the parties having to individually consider and agree to a transaction-specific behavioral code. However, the parties to particular agency relationships may have a different view of what is best for them than the default rules the law offers. If the barriers to arriving at a superior set of specifications are not insurmountable (including adequate understanding and bargaining parity), agency cost theory favors those restrictions that individuals negotiate over those the law imposes, so long as such arrangements do not harm anyone who is not a party to the agreement.[46]

This analysis brings us to the point that is most critical to the present exposition: whether legal and ethical rules that address agency cost problems should be subject to individual exception. Agency cost theory answers a resounding "yes." "Because the fiduciary principle is a rule for completing incomplete bargains in a contractual structure, it makes little sense to say that 'fiduciary duties' trump *actual* contracts."[47] Indeed, the very reason that fiduciary rules can afford to be so stringent and categorical on first inspection is that individual beneficiaries concerned about the law's overprotective slant are free to alter these legal norms. If the obligations were unalterable, they would have to be more balanced and much more nuanced at their inception.[48]

Application to Bedside Rationing

"In many respects, the physician-patient relation exemplifies the principal-agent relation almost perfectly";[49] therefore, agency cost theory "offers powerful insights into the evolution and current organization of the health care industry."[50]

Insured patients face a double-agency problem. Patients appoint doctors as their medical treatment and spending agents because they lack sufficient skill and training and do not wish to bear the anxiety of making these decisions themselves.[51] But delegating a large degree of authority[52] over such a critical matter creates serious problems in accurately pursuing patients' treatment interests— a *medical* agency problem. The full panoply of techniques and mechanisms just surveyed are employed to reduce these agency costs.[53] Direct patient monitoring occurs via informed consent, which is an individual contracting mechanism. Incentives are used in the form of fee-for-service reimbursement to encourage optimal patient care. Bonding occurs through physicians' adherence to an ethical code, and malpractice and fiduciary law applies collective norms for quality of care and patient loyalty.

The adoption of fee-for-service reimbursement to solve the *medical* agency problem, however, creates a new, *economic* agency problem: the distortion of physicians' spending decisions. Under the influence of insurance, physicians do more than what patients would have decided is cost-effective were they willing and able to pay out of pocket. Motivating physicians to consider the costs of their treatment decisions addresses this, a quintessential agency cost problem. The alternatives for correcting this abuse are less acceptable than bedside rationing. Avoiding resource allocation altogether prevents a number of people from being able to afford any agency relationship whatsoever. For others it means that the relationship will be less extensive and therefore less beneficial than it could otherwise be. This wholesale sacrifice of agency benefit is a more severe cost than the decreased autonomy or reduced medical benefit that comes from trimming marginally beneficial care interstitially.

Once some rationing is accepted, the next step is to choose the appropriate rationing mechanism: internalized incentives or external monitoring. Under agency cost theory, there is no single best approach to reducing agency costs; each technique has strengths and weaknesses and so inevitably a mix will be crafted. Therefore, a rule barring bedside rationing would increase agency costs by foreclosing a constructive solution to the inflationary effects of insurance and forcing the adoption of less desirable forms of monitoring such as bureaucratic rules.

At this stage, objections are raised that, even if physicians should consider costs, financial incentives may not be used to induce this role. Agency cost theory trivializes this objection when made in the absolute form. It characterizes financial inducement as merely one of a large menu of motivational techniques, neither intrinsically optimal nor unvaryingly despicable. From a perspective of agency cost theory, the only question is what combination and strength of techniques work best to achieve the client's ends with the least cost and sacrifice of agency benefit. Agency cost theory takes seriously the objection that a financial conflict will erode the trust and confidence that is vital to the treatment relationship, but the theory allows a modulated and differentiated response depending on the actual strength and pervasiveness of these concerns rather than insisting on a prophy-lactic bar.

As a consequence, agency cost theory instructs us that fiduciary law's prohibi-tion of conflicts of interest is not an absolute one. This baseline rule merely sets a presumption which individual subscribers may choose to depart from by electing an alternative form of insurance. In deciding how the baseline rule should be set, however, agency cost theory instructs us to consider the transaction costs of opt-ing out. Where bargaining positions are uneven, and where only a single individual is affected—as with ordinary trusts—a strong presumption against conflicts is war-ranted. Concerns about high pressure bargaining are minimized, however, where the rule affects the interests of a large group of beneficiaries. Moreover, the costs of contracting out of the rule increase with the size of the group; providing de-tailed disclosure to each individual is costly, coordinating a group deliberation and decision is difficult, and obtaining unanimous agreement is impossible. Ac-cordingly, fiduciary law takes a more accommodating view of conflicted transac-tions in corporations than in trust administration.[54]

Likewise, in the health insurance setting, powerful employers, unions, or gov-ernment regulators negotiate on behalf of large pools of patients. It may be ar-gued that these parties are the subscribers' enemies, not their friends, but they do ultimately pay for the insurance benefit. Therefore, they have at least the subscrib-ers' economic interests at stake. So long as there are adequate safeguards against neglecting subscribers' medical interests, it is appropriate under agency cost theory to set a default rule for physician incentives that reflects the reasonable range of actual contract agreements in existence rather than creating a very high presump-tion against any alteration in the traditional physician's role.

HMO Financial Incentive Plans

The more moderated principles established by agency cost theory can be used to test the complex tableau of financial incentives presently in operation within HMOs and the manner in which federal law regulates these incentives. In 1990, when Congress first addressed HMO rationing incentives for Medicare recipients, it recognized the impossibility of maintaining a blanket prohibition.[55] The legisla-tion bans only direct, patient-specific incentives, leaving all others to the regula-tory oversight of the Department of Health and Human Services. New regulations define certain categories of incentives that are per se safe, and they subject HMOs that exceed these thresholds to more intensive oversight of the particular arrange-ments and the resulting patient care.[56] This section briefly summarizes the major contours of each feature that shapes the strength of existing rationing incentives and how they are likely to be regulated. The results will demonstrate that the legal apparatus under Medicare and, for the most part, the HMO industry's own prac-tices set reasonable bounds on fiduciary contracting while simultaneously leav-ing wide berth for constructive experimentation.

As previously summarized, HMOs use three different forms of base pay—salary, fee-for-service, and capitation[57]—supplemented by a variety of bonus and penalty arrangements calculated according to various complex formulae. The strength and effectiveness of these payment incentives vary according to five dimensions, each of which has multiple components: (1) the type of services covered, (2) the practice setting and base reimbursement method, (3) the size of the incentive, (4) the incentive's immediacy, and (5) the presence of various counterbalancing monitoring mechanisms. Each of these will be examined in turn.

Cost-constraining financial inducements are much less threatening when they affect only a doctor's time and not his income. Accordingly, capitation for a physician's own services, like straight salary, imposes only mild financial disincentives to treat.[58] Therefore, the statute does not seek to regulate these base compensation methods at all. The statute applies only where "the plan places a physician . . . at substantial financial risk . . . for services *not provided by the physician*."[59] Financial disincentives to treat do arise, however, where capitation for primary care services is extended to the costs of outpatient testing and ancillary care services, and so these would be regulated as services "not provided by the physician."

The need for financial inducement also depends on the practice setting and the base reimbursement method. This is illustrated by Independent Practice Associations (IPAs), where physicians are dispersed among their individual offices and where fee-for-service base pay is most common.[60] IPAs are the practice settings most likely to place a portion of the physician's pay at risk by withholding a percentage to cover higher-than-expected costs. However, such "withholds" are uncommon in staff-model HMOs where physicians practice in a group setting and are usually paid by salary.[61] Capitation for primary care physicians is a mixed bag. Its base incentive is more akin to salary, but it often applies in a nongroup setting. Also, it creates an inflationary incentive for excessive referrals to specialists. Accordingly, withholds are much more prevalent in primary care capitation plans than in salaried ones, although somewhat less than in fee-for-service plans.[62]

The strength of a financial disincentive to treat depends also on its size in relation to the physician's base pay and whether any stop-loss protection exists to limit the upper end of risk exposure. The typical amount at risk in a withhold pool ranges from 10 to 30 percent of the physician's or the group's base payment, with 20 percent the most common.[63] This is within a range that is consistent with the bad-debt amounts or negotiated discounts which physicians regularly absorb for non-HMO patients. Therefore, these withholds are unlikely to be inordinately distracting and in fact may garner hardly any attention.[64] A comprehensive analysis of data from a large set of HMOs revealed that none of the more elaborate incentive arrangements presently in use had any discernible effect on the rate of hospitalization.[65] Accordingly, federal regulations set 25 percent as the safe-harbor threshold for "the substantial financial risk" that triggers additional scrutiny and safeguards under Medicare.[66]

At the other extreme, capitating individual physicians for the entire range of medical services is generally recognized as creating too great a risk.[67] This places the physician at risk not just for her own time but for 100 percent of the out-of-pocket costs of specialist referrals and hospitalization.[68] No such total-capitation arrangements for individual physicians are known to exist and they are prohibited by the federal regulations.[69] Such arrangements are increasingly common, however, for *groups* of physicians, and, as discussed below, they cause much greater concern as the size of the group grows smaller.

A final factor determining incentive strength is the presence of any stop-loss mechanism that caps the total risk exposure for a physician or a group, either for a single patient or for a patient pool. The federal statute requires some form of stop-loss whenever physicians are exposed to "substantial financial risk."[70] The proposed regulations opt for a simple, aggregate stop-loss that exposes physicians to no more than 10 percent of the risk above the substantial risk thresholds (which is 25 percent).[71]

The fourth critical factor affecting the strength of financial incentives is the psychological immediacy of the incentive. There are at least four different elements other than raw percentage size that shape a given incentive's psychological impact on a doctor's discrete mental decisions: the time horizon, the size of the physician group, the size of the patient pool, and whether the reward/savings is couched as a bonus or a penalty. A patient-specific penalty applied immediately creates too great an incentive to deny necessary care, whereas a year-end group bonus based on profitability is extremely unlikely to create anything more than a subliminal or background concern for the costs of treatment, particularly for large groups.

Accordingly, federal law prohibits "specific payment[s] . . . as an inducement to reduce or limit medically necessary services provided with respect to a *specific individual*,"[72] language which bans only immediate incentives directed to particular patients, and then only if the incentives result in denying medically necessary care.[73] At the other extreme, legislative history indicates that an incentive does not create any "substantial financial risk" if it is applied to at least five physicians as a group or to a patient panel of 25 and is applied no more frequently than semiannually.[74] However, as with the other dimensions, there is no magic formula that strikes the perfect balance between excessive and insufficient impact. For example, with respect to physician group size, a group too large will induce free rider behavior in which no doctor sees it in his interest to economize since he will receive only a tiny fraction of the savings produced by his own treatment decisions. Therefore, incentive plans that fall below these levels are not banned. They are only subjected to oversight by the agency and the requirement of stop-loss protection.[75]

Finally, incentive payments have greater or lesser effect according to the existence of counterbalancing monitoring mechanisms. HMOs are the practice environment in which physicians are most heavily monitored. In contrast with traditional solo office practice, HMO physicians are subject to grievance procedures, frequent subscriber satisfaction surveys, internal quality assurance and peer review processes, and external quality evaluations.[76] These exist in addition to the other structural oversight mechanisms which apply to all physicians, such as licensing, malpractice suits, market forces, and general ethical codes.

Considering all of the above, it is quite difficult without sophisticated empirical testing to determine the permissible range for even one factor in isolation, much less in combination with other factors. The best that can be done is to describe each factor's direction and relative strength. But even this is exceedingly difficult because none of these factors maximizes just a single value. Rather, they each strike a balance between quality and cost, and they do so in a highly complex and interactive fashion that depends on the compound effects of all of the factors in simultaneous operation. As the Department of Health and Human Services concluded after its lengthy report, "[i]t is this ability to adjust factors to increase or mitigate the strengths of each different financial incentive that makes it impossible to classify, categorically, some factors as being too strong."[77] Lacking such confidence, a legal or ethical prohibition of a particular type of economizing incentive, much less all such incentives, is unwarranted.

On balance, although many medical ethicists are united in opposing financial incentives for bedside rationing, this is not where the ethical battle line should be drawn. The important threshold is whether to allow physicians to allocate resources at all. If individualized physician discretion is to have any role, then a form of conflicted interest has already been introduced, namely, that between cost to the group versus benefit to the individual. If society is willing, as it must be, to take this step despite the threat to individual patient trust, then the manner of motivating physicians is a matter of secondary importance. Whether or not to use financial versus administrative or professional incentives concerns only the technical task of crafting the best strategic mix of motivational forces. There is certainly room for wide disagreement over the specifics, but nothing of intrinsic importance inheres in the use of a financial incentive per se.

Notes

1. For various surveys and analyses of this literature, see Pauly et al. 1992; Eisenberg and Williams 1981; Schroeder 1987.

2. See Hall 1988, at 480–83. For the contrasting view, that financial incentives are ill-suited to the structure and content of physicians' work, see Frankford 1994b.

3. Hemenway et al. 1990.

4. For case studies, typologies, and descriptions of the diverse array of HMO structures and payment methods, Hillman et al. 1992, at 137–38; Welch et al. 1990, at 225; U.S. Dep't of Health and Human Servs. 1990; Physician Payment Review Commission 1995; Gold et al. 1995.

5. Rodwin 1995a, 1993, at 179–211; Healey and Dowling 1991; Boyd 1989.

6. Scott 1949; Frankel 1983; Sealy 1962, 1963.

7. Lockett v. Goodill, 430 P.2d 589, 591 (Wash. 1967).

8. Black v. Littlejohn, 325 S.E.2d 469, 482 (N.C. 1985). For the groundbreaking analysis of fiduciary law as it affects physicians' financial conflicts of interest, see generally Miller 1983, at 153. For other important analyses, see Rodwin 1995b, 1993, at 190–91; Boyd 1989, at 154–59; Healey, Jr. and Dowling 1991, at 1001–02; Mehlman 1990, at 388–416; Morreim 1991a, at 296–301.

9. Clark 1985, at 55, 71. See also Sealy 1962, at 73.

10. For works that address fiduciary principles at this more general level, see Finn 1977, at 15–76; Rodwin 1993, at 179–211; Shepherd 1981, at 21–42; Frankel 1983, at 808–16; Scott 1949, at 541.

11. Sealy 1963, at 125 (quoting Aberdeen Ry. Co. v. Blaikie Bros., 1 Macq. 461, 471 (H.L. Sc. 1854)). The opinion qualifies this stricture, however, by observing that it is subject only to proper disclosure of the conflict. See Aberdeen at 471.

12. Geist 1974, at 1307. See generally Mehlman 1993, at 371.

13. Sealy 1963, at 119–24.

14. Levmore 1993.

15. The only significant exception is for government officials, who are subject to an absolute prohibition.

16. Wheat v. U.S., 486 U.S. 153 (1988). See Model Code of Professional Responsibility DR 5–105(C) (1980); Developments 1981, at 1303–04; Restatement (Third) of the Law Governing Lawyers § 202 (Tentative Draft No. 4, 1991). Rodwin 1989, at 1407. This exception is justified by the lack of an identifiable beneficiary, other than the general electorate, capable of providing consent for the public at large.

17. Restatement of Agency § 390 cmt. a (1933).

18. Revised Model Business Corp. Act § 8.31 (1984).

19. Restatement (Second) of Trusts § 170 cmt. a (1959).

20. Angell 1984, at 1385–87.

21. See Capron 1992, at 26–27 (surveying movement toward favoring families as surrogate decision makers); Rhoden 1988, at 437 (proposing that courts recognize presumptive right of families to exercise discretion over treatment decisions).

22. Somers and Somers 1961, at 460.

23. 42 U.S.C. §1320a-7a(b)(1).

24. Gray 1991, at 168–69; Rodwin 1995b, 1993.

25. Pellegrino 1991. See also Good 1988; Zaner 1991.

26. Somers and Somers 1961, at 459. This work cites the seminal work of sociologist Talcott Parsons (1951).

27. Baier 1986, at 241.

28. Luhmann 1973, at 53; Mechanic and Schlesinger 1996.

29. See generally, Brody 1992.

30. Ibid. at 201.

31. Pellegrino and Thomasma 1993, at 69.

32. Rodwin 1993, at 213–19; Rodwin 1989, at 1406–07.

33. See discussion in Chapter 4 at notes 12–14.

34. See Chapter 4 at notes 47 and 48.

35. U.S. Dep't of Health and Human Servs. 1990, at V-8.

36. See Chapter 4 at notes 49 and 50.

37. Hillman 1990, at 892.

38. Ellsbury 1989, at 698–99.

39. See Brook 1989, at 3028 (estimating from available literature that one-quarter of all hospital spending is wasted); Franks and Clancy 1992, at 425 (summarizing risks of overtreatment); Hillman et al. 1990, at 1606 (finding that doctors with investment in radiology equipment order testing four times more often than those who refer patients to radiologists); Steel et al. 1981, at 638, 641 (finding that 36 percent of patients admitted to one respected hospital were injured in some way by medical treatment, 9 percent suffered major complications, and 2 percent died for reasons related to the treatment they received).

40. Orentlicher 1995, at 161.

41. Relman 1985a, at 750.

42. So far the only work that systematically explores the implications of agency cost theory for ethical problems in the treatment relationship is Buchanan 1988. Much additional work needs to be done, however, to develop Buchanan's introductory insights and to extend this framework to collective insurance arrangements. The summary treatment contained in this chapter is drawn mainly from Arrow 1985, at 32, 37–38; Pratt and Zeckhauser 1985, at 1, 2–3; Stiglitz 1987, at 966–69.

43. Thus, it is wrong, as Buchanan does, to view fiduciary status as opposed to agency cost analysis. Buchanan 1988, at 322. Fiduciary rules help to solve agency cost problems. They are one instance of efficient agency risk reduction in action.

44. Much of the recent work in corporate law analyzes corporate fiduciary principles from an agency cost perspective. For a sampling, see Easterbrook and Fischel 1991, 1986; Symposium 1989; Fischel 1982. For works that extend this perspective to fiduciary law generally, see Cooter and Freedman 1991; Davis 1985; Clark 1985, at 77; Anderson 1978.

45. These are termed "relational contracts." Goetz and Scott 1981; Macneil 1978.

46. Clark 1989, at 1706–08.

47. Easterbrook and Fischel 1991, at 92.

48. Davis 1985, at 47.

49. Arrow 1985, at 49.

50. Dranove and White 1987, at 413.

51. Mooney and Ryan 1993; Blomquist 1991; Ohsfeldt 1993.

52. The delegation is so extensive that British health economist Alan Williams has noted the irony that the actual structure of a treatment encounter often appears more as if the doctor is the principal and the patient is the agent.

53. Robinson 1993.

54. Frankel 1983, at 833.

55. Omnibus Budget Reconciliation Act of 1990, Pub. L. No. 101–508, § 4204(a)(1), 104 Stat. 1388, 1388-108 to -109 (codified at 42 U.S.C. §1395mm(i)(8)(A)-(B) (Supp. V 1993)). This statute rescinded for HMOs the total ban on hospital and HMO financial incentive plans that Congress initially applied to Medicare HMO patients in 1986. See Omnibus Budget Reconciliation Act of 1986, Pub. L. No. 99–509, § 9313(c)(1)(E), 100 Stat. 1874, 2003 (codified at 42 U.S.C. § 1320a-7a(b) (1988)). The 1990 legislation inexplicably left in place the ban on hospital financial incentive plans.

56. 61 Fed. Reg. 13,430 (March 27, 1996) (to be codified at 42 C.F.R. § 417.479(g)).

57. Capitation pays a set amount for each patient under the physician's responsibility, regardless of how much care each patient requires.

58. Hillman et al. 1991, at 207, 211.

59. 42 U.S.C. § 1395mm(i)(8)(A)(ii) (emphasis added).

60. Of all the HMO models using fee-for-service payment, 75 percent are IPAs. Hillman 1987, at 1745. See also Physician Payment Review Commission 1995; Gold, Hurley, Lake et al. 1995.

61. In a survey of all existing HMOs in 1986, with a response rate of only 51 percent, Hillman found that whereas two-thirds of all HMOs withhold a portion of pay from primary care physicians, only 21 percent of plans with salaried physicians do so. The same pattern persisted in 1994. Physician Payment Review Commission 1995; Gold, Hurley, Lake et al. 1995.

62. Hillman 1987 found that 82 percent of fee-for-service plans, 67 percent of capitation plans, and only 21 percent of salaried plans use withholds. See also Physician Payment Review Commission 1995; Gold, Hurley, Lake et al. 1995.

63. Ibid. Cases where withholds are as high as 50 percent are extremely rare. They are situations where the HMO was in such dire financial distress that the doctors most likely had little expectation that the withholds would be returned in any event. See U.S. Dep't of Health and Human Servs. 1990, at V-38.

64. "Physicians considered the 10% risk a cost of doing business." Moore and Martin 1983, at 1402.

65. See Hillman et al. 1989, at 90–91 (finding that only method of base payment—salary or capitation—had significant effect on hospitalization rates but that withholding funds did have some effect on use of outpatient services).

66. 61 Fed. Reg. 13,430 (to be codified at 42 C.F.R. § 417.479(e)). The higher- versus lower-risk threshold percentages apply according to whether the incentive payments are assessed annually or more frequently. The additional safeguards come in the form of requiring patient satisfaction surveys and imposing a stop-loss level of 5 percent above the threshold level.

67. See Woolhandler and Himmelstein 1995. The emphasis is on individual physicians because, as discussed below, if total capitation payments are made to a sufficiently large group, the disincentive to treat is greatly more attenuated and depends more on how profit and loss are distributed within the group than on the capitation payment itself.

68. This percentage figure cannot be compared with the 10–30 percent figure cited above, since the latter figure compares the out-of-pocket risk against the base physician payment amount, not against the total costs of treatment. To make such a comparison, it is necessary to know how to allocate the total HMO premium between primary care and other services. For example, if an arbitrary 50/50 allocation were assumed, the relevant risk percentage here would be 50 percent of the physician's base pay, or the prior risk range would be 20–60 percent of total treatment costs.

69. 61 Fed. Reg. 13,430 (to be codified at 42 C.F.R. § 417.479(e)–(g)).

70. 42 U.S.C. § 1395mm(i)(8)(A)(ii).

71. 61 Fed. Reg.13,430 (to be codified at 42 C.F.R. § 417.479(g)(i)–(ii)).

72. 42 U.S.C. § 1395mm(i)(8)(A)(i) (emphasis added).

73. 61 Fed. Reg. 13,430 (to be codified at 42 C.F.R. § 417.479(d)).

74. H.R. Rep. No. 899, 101st Cong., 2d Sess., pt. 1, at 121 (1990). Group size is also reflected in the regulations, which exempt incentives for any physician panel that covers more than 25,000 patients. 42 C.F.R. § 417.479(e).

75. 42 U.S.C. § 1395mm(i)(8)(A)(ii).

76. See generally Gold et al. 1995.

77. U.S. Dep't of Health and Human Servs. 1990, at V-19 to -20.

6

Informed Consent to Rationing

This chapter explores the extent to which resource allocation mechanisms and decisions must be disclosed to patients. Certainly some disclosure is required, but how much and at what time? These are crucial legal and ethical questions regardless of whether health care spending decisions are made by doctors, insurance companies, or government regulators. In any event, some one other than the patient is deciding, so the patient clearly has a right at least to know, if not to alter, the decision.

The right to know is especially crucial for those rationing mechanisms and incentives whose legitimacy depends on the autonomy rationale. The previous chapter, for instance, develops a detailed defense of using financial incentives to encourage economizing by physicians. This defense is based almost entirely on the principle of patient consent to economic conflicts of interest. If patients are not informed of these incentives, or are given no choice over whether to accept them, the foundational consent is obviously undermined. The disclosure issue is compelling even where financial inducement is absent. Regardless of whether physicians are forced to make rationing decisions by third-party rules, or whether they are induced to do so by educational or professional incentives, the messenger who delivers the news is under a fiduciary obligation of candor which the law of informed consent is designed to enforce.

The individual autonomy justification for various resource allocation mechanisms depends on both adequate disclosure and adequate choice. This chapter is focused on the disclosure issue, and its argument is primarily legal, not ethical.

The following chapter takes up the question of choice, that is, even with disclosure, whether consent to rationing is undermined because no viable options are offered; its argument is primarily one of moral and political theory.

This chapter explores the two distinct points at which disclosure of rationing can occur: the time of insurance enrollment or at the bedside. General resource allocation rules and incentives can be disclosed to subscribers of HMOs and other limited insurance plans as part of the terms of the insurance contract. Alternatively, physicians, at the time of treatment, can disclose specific decisions to decline individual items of potentially beneficial care on account of excessive costs. The chapter begins by summarizing the need for more honest descriptions of rationing rules and incentives at the time of insurance enrollment. It then demonstrates that, at the time of treatment, conventional informed consent law, if given its full logical force, could in theory extend to cover decisions to decline marginally beneficial treatment on account of costs; but the law has not yet done so, and a number of doctrinal currents are opposed to this movement. The law's ambivalence regarding ideal theory and actual doctrine is explained by the severe impracticality of requiring optimal patient self-determination under the constraints of limited insurance.

The fundamental incompatibility of conventional informed consent theory and modern economic reality requires that a new theory of economic informed consent be developed. The final part of this chapter articulates this theory using two concepts: prior consent and waiver of informed consent. The first concept reasons that, when patients make informed decisions to purchase more economical forms of health insurance, they consent in advance to a bundle of unspecified refusals of marginally beneficial care. This advance consent is how patients now consent to a bundle of minor treatment decisions when they enter a hospital and how they consent to a basic standard of care under negligence law when they retain a physician. Alternatively, the enrollment decision can be viewed as entailing an informed waiver of the right to be told of particular nontreatment decisions. Whether the courts will view these characterizations as legitimate turns on the nature of the disclosure that occurs at the time of enrollment and on the range of choice that subscribers have, either within the chosen plan or among different plans.

DISCLOSING RATIONING MECHANISMS
DURING INSURANCE ENROLLMENT

To illustrate the need to disclose rationing mechanisms at the time of insurance enrollment, consider the following hypothetical case:

A healthy HMO subscriber is surprised to discover in her mail one day a notice of an opportunity to join in a class action alleging deceptive trade practices. The suit is prompted by the HMO's failure to disclose to enrollees either (1) that it pays its physicians a bonus for keeping hospitalization and specialist referral expenses under budget or (2) that before primary care physicians can order hospitalization, specialist referral, or certain expensive diagnostic tests, they must obtain the permission of a utilization review director, who is constrained in her decisions by a detailed list of "appropriateness" indications for each of hundreds of possible conditions and treatments.

Apart from the legalities, is a subscriber justified in complaining that she has not been informed of rationing incentives and rules, even where there is no reason to believe she has received bad medical care?

HMOs are the best setting in which to pit the idealized ethical requirements of patient autonomy against the hard economic reality of scarce resources. Since their popularization in the early 1970s, HMOs have epitomized both spartan and utopian visions of health care.[1] Their basic method of payment creates an economizing incentive that causes physicians to be more parsimonious in using expensive, marginally necessary services than are doctors paid under open-ended reimbursement. Capitation payment also promotes the "health maintenance" ideal by creating a positive, prevention-oriented style of medicine, in contrast to the incentives under fee-for-service reimbursement which reward physicians the most for patients who are the sickest. This utopian orientation is reinforced with ideals of community and democracy. Under state licensing laws and the federal HMO Act (which sets qualifications for government support),[2] HMO boards must represent the community at large, HMOs must offer open enrollment on adjusted community-rated terms, and subscribers influence policy-making through numerous planning and grievance-resolution processes.[3]

Part of this intensive state and federal regulation is a host of disclosure requirements unlike anything that applies to other health care institutions. HMOs must describe their coverage benefits and limitations, procedures for obtaining care, rates, grievance procedures, service area, and participating providers.[4] These disclosures encompass many of the resource allocation decisions made through third-party mechanisms such as practice guidelines and utilization review. However, strikingly absent from this otherwise-comprehensive list is any requirement that HMOs describe to their enrollees the manner in which they induce their physicians to either abide by these mechanisms or to make economizing decisions on their own.[5]

The common law likewise has refrained so far from imposing a requirement to disclose rationing incentives, although it may yet yield one. An increasing number of plaintiffs' lawyers are arguing that an HMO physician's decision to withhold treatment, such as a Pap smear or biopsy to detect cancer, was inappropriately influenced by undisclosed financial incentives.[6] No definitive law has yet emerged because most of these cases have been settled or dismissed for technical reasons prior to trial. In one reported decision, however, the court ruled that an HMO incentive plan, even if undisclosed, does not constitute fraud or breach of warranty because such plans are consistent with public policy and do not interfere with sound medical judgment.[7] But in an unreported decision, a trial court refused to dismiss similar allegations, ruling that a jury should be allowed to consider whether an incentive plan contributed to the doctor's alleged negligence.[8]

Both of these cases alleged a duty to disclose rationing incentives when they lead to substandard treatment; therefore, neither case resolves whether nondisclosure is illegal wholly apart from the incentives' contribution to harmful negligence. Such a rule is suggested, though, by the much-noted decision in *Moore v. Regents of University of California*.[9] There a patient sought to recover the profits from bioengineered products that were derived from the cancerous spleen his doctors had removed from his body. The California Supreme Court rejected a property claim to the profits but upheld a tort claim for damages based on lack of informed consent. Suggesting that the eagerness to promote scientific advances might result in an unnecessarily risky operation, the court reasoned that, prior to an invasive surgery, a physician "must disclose personal interest unrelated to the patient's health, whether research, or economic, that may affect the physician's professional judgment."[10] Other courts have held that physicians must disclose their alcoholism or their HIV-positive status,[11] leading some commentators to speculate that there is a generalized right to know all factors that might adversely affect a physicians' judgment or performance.[12]

It remains to be seen whether these precedents will be extended to global disclosure of the method of physician payment at the time of HMO enrollment. In contrast to the cases decided so far, rationing incentives (as illustrated in the hypothetical case at the start of this section) affect decisions *not* to treat, and they do not necessarily lead to identifiable injuries. But whichever direction the law might take in the future, it is clear that no existing source of law—federal or state, statutory or judicial—requires the disclosure of the numerous HMO physician incentive payment plans described in Chapter 5, and such disclosure is in fact unheard of in practice.

These disclosure laws and practices are deceptively mired in the utopian ideal that HMOs provide better care for less money. No hint is given in any of the HMO marketing literature that the basic methods of payment to the corporate entity, or the particular payment formulae for individual doctors, create incentives to trim marginally beneficial treatments. To the contrary, HMOs stress their commitment to optimal health. One study of HMO advertisements concluded that they "tend to create a perception that services are provided in a generous and unlimited fashion . . . [belying] the economic premises of prepaid HMO practice."[13] A survey of HMO enrollees in one well-educated, sophisticated work force found that "the vast majority believed that 'in this plan the doctor is only concerned about my health and not limiting the plan's cost.'"[14] Even more disturbing, some HMOs actively suppress information about financial incentives, using "gag clauses" in their contracts with physicians. These clauses prevent physicians from discussing with anyone, including patients, the compensation terms and utilization review guidelines imposed by the HMO.[15]

There is no plausible justification for failing to disclose to HMO subscribers the manner in which rationing incentives function within the organization. Virtually every commentator to consider the issue agrees.[16] To quote only one:

> It is one thing to entrust your life and health at times of crisis to a physician who is committed to the practical ethics that involves a quest for excellence and who may err on the side of doing too much. It is quite another to entrust your life and health at times of crisis to a physician whose diagnostic and therapeutic interventions are limited by new regulatory constraints or incentives of competitive efficiency that "place the provider at economic risk." If the "provider" does not make the patient aware of the implications of that economic risk, then medical paternalism will inevitably take on a different and even more damning kind of odium.[17]

Although some of this insistence on strict candor is thinly disguised opposition to the entire managed care enterprise,[18] even portions of the managed care industry itself appear to agree with the moral obligation to disclose. The Midwest Bioethics Center convened a community task force to develop recommendations for managed care ethics, with heavy participation from the managed care industry. Task force members were "unanimous in their belief that members of managed care plans need to be made aware of how a capitated model works, . . . that they should be informed about payment methods and incentives to providers, and informed when there are potential conflicts of interest."[19]

Resource allocation incentives deserve disclosure because, unlike fee-for-service incentives, it cannot be presumed that the public is generally aware of how these mechanisms operate. Disclosure of financial conflicts of interest is a basic requirement of the fiduciary nature of the treatment relationship discussed in Chapter 5. Elsewhere, a number of state laws require the disclosure of investment and referral incentives that have a distorting *inflationary* effect.[20] Yet, when Congress considered the legality of incentive plans common in HMOs, it discussed only their regulation, never their disclosure.[21]

Many in the HMO industry are opposed to disclosure of the particular details of their physician incentive arrangements because they view this as sensitive business information.[22] This may be true, but information about the array of incentive arrangements in use is easy to come by, and little investment or creative energy is required to devise a formula such as "$25 a month per enrollee, less 20 percent to offset excessive costs of hospitalization and specialist referral services." In contrast, there are much more compelling reasons to keep medical practice guidelines secret that are used by utilization review organizations. These can be massive, complex systems that entail large amounts of expensive, ongoing research and field testing to keep them accurate and up-to-date. Making the details of these systems commonly available would much more plausibly undermine the competitive incentive to develop them in the first place. Also, utilization review firms fear that disclosure of their screening criteria would facilitate physicians' manipulating their diagnoses in order to circumvent the screens.

Even where trade secret claims are legitimate, they do not support total nondisclosure. The general nature and effect of a rationing mechanism can be sufficiently described without going into excruciating detail about its precise components. This is detail that almost surely would not be read even if it were presented. Some opponents of managed care and rationing have advocated that this disclosure be couched with such cautionary warnings and scare statistics that no sensible person would sign up,[23] much as abortion opponents have tried to stack the informed consent deck to intimidate vulnerable pregnant women with graphic descriptions of aborted fetuses and the like. But even in strict fiduciary contexts, the law does not require the recitation of statistical probabilities and quantified risks.

An unadorned description of how the plan works is all that a sensible disclosure standard requires. Physician ethicists Susan Goold and Howard Brody suggest the following appealing formulation:

At the time of enrollment, potential subscribers should be informed about the way allocation decisions are made in the organization, including delegation of some decisions to physicians and, if applicable, financial incentives physicians have to be cost-conscious. Examples of allocation decisions (e.g., refusing to cover referral to a dermatologist for a mole, decisions to restrict use of some medications) may make this more understandable. Second, at the first doctor-patient encounter, physicians should clearly inform patients that they have some responsibility, owed to the population of members as payers, to be prudent in using plan resources. For instance, a primary care provider, seeing a managed care patient for the first time, could say, "Part of my job, as a physician in this insurance plan, is to try and keep costs down so that premiums do not skyrocket. Now, I think that I can provide you with good, even excellent care even within these cost constraints, but you should know that I will consider costs in my recommendations. I will try and be honest about when there is a more expensive but marginally better option that I am not recommending, and you are always welcome to get a second opinion or to purchase it yourself." Or, "We will work together to get you everything you need, although not necessarily everything you want."[24]

DISCLOSURE AT THE TIME OF TREATMENT

It is easy to make the basic case for some global disclosure of resource allocation mechanisms and incentives at the time of enrollment, even though the details are subject to debate and may vary according to the relevant source of law. It is much more difficult to answer, however, whether physicians must disclose their cost/ benefit trade-off analyses microscopically at the bedside when they make individual treatment decisions. This requires a much more extensive analysis of informed consent law and its underlying moral theory. To better focus the lengthy discussion that follows, consider this set of facts:

A 42-year-old otherwise-healthy male with high blood pressure asks his HMO primary care physician for testing to determine the extent of his possible heart disease. The doctor orders a static electrocardiogram, which is a relatively inexpensive test, done on the spot. The test results are negative. Two months later, the patient suffers a nonfatal heart attack while jogging. His lawyer discovers that many respectable cardiac specialists would have performed a more accurate but much more expensive *exercise* stress test that requires referral to a specialized facility; however, it is also consistent with the prevailing standard of care to do only the simpler test for a younger, asymptomatic patient who is at low-to-moderate risk.

Assuming that the patient has no legal basis to claim conventional malpractice, still, does he have a valid informed consent claim for failing to disclose the existence of the more expensive alternative?

The Uncertain State of the Law

One appealingly simple answer to this question is that no disclosure is required for treatment not covered by insurance because providers have no obligation, absent an emergency situation, to render care for free. Informed consent law requires only disclosures that are material to a patient's possible decisions, and one might think it is immaterial to the patient's legal and practical options to disclose expensive but possibly beneficial care that the patient has no right to insist on payment for.[25] "Should a Mississippi dirt farmer be told of an expensive cancer treatment available at Sloan-Kettering that has a one in a thousand chance of saving his life?"[26] If the patient is unlikely to be able to afford the treatment on his own, disclosure is not only pointless, it can be cruel.

It seems clear, however, that knowledge of a nontreatment decision is still highly relevant to a patient's possible course of action, despite the absence of a legal obligation on the part of an insurer to pay for nonrecommended treatment. As philosophers Paul Menzel and Haavi Morreim have each argued, the patient might choose to pay out of pocket, seek to solicit donations, or attempt to challenge the insurer's decision.[27] Even apart from the possibility of acquiring the immediate treatment, the information might be material to a decision whether to switch doctors within the plan or to swtich insurance plans at the next open enrollment opportunity. Alternatively, the patient, considering the costs he would have to bear, might freely elect to follow the doctor's recommendation, thereby shoring up the doctor–patient relationship by avoiding a potential conflict. Some commentators believe that substantial savings could be achieved simply by telling patients more about the costs of their treatment options.[28] Finally, nontreatment information might be considered material, even if it objectively has no effect on any medical decision, simply because the patient would want to know purely for the sake of knowledge.[29] Few nontreatment decisions would clearly escape these standards of materiality. For these various reasons, we must carefully consider the full application of informed consent law.

Informed Consent Law in Theory and in Practice

On the surface, economically motivated decisions to decline marginally beneficial treatment do not readily fit informed consent law. That doctrine arose from battery law, which is concerned with offensive *touchings*, and its focus has al-

ways been on *medical risks*, not economic costs. Thus, several courts have concluded that informed consent liability is "limited to those situations where the harm
suffered arose from some affirmative violation of the patient's physical integrity
such as surgical procedures, injections or invasive diagnostic tests."[30] And, in actual
practice, only a minority of doctors regularly discuss with patients the economic
consequences of their treatment decisions.[31]

However, as the informed consent doctrine and its rationale have developed, it
has become easily capable of embracing a requirement that physicians disclose
each decision in which they bypass, for economic or other reasons, a potentially
beneficial treatment option. The central purpose of informed consent is to enhance
personal autonomy over decisions that affect physical and mental well-being. The
two classic, and incessantly quoted, judicial statements are: "Every human being
of adult years and sound mind has a right to determine what should be done with
his own body," and "Anglo-American law starts with the premise of thoroughgoing self determination. It follows that each man is considered to be master of
his own body."[32] As law professor Marjorie Shultz has thoroughly and cogently
argued, a treatment choice can be equally vital regardless of which way it is
resolved. "If the key issue is knowledge and choice regarding the fate of one's
body, there is no meaningful difference between a decision that will be implemented by touching the body and one that will [not]."[33] As for the medical versus
economic nature of the information disclosed, the California Supreme Court has
held:

> To be sure, questions about the validity of a patient's consent to a procedure typically
> arise when the patient alleges that the physician failed to disclose medical risks . . . and
> not when the patient alleges that the physician had a personal interest. . . . The concept of
> informed consent . . . is broad enough to encompass the latter. . . . [A] reasonable patient
> would want to know whether a physician has an economic interest that might affect the
> physician's professional judgment.[34]

Accordingly, virtually every commentator to consider the issue has concluded that,
either as a matter of law or as a matter of public policy, "a physician's duty to
disclose should extend to . . . [economically motivated] decisions about the withdrawal of care."[35]

Still, there is a difference between the full, logical extension of the purpose
underlying a body of legal doctrine and the literal requirements of the doctrine
itself. If informed consent law remains tied to its traditional doctrinal moorings,
then it may not be free to shape itself into a fully formed "dignitary tort," one that
would thoroughly protect a patient's right to be involved in all aspects of medical
decision making regardless of the ordinary elements of tort law. Several commentators have argued for such an extension, observing that this is the end point of
the path along which the informed consent doctrine has developed.[36] To better
understand this trajectory, I will briefly trace the path of informed consent law
from its origins to this fullest potential.[37]

Battery law, which first gave rise to informed consent liability, is a source of negative rights—the right to be left alone, absent consent. Battery law's application to medical situations was initially constrained by its lenient interpretation of what constitutes consent. The law absolves a batterer from liability if the victim consents after only a brief and general description of the contemplated "offensive touching." The consent requirement was heightened to its present "informed" status only by importing negligence law, which contains a positive duty to render care that meets professional standards. However, negligence law is constrained by its reference to professional custom. This requires the disclosure of only those elements of risk that most doctors customarily discuss with their patients. Therefore, the courts, simply by brute force of logic, not by reference to any existing precedent, heightened the informed consent obligation using a patient-centered test, which inquires whether the risk information is material to a reasonable person in the position of the plaintiff.

This is the point at which traditional informed consent law presently stands: a hybrid battery/negligence tort. Battery elements are retained by still requiring a harmful touching; the law does not punish every disagreeable withholding of information as negligence doctrine might do. Negligence is still respected by imposing causation and physical injury elements, which do not exist in battery law.[38] The plaintiff must show that the omitted disclosure would have changed her decision on the course of treatment and that this change would have improved the outcome. It is these remaining limitations—touching, causation, and injury—that some commentators seek to remove by casting the right to informed consent as a freestanding "dignitary tort," one that, much like invasion of privacy law does, vindicates a person's psychological interest in the information itself, without regard to the tangible consequences of the information.

Reformulating informed consent law into a free-standing dignitary tort would impose on doctors a positive duty to enhance a patient's medical self-determination to the ultimate extent possible. These commentators argue first that a full legal embodiment of patient autonomy requires the standard of care to be elevated from simple disclosure of risk to one of real understanding of the information conveyed (heightened duty).[39] They also argue that any deviation from this ideal should result in liability for the mere dignitary harm caused by denial of full participation in the medical decision. Thus, plaintiffs would be able to recover damages even though the medical risk did not materialize, and so no physical harm resulted (no injury), even though the patient would not have made any other decision if fully informed (no causation), and, most critical to our analysis, even though the decision was a purely passive one of deciding not to treat at all (no touching).[40] In short, these commentators would cut informed consent law entirely free from its doctrinal moorings, borrowing the most liberating, plaintiff-oriented elements of existing battery and negligence law while discarding all constraining elements and creating whole-cloth a uniquely heightened standard of care.

These arguments for an unprecedented[41] extension of tort law have been partially successful only with respect to the touching element, the one that is most
critical for the present inquiry. Removing the requirement of a harmful touching
obviously opens the door for a legal duty on the part of physicians to disclose
resource allocation decisions at the bedside. A handful of judicial decisions have
recognized a right of "informed refusal." This is a right to be informed of the
medical risks entailed in declining a proposed test or treatment. The leading case
is *Truman v. Thomas*,[42] in which the patient died from cervical cancer that could
have been detected had a Pap smear been administered earlier. The doctor testi-
fied that he had recommended the test several times over the course of six years
but the patient declined, stating she could not afford the cost. Nevertheless, the
California Supreme Court made him stand trial under an informed consent theory
because he failed to disclose all the benefits of the test and the risks of its refusal.
Truman has been followed in a number of other decisions,[43] including one in which
the plaintiff recovered $733,000 when his physician failed to urge him forcefully
enough to see a specialist about a tiny mole on his ear lobe that turned out to be
cancerous.[44]

In jurisdictions that do not go this far, informed consent law can still reach
nontreatment decisions. Even if the touching requirement is retained, a nontreatment option can be viewed as an alternative to the primary course of treatment. Conventional informed consent doctrine requires not only the disclosure of
risks that attend the primary intervention, but also the alternatives to that treatment and their risks and benefits.[45] Unless a physician decides to forgo all treatment, it will almost always be possible to conceive of an omitted test or procedure as an alternative to the affirmative medical intervention that was chosen.[46]
In the example on page 198, one court held that the treadmill EKG is an alternative to the resting EKG.[47] In another case, the court held that the physician violated the duty of informed consent by failing to inform a patient who had suffered
a head injury that performing a CAT scan is an alternative to simply observing
the condition.[48] In other words, the omitted procedure was viewed as an alternative to doing nothing.[49]

Cross Currents in the Law of Informed Refusal

To summarize up to this point, the law has shown itself partially amenable to the
idealists' vision of informed consent, which would extend it to all aspects of every
treatment decision, including treatment refusals for economic reasons. The touching requirement from battery law is not essential, and the absence of any insurance coverage for the nonrecommended treatment does not defeat the materiality
of informed-refusal disclosure. This section demonstrates, however, that despite
this theoretical support for extending informed consent law to reach resource allocation decisions, the law has not yet fully taken this step, and several legal currents flow decisively against such a requirement.

Some jurisdictions retain the battery law limitation that imposes a disclosure requirement only where there is some bodily invasion. Others are cautious about extending the requirement that alternative therapies be disclosed. Liability rarely rests squarely on the failure to disclose alternatives.[50] Courts narrowly construe this requirement to apply it only to entirely different courses of case management rather than to simple variations in the chosen course. For instance, in one case the court dismissed an informed consent claim against a doctor who delayed aggressive treatment for pneumonia, reasoning that prescribing additional antibiotics and hospitalizing the patient sooner were additional, not alternative, treatments. It was unnecessary to disclose them because they would not have altered the more limited, initial steps the doctor had taken. "The doctrine of informed consent does not apply to situations where the patient's decision is whether to submit to treatments in addition to the basic treatment given. Rather, it applies only to situations where the choice is between two or more distinct, alternative [mutually exclusive] methods of treatment."[51] More recently, a federal appeals court ruled that a doctor who treated but failed to detect the cause of a back injury need not disclose the additional diagnostic test that might have been done. The court reasoned that "the doctrine of informed consent [should not be transformed] into a general right to all information which the physician possesses."[52]

Even California and Washington State, the most demanding jurisdictions in enforcing informed refusal law, have drawn back the reins somewhat. *Truman v. Thomas* was decided by the narrowest of margins,[53] and subsequent lower courts have restricted it in a manner that precludes its application to rationing decisions. Several California decisions have ruled that, consistent with the facts in *Thomas*, that precedent applies only to nontreatment decisions made by the patient *contrary* to the doctor's medical advice.[54] This fact pattern characterizes each of the decisions that have followed *Thomas* except for one, *Gates v. Jensen*.[55] Therefore, even California courts have agreed that there is no general duty to inform patients of treatments the doctor is in fact not recommending.

Until recently, *Gates v. Jensen*, a 1979 case from Washington State, was the only significant decision squarely to the contrary, for only it had found informed consent liability where a *physician* declined to recommend additional treatment. The court imposed a duty to inform a patient that an alternate, more exact test exists for detecting glaucoma than the simpler test that was performed.[56] Then, in 1995, without citing to *Gates* or the California line of cases, the Wisconsin Supreme Court held a physician liable for $5 million in damages for failing to inform parents of a child who had suffered a head injury that a CAT scan was an alternative treatment to simply observing the child's condition.[57] The only other authority directly on point is a statute in Oregon under the Medicaid rationing scheme described in Chapter 3; this statute requires doctors to advise patients "of any service, treatment or test that is medically necessary but not covered" under the rationing list if it is the custom of other, similarly situated, doctors to do so.[58]

This statute and these two cases echo in empty solitude, however. As another court has observed, "although almost a decade has elapsed since *Gates* was decided, no evidence exists that it has been hailed by courts or commentators. . . . Our search has failed to reveal any case outside the State of Washington in which *Gates* has been cited as persuasive authority."[59] *Gates* has not fared well inside the state either. Under the same fact pattern as the hypothetical case on page 198 (performing a resting EKG rather than a treadmill test failed to reveal severe heart disease), five of Washington's eight justices refused to follow *Gates*.[60] Thus, while in theory the fully extended rationale for informed consent is capable of reaching physicians' decisions to decline marginally beneficial treatment due to its cost, the law has shown considerable reluctance to actually taking this step.

Prudential Limits on Economic Informed Consent

Judicial ambivalence about holding doctors liable for not informing patients of nonrecommended treatment may be caused by the severe burden informed refusal liability would place on the practical workings of doctor–patient relationships. Taken to its logical extreme, informed consent law would require physicians to engage their patients in elaborate explanations for each discrete step in a complex tree of diagnostic and treatment options for even the most minor of ailments. In deciding to employ just a single test, a physician might explicitly or elliptically pass over a dozen or more options. If some commentators had their way, at each step in an ongoing course of treatment physicians might have to engage the patient in an extensive, 14-point dialogue as to each of these treatment alternatives,[61] periodically stopping to test the patient's full comprehension of what he is being told and videotaping these encounters[62] to ensure proof of a sufficiently "prolonged conversation"[63] and "shared decisionmaking."[64] There are no better words than Justice Clark's dissent in *Truman* to capture the extreme impracticability of enforcing this informed consent ideal:

Carried to its logical end, the majority decision requires physicians to explain to patients who have not had a recent general examination the intricacies of chest examinations, blood analyses, X-ray examinations, electrocardiograms, urine analyses and innumerable other procedures. In short, today's ruling mandates doctors to provide each such patient with a summary course covering most of his or her medical education. . . . [This] onerous duty . . . will result in reduced care for others. Requiring physicians to spend a large portion of their time teaching medical science before practicing it will greatly increase the cost of medical diagnosis—a cost ultimately paid by an unwanting public. Persons desiring treatment for specific complaints will be deterred from seeking medical advice once they realize they will be charged not only for treatment but also for lengthy lectures on the merits of their examination.[65]

Thoroughgoing disclosure at the bedside of each aspect of and influence on every treatment option is impractical for several reasons. First, it is inconsistent with the nature of clinical judgment and the manner in which financial constraints are likely to be considered by physicians. Physicians are humans, not computers. As discussed in Chapter 3, their judgmental processes are often more elliptical and heuristic than they are methodical and calculated. Like any other professional engaged with a complex body of knowledge and experience, physicians are subliminally affected by countless influences. Their practice styles develop more from habit and learned tradition than from rigorous, deductive logic. As resource constraints become more manifest, physicians are likely to alter their practice styles more or less subconsciously so that they engage in what is referred to as implicit rather than explicit rationing.[66] Therefore, physicians often may not overtly consider that they are making marginal sacrifices in optimal medical benefit. As demonstrated by the British experience, they will tend to adjust their views of proper practice to fit within the constraints they face.[67] Since implicit rationing will often occur without conscious deliberation, it is unrealistic to require physicians to disclose thought processes they in fact are not actually engaged in.

Assuming, though, that such disclosures were a practical feasibility, we would also have to consider the consequences for the physician–patient relationship. The upshot of the physician's disclosure is that a margin of safety is being sacrificed out of a concern for costs and perhaps in a manner that will ultimately reward the physician. As Haavi Morreim has observed, the physician would repeatedly be confessing to a slight but tangible compromise of the patient's maximal treatment interest out of consideration for his own or someone else's economic self-interest.[68] It is difficult to see how patient trust could survive ongoing disclosures of this nature, yet it is patient trust that informed consent is designed to foster. One physician reports that, in her experience in an HMO gatekeeping capacity, "the collective impact of these negative encounters, though each in itself might have been minor, created a climate of suspicion, cynicism, readiness to fight, and a sense of being used that permeated my office in a way that I had not known before."[69]

The fact that these disclosures could prove so destructive of trust indicates that the decisions being made and the incentives being used may be pernicious. Physicians should not agree to function under institutional and financial arrangements they are not willing to honestly disclose to their patients. On the other hand, given the paradoxes of the psychological basis for patients' trust described in Chapter 5, it is quite possible that, for some perfectly acceptable decisions and incentives, patients would prefer to be kept in purposeful ignorance, or at least to be told only occasionally rather than being reminded each time they see their doctor. Chapter 2 explains that there may be good reasons not to want to be bombarded by the brutal but unalterable reality of limited resources throughout each treatment encounter, at a time when patients may be emotionally vulnerable and in need of reassurance due to the extreme anxiety of serious illness. People may be much better able and willing to process this information at the time of insurance enrollment.

Morreim hopes to ameliorate the dilemma between preserving physician discretion and undermining patient trust by using specially trained staff to assist physicians in conducting these delicate disclosures in a manner that avoids upsetting patients.[70] This is a sound idea, but it envisions the disclosure of rather vague generalizations that fail to specify the actual treatment options being omitted. Instead, these disclosures more closely resemble the global disclosures at the time of insurance enrollment, which merely put patients on notice of the general incentive structure for resource allocation and their rights to inquire further about specific treatment decisions. Even if this were a sensible hybrid—general, global economic disclosures at each treatment encounter—this type of disclosure would hardly withstand the rigor of courtroom scrutiny, which requires a much sharper degree of detail and description. The simple and innocuous disclosures that seem compatible with daily patient encounters might not protect physicians from liability. Consider, for instance, the following example taken from Goold & Brody 1995:

A physician, talking with a patient with typical migraines, might say, "Your headaches are typical for migraines. In about one of 1,000 cases these types of headaches are due to other abnormalities, which we could find on a CT scan or MRI of the head. There is also a good chance (about one out of three) that an 'abnormality' on a scan would not really be there, and this could cause worry and possibly unnecessary further tests. I don't generally recommend scans for migraines because of this risk of error and because they are expensive."[71]

In comparison, as mentioned earlier, a California court upheld a large plaintiff's verdict for failing to urge a patient forcefully enough to obtain a biopsy on a tiny mole, holding that it was not sufficient for the doctor, a general practitioner, to "strongly recommend [seeing] a specialist" and to warn him that "all pigmented skin lesions are suspicious in nature" until removed and studied microscopically. The court reasoned that the doctor should have specifically mentioned the risk of cancer and its consequences.[72]

A final practical obstacle to thoroughgoing disclosure of economically motivated treatment refusals is the effect on potential contract disputes over the terms of insurance coverage. Health insurance coverage is almost universally defined in terms of "medical necessity," which is interpreted in practice as covering any treatment that is potentially of any medical benefit.[73] Therefore, in order for managed care plans to maintain a legally defensible denial of care, at present they are well advised to contend that the treatment is either harmful or of no plausible benefit. Honest appraisals of health care rationing decisions, however, require physicians to admit that some attenuated, long-shot benefits may be sacrificed and that some other doctors may have a different view. Once this is conceded, however, insurers will be hard pressed in the current legal environment to deny coverage for the treatment. Physicians are caught in the intractable dilemma: Treatment denials should be truthfully disclosed, but an unvarnished disclosure will have the practical effect of undermining their ability to enforce the denial.

This then brings us to the crux of a quandary first posed by philosopher Norman Daniels:

An interesting question now arises. Suppose that the only way for a [health care] ration-ing scheme to remain stable is for the grounds for the rationing to be disguised, and yet there are good prudential reasons for implementing such a scheme. Is the scheme just? . . . It may be that what is ideally just is not feasible under some conditions, that is, if the publicity constraints are adhered to. We then need an account of what is permissible when what ought to be justifiable is politically infeasible. Here philosophers have generally fallen silent, and I shall too.[74]

While philosophers have the luxury of remaining silent, the law does not. It is presented with these concrete dilemmas and must respond in some fashion, for when asked to compensate real injury, silence itself is an answer.

In other, analogous contexts, the law has resolved the conflict between ideal patient self-determination and the practical demands of social necessity by sacri-ficing somewhat the ethical ideal. A distant analogy can be found in the disclosure practices that occur when public health or safety regulations require physicians to breach their patients' confidences. Every state by statute requires physicians to report to the police any patient of theirs suspected of child abuse; they must also report to public health authorities various kinds of contagious conditions such as HIV infection.[75] Similarly, psychiatrists have a duty to prevent their dangerous patients from injuring themselves or others, either by confining the patient or by warning the potential victim.[76] Strict adherence to informed consent theory would require doctors to inform their patients of these conflicted responsibilities either at the outset of the treatment relationship or at the time of reporting. However, the same pragmatic concerns that apply to resource allocation decisions make it inconceivable that informed consent doctrine would actually impose liability for failing to warn of public health and safety disclosures. As Tom Murray explains, "such a warning would be awkward at best, usually unnecessary, and it might make the establishment of an open, trusting relationship difficult. . . . Practically, then, 'Miranda'-type warnings are likely to create as many problems as they solve."[77]

The compromise of informed consent ideals to meet real-world prudential con-cerns can be seen in a host of other, more prosaic, aspects of legal doctrine and actual practice.[78] Most telling is the obvious fact that informed consent is rou-tinely sought only for invasive procedures and at major junctures in the course of treatment, such as at the point of hospital admission. Despite the doctrine's literal application to every single treatment or nontreatment decision, and despite the defensive behavior caused by physicians' hypersensitive liability concerns, rarely is written informed consent obtained to prescribe medication or perform a rou-tine test.[79] Never is it obtained for the multitude of injections, bodily inspections and manipulations, midnight awakenings, and other personal invasions one en-counters during the course of hospitalization. It is simply felt that, in practice, it is not worth carrying informed consent requirements to their logical extreme for minor, routine steps, even on pain of the physician's liability or the patient's risk of harm.

This practice is consistent with legal doctrine, which presumes that, by submitting oneself to treatment, a patient consents, absent any objection, to the many minor bits and pieces that make up the entire treatment encounter. This "bundling" concept of informed consent arises by legal implication even though the patient receives no risk/benefit disclosure about each of these component parts. For instance, one court ruled that no special informed consent is required for use of forceps during delivery, since this is simply a tool for carrying out the general treatment plan that the patient agrees to upon admission to the hospital.[80]

The law regularly compromises pristine informed consent to practical reality in other ways. The unique core of informed consent, which separates it from ordinary battery law, is its requirement that patients comprehend, not simply consent to, the risks entailed in a medical decision. In theory, the emphasis is on substantive understanding gained through meaningful conversations rather than on procedural formalities such as signing paperwork. But if full comprehension were the literal standard, much beneficial medical care could simply not be rendered. Dozens of empirical studies have documented the frustrating reality that some people will never sufficiently comprehend the medical options they face regardless of how thorough the explanation. They simply lack the intellectual capacity, the personal motivation, or the experiential base to come to grips with any form of disclosure.[81] The law, recognizing the frailty of human intelligence and communication skills, does not in fact require actual understanding, only adequate disclosure. Informed consent requirements are satisfied simply by a recitation of the material risks in language that ordinary people *should* understand; it is not necessary to demonstrate the actual comprehension that informed consent ideally is intended to foster.[82]

The law also compromises informed consent ideals in the core elements of causation and materiality of risk. Despite trenchant criticism from academic commentators, about half the states retain an objective, reasonable-person standard for what information doctors must disclose rather that the subjective, individual-patient standard that logically is necessary to fully promote the value of individual autonomy.[83] This dichotomy is even more striking for the causation element of whether disclosure would have changed the patient's mind. Again, although a subjective standard best fits with informed consent theory,[84] all states enforce an objective, "reasonable person" test for proving what decision the patient would have made if properly informed. Courts and legislatures have been persuaded to set aside theoretical niceties in favor of administrability after considering the difficulties that physicians would have in defending against the resulting accusations in front of juries sympathetic to the plight of unfortunate victims.[85] The latest example of this pragmatic restraint can be found in the California Supreme Court's 1993 decision in *Arato v. Avedon*. There, the court held that doctors need not specifically disclose the low chance of success of a demanding treatment regimen for cancer that ultimately failed. The court rejected the family's claim that the patient was put through needless suffering, stating:

The [clinical contexts] in which physicians and patients interact and exchange information . . . are so multifarious, the information needs and degree of dependency of individual patients so various, and the professional relationship itself such an intimate and irreducibly judgment-laden one, that we believe it is unwise to require as a matter of law that a particular species of information be disclosed.[86]

Analogous prudential concerns counsel that pristine informed consent be compromised in the resource allocation situation as well. This is the path that Great Britain has taken,[87] partly out recognition that "the economics of the British National Health Service could not tolerate" total patient sovereignty.[88] Similarly, in our much richer but still constrained health care financing system, the scope of a physician's obligation should be shaped by a realistic sense of what is feasible within a managed care treatment relationship. Even some of the commentators who advance the most utopian versions of informed consent ethics concede that the law is too blunt an instrument for behavioral control to enforce an ethical ideal through liability rules.[89] But as convincing as this pragmatic reasoning might be, it still fails to supply a principled basis for abruptly suspending all informed consent requirements in a resource-constrained environment. Specifying exactly what disclosures should and should not occur requires filling in this analytical void with a new theory of economic informed consent.

A THEORY OF ECONOMIC INFORMED CONSENT

Ethics and Economics in Fundamental Conflict

The full, unfettered autonomy model that is embodied in the idealist version of informed consent has its roots in the broad-based social movement known as bioethics which arose in the 1960s and 1970s. In the spirit of the civil rights movement, seminal decisions such as *Quinlan* and *Canterbury*[90] invoked the doctrine of informed consent as a legal tool to empower patients and to counter the deeply entrenched paternalism of the medical establishment. These developments occurred during an era of unconstrained financing, when private insurance deferred absolutely to individual physician and patient desires and Medicare and Medicaid had just been formulated on the same laissez-faire reimbursement model.[91] Vigorous enforcement of informed consent law fit hand-in-glove with open-ended, charge-or-cost-based reimbursement with free choice of physician. This blank check form of insurance was fully compatible with eliciting and effectuating the full range of patients' personal values and preferences at every stage of medical care. With insurers hardly raising an eyebrow, patients could afford to demand as many and whichever doctors they wanted, and they could become active and informed participants in each stage of treatment decision making, ordering every conceivable test and procedure that offered some plausible benefit.

Paradoxically, informed consent ethics and health care economics are also fully compatible with a time earlier in the century, prior to the spread of health insurance, when patients paid almost entirely out of pocket. Then, too, patients had a right to demand all the care they could afford to pay for, but physicians and hospitals could decline patients unable to pay. Although informed consent law was not then fully enforced, had it been, autonomy would be fully respected on both sides of the treatment relationship, within the constraints of available resources.

Now, we find that neither state of affairs is acceptable. Comprehensive, unlimited insurance is no longer affordable, and the state of medical science is such that patients should not be forced to pay primarily out of pocket. Health insurance is both desirable and affordable, but the form of insurance that is most affordable does not allow us to demand all the care that conceivably is of any benefit regardless of cost. Therefore, we must adopt what I refer to as the patient welfare compromise of insured-but-rationed health care. This patient welfare compromise creates an ethical bind: In order for affordable insurance to exist, some degree of financial autonomy must be relinquished to physicians or others.

Perfect autonomy would be achieved if insurance were banned and patients were forced to pay for all of their care out of pocket, for then the cost/benefit trade-off for each discrete treatment decision would be authorized by each patient. But we have a strong desire for some form of insurance in order to guard against the exigencies of poor health and the anxiety of having to think about money during the stress of illness. Some sacrifice of legally enforceable autonomy is necessary if a system of comprehensive but affordable insurance is to be maintained. The very nature of insurance makes it impossible to carry out all patient preferences at the time of treatment and still preserve the patient welfare compromise. After purchasing insurance, a patient no longer has the incentive to fully evaluate the cost-effectiveness of various treatment options. Insured patients have a strong free rider incentive to order more care than they would be willing to insure against if the choice were put to them at the time they were making the enrollment decision. It is for this reason that we can no longer give full force to the notion of patient autonomy as it has been conceived of by conventional bioethics—from the perspective of the presently ill but fully-insured patient.

The desire to preserve an affordable form of insurance demands that we formulate a new brand of ethics, one that is sensitive to the patient welfare compromise entailed in rationed insurance. The patient's choice to assign resource allocation decisions to others so that she does not have to pay for all care out of pocket necessarily diminishes her role in making the resulting medical spending decisions. For ethics or law to insist that all beneficial medical treatment must continue to be ordered regardless of the cost is to force patients to purchase a brand of insurance they may no longer afford. And for patients under rationed insurance to insist on treatment whose costs outweigh its benefits is to demand more comprehensive insurance coverage than they have paid for (or than voters through their legislators have agreed to fund).

This reasoning, however, only goes so far as to reject the furthest reaches of individual rights-based bioethics. It does not resolve what bounds may properly be set on the level of participation patients may continue to expect in resource allocation decisions. Even if patients can no longer insist on all treatment for free, can they at least insist on being told of each treatment that is being denied? To answer this, we must construct a new theory of economic informed consent, one that reconciles legal idealism with practical necessity. I propose to do this through the analytical devices of prior consent and waiver of consent.

This theory of economic informed consent reasons that when consumers make fully informed purchasing decisions to join a constrained insurance plan rather than an unlimited one, they knowingly opt into an economizing style of medicine in exchange for lower premiums or more comprehensive coverage. Inherent in this informed purchasing decision is acquiescence in a system for rationing marginally beneficial care, either through centralized rules or by individualized discretion. This rational choice of a cost-sensitive practice style, if properly disclosed in advance, can entail either prior consent, or waiver of informed consent, to giving up particular items of treatment on account of their costs. Thus, if the global disclosure of rationing rules and incentives occurs that is recommended at the start of this chapter, this can be taken as, in itself, fully satisfying the theoretical requirements of informed consent law without necessitating further treatment-specific disclosures when the individual medical spending decisions are made or enforced at the bedside.[92] More detailed disclosures are required only in response to questioning by the patient.

Prior Consent To Rationing

Actual versus Presumed Consent

I am not the first to suggest the concept of prior consent to health care rationing as a way to reconcile the demands of patient autonomy with the need to preserve an affordable form of insurance. Paul Menzel[93] and others[94] have developed the general reasoning that patients can be bound at the time of treatment to decisions made when they purchase insurance. In my own way of putting it, prior consent reasons that enrolling with an HMO constitutes blanket advance consent to the subsequent denials of marginally beneficial care brought about by the rules, procedures, and incentives disclosed at the outset (and periodically affirmed through annual open enrollment decisions); thereafter, additional disclosure at the time of treatment is unnecessary.

Prior consent should not be confused with the separate concept of presumed consent, which Menzel also develops.[95] Presumed consent reasons that consent requirements are satisfied if it can be shown that *had* the patient been asked she would have consented. Menzel argues that presumed consent is an adequate substitute when actual consent is impossible or prohibitively costly; for instance, actual consent is not required from a patient in an emergency condition. He extends this absolute incapacity argument to the relative disabling effect that insurance has on economic rationality. The inability of insured patients to rationally assess which medical benefits are worth the costs paid by insurance is a form of incapacity that allows the invocation of presumed consent. Since the proper vantage point from which to gauge patients' cost-sensitive treatment preferences is when they choose how much to spend on an insurance premium, Menzel argues that resource allocation decisions are legitimate when they reflect what the patient would have agreed to if asked before she was sick, at the time of enrollment.

This controversial position raises a number of empirical and normative difficulties. The main empirical difficulty is knowing what patients actually would have agreed to. The normative difficulty is that the moral significance of presumed consent is far inferior to that of actual consent in satisfying the personal autonomy values that underlie the informed consent requirement. As Menzel recognizes, presumed consent carries moral weight only where it is impossible or prohibitively expensive to obtain actual consent. The problem is that "prohibitive" cost is defined as costly enough that the person in question would, if asked, prefer not to be consulted. Since it is often not feasible to actually ask this, we are forced to speculate whether and when patients would find presumed consent acceptable.[96]

Fortunately, we need not resolve these difficulties created by presumed consent since my argument is that a fully informed decision to enroll in a limited insurance plan constitutes *actual* consent to the subsequent treatment decisions. Under proper enrollment procedures, there is nothing fictitious about the consent. Obtaining actual consent to rationing is not infeasible if one relinquishes the notion of consenting to discrete treatment decisions and instead adopts the concept of consent to a decision making *mechanism*. Actual informed consent is given, even if all of the multitude of possible nontreatment decisions and their particular risks and benefits are not described to the patient, because the patient is informed of and consents to the broad parameters contained in a set of resource allocation rules or implemented by a set of economizing physician incentives. By agreeing in advance to these rules and incentives, a subscriber is bound by the treatment decisions that result from these mechanisms, much as a principal is bound by the commitments his chosen agent makes for him, even though he is unaware of them.[97]

Bundled Consent to a Diminished Standard of Care

Prior consent to a treatment refusal mechanism is precisely the basis on which surrogate decision making is founded for refusing life-sustaining treatment using a "durable (or medical) power of attorney." The patient's informed appointment of a health care agent satisfies consent requirements even for decisions as monumental as withdrawing life-support. In essence, the argument here is that an informed enrollment decision constitutes prior explicit consent to appointing the HMO medical director and the primary care physician as agents for a bundle of less significant but equally (or more) nonspecific treatment refusal decisions.

Bundled consent is also how we now view a single decision to be hospitalized or operated on. These decisions are taken as entailing consent to hundreds of discrete events of testing, medication, and bodily examination during the course of what may be a rather long and complex episode of treatment.[98] We would think it frivolous for a hospital patient to argue that his privacy was invaded because he never gave specific consent to be woken countless times at night for blood pressure and temperature checks, or that nurses committed battery by injecting an I.V. needle to administer fluids or antibiotics ordered by the doctor. These low-profile intrusions are so second nature that doctors, nurses, and even patients do not conceptualize them as discrete decisions requiring consent.[99] Likewise, bundled consent should apply to economically motivated refusals of marginally beneficial treatment because, when an insurance subscriber knowingly enrolls in a constrained system of financing, he buys into an entire cost-constrained medical philosophy and set of practices.

This bundling concept is also the analytical foundation for the conventional malpractice standard of care. The strongest justification for using professional custom as the basis for malpractice liability is that this is the duty that a provider implicitly undertakes when a treatment relationship is formed.[100] Modern "relational contracting" theory explains that it is unrealistic to impose on patients and physicians the impossible burden of specifying the minutiae of an explicit contractual standard of medical practice. Instead, the law assumes that doctors, when they take on the care of a patient, automatically promise the bundle of unspecified treatment obligations entailed in customary professional practice. Patients cannot assert that they are not governed by the conventional practice standard simply because they lack specific notice of its content. When patients choose generalists over specialists, or choose non-physician-allied health professionals or practitioners of holistic medicine, it is taken for granted that a lower or different standard of care applies without the need to specifically warn patients that superior care may be available elsewhere.[101]

As economic constraints induce practice styles to shift, one or more cost-constrained malpractice standards will emerge as respectable alternatives to the inflated, fee-for-service standards that historically prevailed.[102] Thus, commentators envision that a separate HMO custom will govern negligence suits brought by HMO patients.[103] Where that standard is explicitly disclosed (in general terms) at the time of enrollment, informed consent requirements should not be allowed to negate it.

This line of argument does not quite hit the mark, however. It only establishes that informed consent is not necessary to alter the malpractice standard of care. More relevant is whether, within the range of acceptable treatment decisions, informed consent requires disclosure before opting for one minimally acceptable treatment over a possibly superior alternative. The conventional understanding of the fit between malpractice law and informed consent is that, even though the malpractice standard is set globally at the time the relationship is formed, the disclosure requirement still must be met when individual, nonnegligent[104] treatment decisions are made. Similarly, here, the objection would be that global disclosure of rationing mechanisms is sufficient only to set the outer contractual bounds of a lower, cost-sensitive standard of customary practice; it does not exonerate physicians' informed consent obligations at the bedside, which are based on the fiduciary character of the treatment relationship.

The same result can be accomplished through another route, however. Even applying informed consent at the bedside, about half the states apply a professional custom standard to determine what information must be disclosed and for what events. In these jurisdictions, physicians would not have to disclose specific nontreatment decisions if a respectable number of doctors in similar practice settings routinely did not do so. Admittedly, most academic commentators reject the professional standard in favor of a patient-specific standard for disclosure, but even in many of the more liberal jurisdictions that accept this argument, treatment-specific consent is required only for the most dramatic, invasive, and high-stakes medical decisions such as surgery.[105] Otherwise, routine treatment decisions are judged only by the baseline professional custom standard provided by malpractice law.

Similarly, in the context of our inquiry, even if informed consent law were to be liberalized to reach nontreatment decisions that are consistent with a cost-constrained standard of care, they should reach only the most dramatic, high-stakes nontreatment decisions, such as pulling the plug on life-support or declining a life-saving operation for a terminally ill patient. Otherwise, everyday, small-ticket, and low-stakes decisions made at the margin of conventional treatment patterns are simply consented to in advance as part of the basic agreement to a cost-constrained standard of care. Therefore, the law should require bedside disclosure in the former situations despite the difficulty that arises in drawing a justiciable line between dramatic versus routine treatment refusals. It may be, though, that legislative enactment or regulatory oversight would do a better job than the common law in crafting a suitable distinction.

The Transparency Standard and Clinical Judgment

Further support for the bundled-consent concept can be drawn from the academic literature that critiques informed consent law. Critics complain that this body of law is incompatible with medical practice because it arises from legal principles that were developed in an adversarial setting between strangers. Attempting to fit legal rights into this mold results in breaking a caring, trusting, and interactive relationship into unnaturally discrete and confrontational decision points. "The law views the transaction cross-sectionally (there is disclosure and there is agreement) . . . rather than [as] an on-going organic process."[106] For this reason, bundled consent at the outset of the physician–patient relationship is more consistent with the nature of medical practice than are discrete and sporadic disclosures throughout. It occurs at the point the relationship is being formed or renewed, and in a setting that unavoidably is already contractual in nature.

The bundling concept is also consistent with the manner in which doctors are likely to factor cost constraints into their clinical thought processes. As discussed above, doctors are likely to consider costs only subliminally, as their practice styles gradually evolve to accommodate reimbursement constraints or clinical guidelines. Such unconscious thought processes are not the primary target of informed consent law. Instead, it applies mainly to decisions deliberately made. Accordingly, Howard Brody advocates the adoption of a "transparency standard" that requires doctors to disclose "precisely those [factors] that the physician weighed seriously before deciding what intervention to recommend,"[107] leaving to the patient the obligation to ask questions when clarification and elaboration are desired.[108] This is consistent with the view that the main purpose of informed consent law is to require the doctor to disclose what she is thinking; its primary job is not to force her to think and practice differently than she actually does. That is the job of professional negligence law.

It is highly questionable whether this transparency standard would survive judicial scrutiny when applied to invasive procedures. The leading case specifically "discard[s] the thought that the patient should ask for information before the physician is required to disclose. . . . Caveat emptor is not the norm for the consumer of medical services."[109] This transparency standard has greater legal support in the context of treatment refusals, however. Several courts have held, for instance, that where the heart of a complaint is negligent nontreatment or misdiagnosis, informed consent does not apply because no actual treatment decision was made to which an informed consent requirement could attach. Instead, the doctor's (in)actions must be judged under the ordinary malpractice standard of care.[110]

One particularly notable instance of this negligent nontreatment reasoning is found in the "wrongful birth" suits brought by the parents of severely deformed infants. These suits seek to hold obstetricians liable for failing to recommend diagnostic tests that might have revealed a birth defect or genetic risk in time to avoid conception or obtain an abortion.[111] Even though the heart of the patient's complaint is inadequate information, wrongful birth cases are not reasoned on "informed refusal" grounds. Rather, proper genetic counseling is considered to be simply part and parcel of the obstetrical standard of care, governed by professional custom.[112] Similarly, when genetic testing is performed, Sherman Elias and George Annas recommend that the risks of genetic screening be disclosed in a generic fashion that obtains blanket consent to a bundle of tests at the outset of the endeavor. Even these strong advocates of patients' rights see no need to specifically inform patients of each of the particular abnormalities that might be detected or to warn them of the tough pregnancy or family planning decisions they might have to make.[113]

An even more direct application of this reasoning that is widely accepted in bioethics and the law applies to so-called "futile" treatment—care that falls outside the prevailing standard of care more from its lack of medical benefit than its medical risk. The conventional thinking is that informed consent law cannot be used to force physicians to provide care that, in their view of medical benefit, has no utility whatsoever, such as laetrile for cancer patients, antibiotics for a viral respiratory infection, or megadoses of vitamin C for a common cold. No one even considers that doctors should inform patients as they silently bypass such generally disapproved alternatives, even though some other doctors indeed believe in the utility of these treatments.[114] Physicians are free to limit themselves to their chosen school of practice so long as that school is accurately reflected in their representations to the general patient community.

However, it is much more controversial whether this same thinking should apply if the concept of "futility" expands to cover care that is of *marginal* benefit. Some bioethicists and physicians increasingly are arguing that very expensive and invasive treatment for terminally ill patients should be declared "futile," even if it provides rare or temporary relief, so long as the treatment has almost no chance of reversing the patient's underlying condition. For instance, they argue that *physicians and nurses* may refuse CPR even though it may in fact revive the patient, if statistics show he is very unlikely to survive to leave the hospital.[115] It is disturbing how common this practice is.[116] Relying on the traditional applications of the futility concept, some of these commentators go further and argue that futile treatment of this sort can be declined even without informing the patient or his family.[117] That some highly respected clinical ethicists believe that treatment-specific disclosure is not required even for dramatic, life-and-death nontreatment decisions that are deceptively labeled as "futile" certainly causes some concern about expanding physicians' authority over resource allocation decisions. The willingness on the part of some thoughtful commentators to go this far does indicate by contrast that it is not ethically extreme to lift disclosure requirements for much more routine and low-visibility treatment refusals, particularly where patients are informed in advance that they are subject to these resource allocation decisions.

Waiver of Informed Consent

It is perhaps easier to characterize an informed enrollment decision not as advance consent to medical spending decisions but as a waiver of the right to be informed when such decisions are made. Actual prior consent justifies silent rationing by arguing that global disclosure satisfies the primary duty; waiver invokes an affirmative defense to a prima facie violation of that duty. Under the waiver characterization, informed consent requirements are not met; they are dispensed with at the patient's request. A number of legal authorities and commentators have observed in passing that informed consent can be waived, for to rule otherwise would undermine the very value of personal autonomy that the doctrine is intended to enforce.[118] Allowing waiver is perfectly consistent with informed consent doctrine since the principal effect of consent is itself a waiver—of the right not to be touched. The law is not foolish enough to hold that the primary right of bodily integrity can be waived but that the secondary informational right cannot.

Waiver of informed consent is commonly practiced in even the most ethically scrutinized of treatment settings—medical research. Despite the rigorous application of informed consent principles that is necessary to meet federal funding requirements,[119] research subjects routinely are allowed to waive full disclosure in the interests of science when they participate in double-blinded studies that require some of them to receive placebos.[120] Even more potent is the form of waiver inherent in research that involves mild forms of deception, as is common in psychology. In order to produce certain behavioral effects or avoid certain biases, study participants are sometimes actively misled about the object of the study and the identities and roles of the various participants. In these circumstances, informed consent is dispensed with not by the individual participants but by the "Institutional Review Board" that approves the study.[121]

Some academics argue that proper respect for personal autonomy prohibits enforcing waivers of informed consent.[122] These strict autonomists sometimes characterize informed consent as an "inalienable" right.[123] Because the law clearly does not accept this misapplication of the concepts of autonomy and inalienability,[124] I will summarize in only the briefest fashion the flaws in this argument, grouped around the purposes informed consent is intended to serve. As with most ethical dictates, the purpose of informed consent may be framed in either instrumental or intrinsic terms:[125] Patient participation in medical decision making may be necessary to achieve some other, ultimate purpose (such as better patient health), or instead informed consent may be a good in itself because it enhances personal autonomy.

An instrumentalist must honor valid waivers of informed consent because patients might decide that full disclosure causes them excessive anxiety, is too time-consuming, or is otherwise not, in their own view, in their overall best interests.[126] The very act of consulting a doctor and submitting to treatment entails a waiver of some rights to bodily integrity, yet the relinquishment of these fundamental rights for the patient's greater good is never questioned. For economic informed refusal, the patient may likewise view it in his best medical and economic interests to relinquish decisional and informational rights in order to facilitate cost-effective treatment and affordable insurance.

The argument against waiving informed consent is equally unavailing for those who attach intrinsic value to patient knowledge. It would convert informed consent from a liberating and empowering right to a confining and burdensome duty to demand that patients must always listen to a comprehensive recitation of their treatment risks and alternatives. Therefore, it is really a form of paternalism, not respect for autonomy, that leads some theorists to give absolute value to full disclosure.[127] Under the correct view, it is an *exercise* of autonomous decision making, not its defeat, to waive full disclosure. However much or little a patient might desire to participate in medical decision making, he is exercising an autonomous choice so long as his informational options and their consequences are sufficiently disclosed.

Naturally, it is possible to take this entire line of argument too far. If applied too freely, these bundling and waiver characterizations could result in dispensing with all informed consent requirements forevermore with only the briefest and most obscure of legal boilerplate buried in the fine print of an insurance contract. Certainly, for these characterizations to be fairly and reasonably applied, some meaningful choice and understanding is necessary, topics to which I now turn. But, before doing so, I stress that this line of argument does not seek to eliminate the entire range of informed consent law. I still view this law as largely intact at its core: as it applies to the medical risks of invasive treatment. It is only at the outer periphery of economic influences on nontreatment decisions or treatment alternatives, where the law applies only foggily at best, that we can with comfort use waiver and bundling concepts to define or limit the application of informed consent principles based on terms in a health insurance contract.

The Inability to Understand Economic Disclosure

So far, we have sketched the analytical basis on which the law might permit disclosures of rationing incentives and rules at the time of insurance enrollment to substitute for the bedside disclosures that informed consent theory ideally would like. Some critics object, however, that these simple advance disclosures are insufficient to satisfy even minimal informed consent requirements because patients have great difficulty accurately and rationally assessing the probabilistic, risk-based information that is relevant to understanding resource allocation mechanisms.[128] Most laypeople (and even many doctors) suffer from a number of cognitive biases and limitations in comprehending statistical probabilities. They:

- Give disproportionate weight to memorable, personalized anecdotes—that Uncle Fred died from heart surgery is more important than all the other information
- Exaggerate risk information by disassociating it from its base rate of prevalence—harm to 40 percent of people with condition X is viewed as a high risk, even though condition X is very rare
- Underestimate disjunctive probabilities and overestimate conjunctive ones—where there is a 50 percent chance of harm A and a 50 percent chance of harm

B, people fail to perceive that the probability of A *or* B occurring is 75 percent, but the probability of A *and* B occurring is only 25 percent
* Have different perceptions of the same odds depending on whether they are framed in positive or negative terms—5 percent chance of failure versus 95 percent chance of success[129]

These biases and cognitive limitations are particularly severe where patients lack the knowledge that comes from having experienced the relevant risks themselves. Thus, the HMO subscriber who thinks that it makes sense when he is healthy to sacrifice a margin of ultimate safety may later come to regret this decision if he cannot choose the specialist or the high-tech treatment he wants when he is suffering from a serious illness later on.

It is important to appreciate these inevitable failures to convey complete understanding, but equally important to realize that enrollment disclosures have at least some success. The types of disclosures I envision are similar to the terns now used to inform subscribers of the basic scope of their insurance coverage. Testing has shown that these terms are reasonably successful in conveying basic understanding to most people. "The vast majority of families understand insurance policies that specify one or two parameters in their benefit provisions."[130] Only for specialized populations that face complex, overlapping coverage, such as elderly subscribers to Medicare supplemental policies, is there well-documented evidence that consumers fail to understand in general terms what their health insurance covers.[131]

Whether something more than basic understanding by most people is required—full and detailed comprehension by virtually everyone—depends on whether one attaches instrumental or intrinsic value to informed consent. The instrumental justification for informed consent law is that individuals know better than physicians or others what best fits their personal values; therefore, following patients' wishes will result in more beneficial results.[132] Beneficial results here are not defined narrowly in terms of just medical benefit; informed consent allows other personal values—religious, aesthetic, and economic—to be factored into medical decision making. For the very reason that informed consent law serves instrumental and nonmedical purposes, it is subject to pragmatic limitations in its own enforcement. One of these limitations is consumers' capacities for understanding. As Clark Havighurst has argued, "for courts to insist on perfect consumer knowledge . . . and fully individualized choice as prerequisites of an enforceable contract for health coverage would effectively destroy private contracts . . . in the interest of the very insureds whose interests the legal system purports to protect."[133]

The argument that subscribers cannot understand bundled consent is more compelling when considering the intrinsic basis for informed consent. The intrinsic value at stake is individual choice in matters of ultimate importance such as life and disability. The relativist version of this intrinsic value is that the more patient understanding and participation the better, regardless of the costs to other values entailed in achieving greater autonomy. The absolutist position is even stronger: No valid consent is obtained unless understanding is perfect. But both versions are merely assertive argumentation. For the very reason that the value is intrinsic, there is no subsidiary argument or external point of reference to determine when, and at what level, the value is ideally or minimally satisfied. Therefore, it is equally plausible to argue, as others have, that no particular level of comprehension is demanded even by an intrinsic justification for informed consent. For instance, some have argued that the value of individual choice is most satisfied when decisions are the least rational. Personal autonomy in the view of many people has its greatest force against collective, externally imposed decisions in the very cases where individual choice is the most idiosyncratic and emotionally biased—in other words, where there is the greatest divergence between external and internal values. "Individual freedom here is guaranteed only if people are given the right to make choices which would generally be regarded as foolish ones."[134] Therefore, rational understanding of the relevant risks and benefits is largely irrelevant to the intrinsic worth of being given the information.

Viewed from a more pragmatic legal perspective, flaws in comprehension cannot automatically vitiate consent, whichever value base might be considered. This is because the law assumes that the default position for failed consent is no consent. Since the law takes the absence of consent to be equivalent to the refusal of consent, the objection that imperfect comprehension undermines consent would absurdly prohibit medical and economic choice altogether in the name of autonomous control of medical decision making. Informed consent theory presumes an ideal level of individual participation and control that rarely, if ever, is achieved in real-world settings. Therefore, for proposed medical interventions, the only sensible default to the inevitable failure of comprehension—other than abandoning the effort altogether—is to respect the autonomous exercise of consent nevertheless. Imagine the rule that told a patient, "we may not operate to remove your infected appendix unless you pass an informational exam, because unless you really understand all the complexities of the risks entailed, the law declares that you have not given valid consent." Even more ludicrous, where the best medical judgment is *not* to operate, imagine saying, "we *must* operate because you cannot truly comprehend the medical benefits of *refusing* the operation."

To avoid these absurdities, informed consent law does not blindly default to the opposite of what is medically proposed simply because disclosure fails to produce adequate comprehension. The law declares that adequate disclosure alone is sufficient, and devises objective and theoretical, not subjective and empirical, tests for when disclosure is deemed adequate. We hold that simple disclosure of these conventional risks is sufficient to subject patients to extraordinarily invasive, experimental procedures that roll the dice on life-and-death stakes. We do so despite the patient's deficits in comprehension, because a decision still must be made one way or the other. To insist that the patient's and physician's preferred course cannot be followed absent full comprehension is to mandate the worst alternative by default.

There is no basis for departing from this reasoning when economic cost/benefit trade-offs are made in addition to medical risk/benefit trade-offs. When economically influenced nontreatment decisions are at stake, there is no more principled basis for setting the opposite default rule.[135] When the issue is whether to treat, we accept the validity of disclosure despite actual deficiencies in patient understanding because the only alternative is to withhold desired treatment. When the issue is whether to decline treatment, this solution is equally compelling because the only alternative is to force unwanted treatment. It is only when we confront whether to bundle or waive the required disclosure that some ethicists impose their prickly objections to the effectiveness of consent. It is self-defeating to require that, in order for bundled consent or waiver of consent to be informed, the person must be told and must understand all the detailed information that he is asking not to be told.

To illustrate the inconsistency of such a position, consider how convincing the following objections are to the adequacy of a global enrollment disclosure when they are also applied to bedside rationing decisions. To make this point, I have rephrased Paul Appelbaum's objections to my argument by substituting his desired disclosures (at the point of treatment) for mine (at the point of enrollment):

> Note that postulating an effect of disclosure at the time of [treatment] depends on an interrelated set of highly questionable propositions: that disclosure is made in language sufficiently clear for a lay person to understand; that [patients] are alerted to the importance of the information, such that they attend to its presentation, whether oral or written; [and] that persons unsophisticated about medical concepts are able to appreciate the implications of the information for their [present] medical conditions. . . . Even were all these desiderata to be achieved—an accomplishment students of informed consent in the real world would recognize as little short of miraculous—considerable doubt would remain as to whether patients still would grasp the impact of economic factors on their care. . . . Only a cockeyed optimist is likely to respond to these queries in the affirmative. . . . I conclude, therefore, that disclosure at the time of [treatment] of an insurer's limitations on coverage based on economic considerations is unlikely to leave subscribers meaningfully informed about the ways in which their doctor's recommendations are being affected by concern over costs.[136]

If real-world constraints on patients' attention spans, analytical abilities, and experience base limit the effectiveness of disclosure at enrollment, so will they at the bedside. What are we to do? We cannot just prohibit doing that which is being disclosed. We can attempt to improve the disclosure, but when those improvements meet their inevitable practical limits, our only choice is to proceed in the face of epistemological imperfection.

Constraints on Choice

The success of this argument still depends on whether in fact patients would prefer not to be told of long-shot, expensive treatment options that aren't covered by their insurance. Nothing I have said proves that they would. If not, treatment-specific disclosures must be given at the bedside. A variety of opinion surveys have explored fully insured patients' desires to be informed of treatment being performed on them. These surveys generally support the conclusion that doctors should initiate at least some discussion, if not the full-bore exegesis the law seems to demand.[137] However, none of these surveys examines the point of inquiry here.[138] Even if they did, the possibility that people would have mixed preferences tells us that the best course is simply to put the choice to actual insurance subscribers.

Whether patients in a real-world setting will give bundled consent to resource allocation mechanisms or will agree to waive informed-refusal disclosures at the bedside naturally depends on what their options are at the time. Quite a few more will demand full disclosure if that option comes at no cost or inconvenience to them in their choice of insurance plans, but they will have to think about it much harder if they learn that the least-expensive or most-extensive insurance (or both) demands this concession. Can it be said that informed consent is freely given or waived if the decision is made on pain of a substantial sacrifice in health benefits or increase in premiums? What if the *only* insurance available requires waiver of informed refusal, so that the only means to obtain full disclosure of nontreatment decisions is to pay out of pocket?

In the next chapter I address constraints in choice under the rubric of coercion, employing moral and political theory. There, I conclude that some restrictions in choice do not undermine consent. However, the main issue in the next chapter concerns what items of treatment insurance is morally obliged to cover, not what are the legal limits on the style of physician communication. The scope of insurance coverage is decided in an arms-length commercial transaction. The present inquiry imposes a much more demanding standard. The right to be informed springs from the fiduciary character of the treatment relationship, which removes the issue from the ordinary rules of the marketplace. As comprehensively surveyed by Professor Maxwell Mehlman, the more exacting rules of fiduciary contracting require not just minimal fairness, but (1) full disclosure, (2) fair substantive terms, and (3) a reasonable range of choice.[139]

Based on the prior discussion, I will presume that subscribers are given adequate notice of a treatment disclosure rule that is objectively reasonable. This satisfies the first two of these fiduciary requirements (full disclosure and fair terms). My purpose here is to inquire, by referring to analogous legal contexts, how unconstrained the subscriber's choice over this disclosure rule must be in order to satisfy the legal concerns that attach to limited disclosures. I will explore both a range of disclosure options *within* the chosen insurance plan and a range of choice *among* insurance alternatives.

Ideally, patients would be allowed to pick precisely the degree of disclosure they desire from any provider with no consequence to themselves. This could be accomplished as Tristram Engelhardt suggests, by asking "subscribers to insurance programs . . . to check which standard of disclosure they wished used in their treatment . . . [and to] review their choices semiannually or annually."[140] However desirable this approach may be, it may not be feasible and it is not required by the law. Clark Havighurst warns against the temptation to enforce a "supermarket paradigm" of choice that requires nearly infinite variation among all options. He observes that the realistic objective is political and social legitimacy, not perfect autonomy, and legitimacy usually attaches to an adequate but constrained range of choice.[141] In the words of Ruth Faden and Tom Beauchamp, "to chain informed consent to *fully or completely* autonomous decision making stacks the deck of the argument and strips informed consent of any meaningful place in the practical world, where people's actions are rarely, if ever, fully autonomous."[142]

What constitutes an adequate or legitimate range of disclosure options will differ depending on whether a patient is choosing an individual doctor or an overall health plan. Individual doctors may find it difficult to offer multiple disclosure standards among their many patients and still satisfy the burden of proof required if their decisions are challenged in court. Doctors' bedside manner, like their basic medical practice style, tends to be fairly uniform across patients. Therefore, fiduciary law is probably lenient enough to allow a doctor to employ a single disclosure standard for all of his patients so long as it is a reasonable one and is declared at the outset of the treatment relationship. The presumed ready availability of countless other doctors should permit a single physician to offer a reasonable but nonstandard disclosure style on a take-it-or-leave-it basis.[143] Even as forceful an advocate of ideal informed consent law as Marjorie Shultz would allow a liberal waiver rule for a single physician, observing that

[t]he danger that doctors would use their power to insist that patients give them broader decisionmaking authority than the patient might wish would be forestalled by [the fact that] . . . doctors are increasingly having to compete for health care dollars. Patients wishing more authority in decisionmaking are likely to have the bargaining power to achieve this goal.[144]

Can the same be said for a patient who faces a group of doctors organized into an insurance plan? Choice might still be preserved, if not within the plan, then among plans. A private employer might offer a range of insurance options or a government program might be administered through a voucher system. We have already observed that a hospital can, without violating fiduciary principles or being accused of coercion, insist that a patient cooperate with certain administrative and patient care protocols if they wish to receive treatment in the facility, even though some of these may be bothersome or unpleasant. Likewise, an HMO should be able to offer its services contingent on agreement to a reasonable disclosure standard, even one that is lower than the law ordinarily sets, so long as the HMO does not dispense with informed consent requirements entirely. Restricting informed consent to major, invasive treatment decisions is only a specification and limitation of the right, not a complete waiver.

Some limitation of individual choice is particularly appropriate given the collective nature of insurance. An insurance subscriber joins a community of interest when he pools his risk with others. This necessarily requires a collective agreement on certain terms and conditions of coverage since demanding tailor-made insurance would destroy the economies of scale that make insurance a desirable product in the first place. Where the treatment function is integrated with the insurance function, as in HMOs, subscribers necessarily must be bound by a collective agreement on certain aspects of the treatment relationship as well.[145] For one subscriber to insist on a greater degree of disclosure than the rest of the pool is willing to tolerate is no more ethically compelling than insisting on more treatment than the subscriber has paid for. This is why individual rights-based informed consent principles derived from a solo-practice, third-party reimbursement setting do not automatically apply to the new forms of health care delivery.

Still, what if silent rationing is the *only* form of insurance an employer or government program offers? Can it be said that the patient gives free consent or makes a willing waiver if he is unable in practical terms to say no? The closest legal guidance[146] lies in the small collection of cases concerning agreements to arbitrate rather than litigate HMO malpractice suits. The leading decision, *Madden v. Kaiser Foundation Hospitals*,[147] enforced a clause in a standardized HMO enrollment form that requires disputes to be submitted to binding arbitration, despite the subscriber's claim that she was unaware of the provision and never agreed to it. The court noted that the subscriber was offered a number of health plans by her employer, some of which did not require arbitration.[148]

It is a matter of speculation whether the option to select nonarbitrated insurance was an essential element of this decision,[149] but it is reasonable to conclude that many courts will be hostile to informed consent waivers if no other option is readily available to the subscriber.[150] On the other hand, it is also reasonable to conclude that a partial waiver (one relating only to economic informed refusal), negotiated as part of an employer-provided health plan, fully comports with fiduciary contracting rules if the subscriber is given some choice, either within the plan selected or among other available plans. Choice exists within the plan if the subscriber need not accept the waiver, even on pain of paying a higher premium. Choice exists outside the plan if other plans are available that do not contain the waiver, again even if they come at a higher cost or with lower benefits. Nothing in fiduciary contracting law prevents charging subscribers the fair price of the actuarial risks they choose to insure.

CONCLUSION

This chapter has mounted a rather relentless attack on full-bodied application of informed consent law to all medical spending decisions. In doing so, I do not mean to argue that no legal duty exists or that consent (or waiver) should be blithely found to exist in any enrollment decision. Instead, I mean to sketch a theory of economic informed consent that articulates the conceptual parameters for constructive debate about the precise circumstances and extent of disclosure. Some global disclosure of rationing incentives, rules, and mechanisms is required at the outset of enrollment, although this presently is not done. If such a disclosure can be accomplished, it would validate at least some subsequent resource allocation decisions without the need for doctors to make (non)treatment-specific disclosures at the bedside. This results from either a bundled-consent conception or from a waiver of consent conception. For either of these characterizations to hold, however, some meaningful choice must exist at the time of insurance enrollment, which also does not presently exist for many—perhaps the majority—of subscribers to managed care plans. Therefore, a silent rationing scheme is not legitimate in the present marketplace with its existing enrollment practices. In particular, I want to stress that I do not support the use of "gag clauses" as they are currently used in some managed care contracts between physicians and HMOs.[151]

I am not content to leave this intricate and rather abstract analysis at such an inconclusive and inchoate stage. It is incumbent on me to at least trace how the theory of economic informed consent would ideally shape disclosure practices at enrollment and at the bedside were it to be implemented. In my view, subscribers to HMOs and other limited insurance arrangements should be explicitly told, at initial enrollment and at each periodic reenrollment, of the framework and incentives for making resource allocation decisions, both through centralized rules and through individualized discretion. This would entail the following, in addition to the items of disclosure that are presently made concerning the scope of coverage, grievance and appeal rights, etc.:[152]

1. *A common sense explanation of the goal of economical insurance*, namely, to eliminate expensive treatment that has slight or questionable benefit in order to make health care coverage more comprehensive and more affordable.
2. *A general description of who exercises authority over medical spending decisions*, such as the role of the primary care physician and the supervising medical director in approving specialist referrals, expensive testing, and hospitalization.
3. *A specification of the sources, but not necessarily the complete content, of rules that govern these decision makers.* Such rule-based authorities might include various internal committees, or guidelines set by certain external groups.[153] Copies of existing rules of this nature should be available for inspection at the patient's request, and a sampling of easy-to-understand examples from representative situations should be prominently mentioned.
4. *A fairly specific description of the financial incentives that influence physicians' decisions.* Exact dollar figures and intricate formulas are not necessary, but subscribers should know of the general structure of both the base payment method (salary, capitation, or fee-for-service) and of supplemental bonus or

penalty incentives. Unless the general tendency of an incentive is obvious, it should also be described, but not necessarily in apprehensive or pejorative terms. For example, subscribers might be told that a bonus pool is intended to make physicians more aware of the costs of expensive treatment they order.

5. *An explanation of what patients can expect to be told when potentially beneficial treatment is not recommended due to its costs.* The following is one possible version:

> Our medical professionals will provide a range of treatment options that is reasonable and standard for this kind of insurance in this part of the country and this practice setting. However, they will not always point out where their professional judgment differs from those who practice under more expensive forms of insurance or who following different styles of medical practice. Patients are always free to ask questions about their course of recommended treatment. Those questions will be answered honestly and thoroughly, including suggestions for where to obtain second opinions or where to obtain treatment that is not available under this insurance plan. However, patients may not demand treatment that is more expensive than this plan allows or that, in the view of our medical professionals, exceeds appropriate medical standards.

Despite these disclosures at enrollment, not all resource allocation decisions should be made silently. The most difficult aspect of economic informed consent is specifying what nontreatment decisions doctors still must disclose at the bedside. Law professor Peter Schuck advocates that, instead of a unitary doctrine of informed consent, we should develop several doctrines that are specific to different treatment contexts and to patients' varying informational needs.[154] Adapting this idea to the present analysis, some nontreatment decisions are so high-stakes or value-laden they should never be relegated to silent rationing or left to patient initiative to uncover. Obvious examples include pulling the plug on life-support or declining a lifesaving operation for a terminally ill or comatose patient. Other less dramatic nontreatment decisions should also require direct patient participation if they might have unique importance to some patients. For instance, a low risk of a slight physical impairment might be of such fundamental importance to an athlete, musician, or performing artist that it is imperative to give them the option to pursue more aggressive or specialized treatment than is appropriate for ordinary patients.

Defining and policing these categories of mandatory disclosure will be extremely difficult conceptually, but nevertheless essential to maintaining an acceptable system of resource allocation.[155] Some of these difficulties might be handled by addressing more dramatic, life-and-death resource allocation decisions through very public and participatory rule-based mechanisms. Others might be handled by providers periodically conducting an explicit "values inventory" of their patients so that there is some objective basis for knowing when clinicians should be aware of areas of unique importance to particular patients. There is ample room for creative thought and innovative techniques as these issues are fleshed out in practice.

The first step in undertaking this effort is to correct the deficiencies in existing economic disclosure practices at the time of insurance enrollment. Although these economic disclosures will be vigorously resisted by some (but not all and perhaps not even most) elements of the insurer and provider communities, this approach to making health care spending decisions is necessary in order to satisfy a balanced, pragmatic view of the present requirements of informed consent law. Nevertheless, this theory of economic informed consent is subject to a major disabling limitation: It requires for its legal and ethical justification some reasonable range of consumer choice among insurance plans so that silent rationing is not forced on anyone by their dire need to remain insured. This limitation reaches much further than simply the need to enhance and clarify disclosure practices. It requires that private employers offer more than a single health insurance option and, more radically, it demands that public programs be run under principles of consumer choice that are common only in private markets. How this might be accomplished and the extent to which it is morally (as opposed to legally) required are addressed in the next chapter following a summary of the book's major conclusions.

Notes

1. On the somewhat divided and contradictory public policy roles of HMOs, see Havighurst 1978, at 130–36.

2. 42 U.S.C. 300e et seq. (1988 & Supp. V 1993).

3. See generally Emanuel 1991, at 204–11; Garvin 1996.

4. 42 C.F.R. 417.126 (1994).

5. A few states have considered bills that would require HMOs to disclose financial incentive plans, but to date only Arizona has enacted one. See 4 Health Law Rep. (BNA), at 768 (May 18, 1995), (discussing SB 1297, which requires "a description of any incentives or penalties associated with influencing plan providers to withhold services"). A brand new Medicare regulation requires disclosure, but only if subscribers request it. 42 C.F.R. 434.70.

6. See sources cited in Chapter 4 at notes 12–14. The legal causes of action range from standard breach of contract, to negligence and fraud counts, to more innovative conspiracy and tortious interference theories. Most of these are instances of supplemental counts that elaborate on a basic malpractice cause of action. However, one case is unique in that it involved no direct patient injury and it focused solely on disclosure, not negligence. Teti v. U.S. Healthcare, Inc., C.A. No. 88–9808 (E.D. Pa.) (filed Dec. 27, 1988; dismissed Nov. 21, 1989). *Teti* was filed under RICO, the federal racketeering law, 18 U.S.C. § 1961 et seq. by one of the plan's subscribers who complained of her doctor's refusing a requested specialist referral. Meyer 1989, at 4. The case was dismissed from federal court for failure to state grounds for relief under federal law, but, at last word, the plaintiffs had refiled in state court. Rodwin 1993, at 168. See also Anderson v. Humana, 24 F.3d 889 (7th Cir.

1994) (ERISA preempts state law claim of fraud against HMO for failing to disclose physician incentive structure).

7. Pulvers v. Kaiser Foundation Health Plan, 160 Cal. Rptr. 392, 394 (Ct. App. 1979). The court observed that the jury found under the malpractice count that no negligence was committed. Another court ruled that it was proper to exclude evidence that profit motivation might have caused an HMO physician to fail to hospitalize a patient with labor complications, observing that such evidence "was only marginally relevant [to malpractice] and potentially very prejudicial." Madsen v. Park Nicollet Medical Center, 419 N.W. 2d 511, 515 (Minn. Ct. App. 1988).

8. On the other hand, the court also ruled that financial incentive plans are not per se in violation of public policy. Bush v. Dake, No. 86–25767 (Mich. Cir. Ct., Saginaw County, April 27, 1989), summarized in 17 *Health Law Digest*, No. 8, at 16. The case was subsequently settled. It is possible to reconcile this conflicting decision with *Pulvers* by observing that, where negligent treatment exists, a financial inducement can be found to be a contributing factor, but, standing alone, it does not constitute an independent tort.

9. 793 P.2d 479 (Cal. 1990).

10. Ibid. at 483.

11. Hidding v. Williams, 578 So.2d 1192 (La. Ct. App. 1991); Behringer v. Princeton Medical Center, 592 A.2d 1251 (N.J. Super. Ct. 1991).

12. For a thorough analysis of these cases and a review of the secondary literature, see Bobinski 1994, at 362–69. See also Twerski and Cohen 1992 (discussing whether there is a duty to disclose statistics about individual physicians' success/failure rates).

13. Brett 1992, at 1355.

14. Mechanic, Ettel, and Davis 1990, at 22. See also Stephens 1989, at 703 (describing HMOs' sales pitch as "the big lie").

15. Pear 1995.

16. Anderson 1988; Physician Payment Review Commission 1989, at 275; Levinson 1987; Hirshfeld 1990, at 118, 142–43; Figa and Figa 1990, at 152–54; AMA Council 1995b, at 330–35; Sanders 1991; Fleck 1990, at 117; Bobinski 1994; McGraw 1995.

17. Stone 1985, at 312.

18. For instance, the AMA's "Patient Protection Act," which is pending in Congress and in a number of states, and whose purpose is widely viewed as being hostile to managed care insurers, contains a provision calling for disclosure of "financial arrangements . . . that would limit the services offered, restrict referral or treatment options, or negatively affect the physician's fiduciary responsibility to his or her patients, including but not limited to financial incentives not to provide medical or other services." § 2(b)(1)(iii) (version dated May 23, 1994).

19. Christopher, Biblo, Johnson and Potter 1995, at 89. The task force disagreed, however, over how and when such discussions should occur, particularly, over whether they are the responsibility of the physician in a clinical setting at the commencement of treatment.

20. Bobinski 1994, at 360.

21. 42 U.S.C. § 1395mm(i) (1988 & Supp. V 1993); H.R. Rep. No. 899, 101st Cong., Committee on Ways and Means, Oct. 18, 1990. Implementing regulations do require disclosure, but only when a patient requests it. 42 C.F.R. § 434.70.

22. See Friedman 1986, at 219.

23. See Levinson 1987; Rodwin 1995b. For instance, Mehlman 1990, at 392, in discussing the waiver of the right to sue for malpractice, argues that "patients need to be told of risks like the possibility of greater carelessness by a provider . . . [and] be given estimates of both the magnitude of the benefits and risks, and their probability of occurrence."

24. Goold and Brody 1995, at 141. Havighurst 1995, at 187–90 also offers another, somewhat more detailed and formalized, version that is better suited for contractual language. See the Conclusion to this chapter for additional suggested approaches to formulating the disclosure.

25. By way of analogy, one court has ruled that there is no duty to disclose the availability of an abortion procedure that was illegal in the state but could be obtained in another state. Spencer v. Seikel, 742 P.2d 1126 (Okla. 1987). This suggests the general absence of a duty to disclose treatment that is not readily available. See generally Terrion 1993 (arguing that such a duty should exist, but only to provide bare notification of the procedure, not to provide detailed information, unless requested).

26. Bailey 1986, at 20.

27. Morreim 1991b, at 115 (disclosure requiredif there is "any realistic possibility" that patient could arrange for treatment, even by soliciting donations); Menzel 1990, at 145.

28. See, e.g., Turner et al. 1995 (half of patients who recieved intensive care at one hospital would have declined this care had they been told of the costs and required to pay a portion).

29. See Moore v. Regents of the Univ. of Cal., 793 P.2d 479, 484 (Cal. 1990) ("The possibility that an interest extraneous to the patient's health has affected the physician's judgment is something that a reasonable patient would want to know in deciding whether to consent to a proposed course of treatment. It is material to the patient's decision and, thus, a prerequisite to informed consent."). Several surveys reveal that most patients, even those with full insurance, want to be told about the costs of their treatment options. See Turner et al. 1995; President's Commission 1982, vol. 3 at p. 79.

30. Karlsons v. Guerinot, 394 N.Y.S.2d 933, 939 (N.Y. App. Div. 1977) (no liability for failing to recommend amniocentesis or warn of risk of giving birth to deformed child). See also Atlanta Obstetrics and Gynecology Group v. Abelson, 392 S.E.2d 916 (Ga. Ct. App. 1990) (same as *Karlsons*); Roark v. Allen, 633 S.W.2d 804, 808 (Tex. 1982) (no liability for failing to warn of possible complications after difficult childbirth); Kalsbeck v. Westview Clinic, 375 N.W.2d 861, 869 (Minn. Ct. App. 1985) ("The doctrine of informed consent does not apply to situations where the patient's decision is whether to submit to treatments in addition to the basic treatment given") (dismissing claim against physician who delayed aggressive treatment for pneumonia); Madsen v. Park Nicollet Medical Center, 431 N.W.2d 855, 859 (Minn. 1988) (same, for delay in hospitalizing patient in premature labor); Moure v. Raeuchle, 604 A.2d 1003, 1008 (Pa. 1992) (informed consent law is limited to invasive procedures); Shultz 1985, at 234–40 (collecting and discussing cases).

31. Hastings Center Report, June 1988, at 45 (71 percent of patients report their doctors seldom or never discuss the costs of the medical treatment); Am. Med. News, Dec. 21, 1990 (only 25 percent of doctors report usually discussing fees before treatment); President's Commission 1982, at 79 (only 38 percent of doctors initiate discussion on the costs of treatment); Rosoff at 342 (over half of physicians do not commonly disclose treatment costs and insurance coverage, and over two-thirds do not discuss costs and coverage of treatment alternatives).

32. Schloendorff v. Society of New York Hosp., 105 N.E. 92, 93 (N.Y. 1914) (Cardozo, J.); Natanson v. Kline, 350 P.2d 1093 (Kan. 1960).

33. Shultz 1985, at 232. Accord Gates v. Jensen, 595 P.2d 919, 922–23 (Wash. 1979) ("The patient's right to know is not confined to the choice of treatment. . . . Important decisions must frequently be made in many non-treatment situations"); Truman v. Thomas, 611 P.2d 902, 906 (Cal. 1980) ("The duty to disclose was imposed . . . so that patients might meaningfully exercise their right to make decisions about their own bod-

ies. The importance of this right should not be diminished by the manner in which it is exercised").

34. Moore v. Regents of the Univ. of Cal., 793 P.2d 479, 483 (Cal. 1990). Observe, though, that *Moore* concerned the disclosure of risks prior to undertaking an operation, not, as in our present concern, prior to declining treatment.

For additional analysis of the disclosure of nonmedical factors, see Bobinski 1994.

35. Blumstein 1981, at 1394. Others who have reached the same conclusion (often without citation), include President's Commission 1982, Vol. I, at 77 ("a physician ought not withhold information about a treatment from a patient simply because the physician judges its potential benefits not to be worth its costs. . . . [A]lternatives should still be described, even though they would not be covered by a patient's insurance plan . . . lest the patient be deprived of the opportunity to seek other avenues for paying for the treatment"); Morreim 1991b, at 115–23; Menzel 1990, at 145–46, at 287–92; AMA Council 1995b, at 330–35; Kapp 1984, at 251 (suggesting that informed consent law may require "frank discussion concerning the quality, cost and resource allocation implications of the various alternatives"); Mehlman 1986, at 861–62 & n.336; Glover and Povar 1991, at 13, 17, 20 ("It seems a particularly pointed corruption of the physician's promise if he or she deepens the patient's vulnerability by way of hidden omissions. . . . Since truth-telling is such an essential component of both autonomy and the patient-physician relationship, thorough disclosure of the reasons for physicians' recommendations would seem to be required"); Miller 1992, at 70–71 ("If physicians withhold the information that potentially beneficial treatment is being denied their patients for economic reasons, they not only usurp the possibility of patient choice or self-help on the matter, but they assume a staggering moral burden. . . . To deny patients such information is to compromise the exercise of personal autonomy, the *raison d'etre* of the informed consent doctrine"); Lu 1993, at 550; Rodwin 1995a, at 604–06; Fleck 1990, at 117 ("the publicity condition would require HMO physicians to present to patients all treatment options for their condition that were medically reasonable, including those that were not cost-effective and those that would not be covered by the terms of the HMO plan"); Perry 1994, at 375–80; Jonsen, Siegler and Winslade 1986, at 150; Newdick 1995, at 297–303 (analyzing British law).

To date, the only published American authority squarely taking an opposing view is Jacobson and Rosenquist 1988, at 1589 ("alternatives that are prohibitively expensive or restricted to certain high-risk categories should not be a part of informed consent. . . . That result stretches the concept of informed consent well beyond what is necessary for a patient to evaluate the range of medical practice decisions and to maintain self-determination."). This article argues that doctors need not inform low-risk patients of a new solution available for use in angiography, which is a diagnostic technique to detect restricted arteries. The new solution avoids a one-in-40,000 chance of an allergic reaction, but at a cost 12–15 times greater than the old one. See also Havighurst 1992, at 1787 n.80 ("the informed consent principle should be irrelevant, as such, in assessing insurance contracts"); McGraw 1995 (expressing hesitancy about requiring bedside disclosure of rationing incentives).

Professor Mary Anne Bobinski takes a more complex look at this issue, observing that informed consent law possibly applies but is unlikely to require disclosure due to the complications discussed below, but arguing that disclosure should be required nonetheless. She fails to clarify, however, whether disclosure should be the global one at enrollment or the treatment-specific bedside version considered here. Bobinski 1994.

36. The leading account is Katz 1984, at 69–79; Katz 1977. See also Capron 1974, at 419–22; Shultz 1985, at 278; Meisel 1988.

37. The following survey is drawn generally from all of the legal literature cited in this and the following sections, as well these excellent treatises: Rozovsky 1990; Rosoff 1981.

38. Battery law does not require injury or causation in order to impose liability. Therefore, it potentially punishes any touching without consent without regardless of the degree of tangible bodily harm or any objective evidence of whether the plaintiff would have given consent if it had been sought. Shultz 1985, at 225.

39. Comment 1981; Jones 1990.

40. See Katz 1984, at 79 ("What patients might or might not have agreed to, if properly informed, is beside the point"); Twerski and Cohen 1988, at 621 ("if a failure to disclose violates the interest of autonomous choice, the damage to that interest is the same regardless of the success or failure of the medical procedure which followed the uninformed choice"); Shultz 1985, at 290–91 (acknowledging that damages would be awarded for informed-refusal violations even if the omitted test would have been negative).

41. The dignitary (nontouching) aspect is reflected in several other places in tort law; what is unique to these arguments is dispensing with injury and causation in the context of a very demanding duty. The closest analogy is to cases that compensate for deprivation of the right to vote without showing that the election's outcome would have been altered (injury). Twerski and Cohen 1988, at 651. However, these cases do not impose any particularly heightened standard of care, and they still require a showing that the plaintiff would in fact have voted (causation).

42. 611 P.2d 902 (Cal. 1980).

43. The second-most-prominent decision is Gates v. Jensen, 595 P.2d 919, 923 (Wash. 1979), which sustained an informed consent cause of action against an ophthalmologist who failed to follow up aggressively enough on inconclusive results from a glaucoma test. The court ruled that "the existence of alternative diagnostic procedures to conclusively determine the presence or absence of that disease are . . . facts which a patient must know in order to make an informed decision on the course which future medical care will take." See also Chrisher v. Spak, 471 N.Y.S.2d 741 (N.Y. Sup. Ct. 1983) (failure to fully explain reasons for recommending surgery to relieve pinched nerve in foot, which turned out to be caused by a tumor); Battenfeld v. Gregory, 589 A.2d 1059 (N.J. Super. Ct. App. Div. 1991) (failure to explain why it is advisable to remain in hospital until temperature has normalized for 24 hours could have caused injuries resulting from ruptured appendix).

44. Moore v. Preventive Medicine Medical Group, 223 Cal. Rptr. 859, 861, 863–64 (Cal. Ct. App. 1986). Incredibly, the court held that it was not sufficient for the general practitioner to "strongly recommend [seeing] a specialist" and to warn him that "all pigmented skin lesions are suspicious in nature" until removed and studied microscopically. The court reasoned that the doctor should have specifically mentioned the risk of cancer and its consequences.

45. Annotation 1985.

46. Faden and Beauchamp 1986. In one remarkable decision, the court found that *doing nothing* is an alternative whose benefits and risks must be specifically disclosed. Archer v. Galbraith, 567 P.2d 1155, 1161 (Wash. Ct. App. 1977). The patient's voice was impaired by removal of a tumor from her thyroid gland that turned out to be benign. She prevailed in the argument that the doctor should have informed her that waiting and watching was an alternative.

47. Keogan v. Holy Family Hospital, 622 P.2d 1246 (Wash. 1980). See also Logan v. Greenwich Hosp. Ass'n, 465 A.2d 294 (Conn. 1983) (where needle biopsy punctured gallbladder, there was a duty to inform of possible alternative surgical procedure, even though it was more hazardous). But see text below at note 52.

48. Martin v. Richards, 531 N.W.2d 70 (Wis. 1995).

49. See also Doe v. Johnston, 476 N.W.2d 28 (Iowa 1991) (a patient infected by the AIDS virus from a blood transfusion following planned surgery had a right to be informed

that an alternative existed of "autologous transfusion," that is, drawing, storing, and reinfusing the patient's own blood).

50. See generally, Annotation 1985; Prillaman 1990, at 56–57; Shultz 1985, at 241–42.

51. Kalsbeck v. Westview Clinic, 375 N.W.2d 861, 869 (Minn. Ct. App. 1985). This reasoning was carried even further in Madsen v. Park Nicollet Medical Center, 431 N.W.2d 855, 859 (Minn. 1988), where a doctor chose to manage premature labor by monitoring at home rather than hospitalizing.

52. McGeshick v. Chouchair, 9 F.3d 1229, 1233, 1235 (7th Cir. 1993). See also Parris v. Sands, 25 Cal. Rptr. 2d 800 (Ct. App. 1993) (no duty to disclose antibiotics as alternative treatment for upper respiratory infection; no general duty to disclose treatment the doctor does not recommend); Moore v. Baker, 989 F.2d 1129 (11th Cir. 1993) (no duty to inform patient of medication therapy as alternative to surgery).

53. The Supreme Court decision was 4-to-3 with a vigorous dissent by Justice Clark, while the court of appeals went the other way 2-to-1, as did the trial judge. Shultz 1985, at 246.

54. Munro v. Regents of the Univ. of Cal., 263 Cal. Rptr. 878, 885 (Ct. App. 1989); Scalere v. Stensen, 260 Cal. Rptr. 152 (Ct. App. 1989); Jamison v. Lindsay, 166 Cal. Rptr. 443, 446 (Ct. App. 1980); Parris v. Sands, 25 Cal. Rptr. 2d 800 (Ct. App. 1993).

55. 595 P.2d 919 (Wash. 1979).

56. Ibid.

57. Martin v. Richards, 531 N.W.2d 70 (Wis. 1995). The physician diagnosed the child's symptoms as only a concussion, where in fact she had suffered internal bleeding. The jury found that the doctor adhered to the standard of care and therefore there was no negligence, but it imposed liability anyway for failure to disclose the option of obtaining a CAT scan and transferring to a larger hospital.

58. Or. Rev. Stat. § 414.745 (1991).

59. Madsen v. Park Nicollet Medical Center, 431 N.W.2d 855, 859 n.9 (Minn. 1988).

60. Keogan v. Holy Family Hospital, 622 P.2d 1246, 1260–61 (Wash. 1980). Peculiarly, the opinion by the three justices in the minority on this issue was labeled as the "majority" opinion. This confusion resulted because most of the five agreed with the other three that the case was sustainable under another legal theory.

61. One frequently cited commentator provides an exhaustive three-page, 14-point list of guidelines that require physicians to describe the procedure in detail, why the patient's condition might necessitate it, all risks the patient would consider material, the factors used to determine which risks to disclose, the potential benefits of the procedure and the efficacy of the treatment in achieving those benefits, alternative treatments and their risks and benefits, and why the physician thinks one course is preferred. The doctor then must make special efforts to encourage patient inquiries or have information repeated, he must frequently ask whether the patient understands, and he must inform the patient of the right to disagree and choose any alternative and the right to change his mind at any time. This commentator encourages long and multiple disclosure sessions of this nature throughout the course of treatment to ensure the patient still retains all of this information. Comment 1981, at 192–95.

62. Jones 1990, at 412.

63. Burt 1979, at 124.

64. Katz 1984.

65. 611 P.2d 902, 910. See also Schuck 1994, at 899–959 (contrasting idealists' and realists' versions of informed consent, and advocating a cost/benefit analysis for reconciling the two); Fajfar 1992 (advocating generally a cost/benefit analysis of required disclosures).

66. Luft 1982.

67. Aaron and Schwartz 1984a.

68. Morreim 1985, at 35 ("unfortunately, the solution is virtually as pernicious as the original conflict of interest. A truly full disclosure of the conflict would require that the physician tell the patient not only the financial facts, but also their implications. . . . The trust between physician and patient could be devastated. The patient . . . [w]ould entertain a pervasive suspicion"); Morreim 1991b, at 329 ("Conversations of economic disclosure can be exceedingly awkward. Neither patients nor physicians are accustomed to putting a price tag on health. Parents may be loath to say, 'No, we can't pay for that level of care for our child,' while physicians may be equally reluctant to say 'I'm sorry, but because you're poor we really can't make that expensive therapy available to you.'"). Despite these difficulties, Morreim, unlike me, argues that these disclosures must be made at the bedside.

69. Stephens 1989, at 702. See also Gillon 1988, at 125–26 (documenting the destructive effect of saying no to a patient who came seeking an expensive antiinflammatory drug for arthritis when she had not yet tried aspirin); Hardwig 1987, at 51 ("Such conversations . . . would . . . cause great suffering and outrage on the part of patients, . . . [and] would take an enormous toll on the fiduciary relations between doctor and patient"); Stone 1985, at 312 ("[I]f it is ethically wrong to conceal these new economic incentives and the medical profession's response to them, to reveal them may threaten the trust and confidence of patients even in 'caring physicians.' 'Caveat emptor' will be more relevant than 'primum non nocere' in doctor-patient relationships.").

70. Morreim 1991b, at 121.

71. Goold and Brody 1995, at 141.

72. Moore v. Preventive Medicine Medical Group, 223 Cal. Rptr. 859, 861, 863–64 (Cal. Ct. App. 1986).

73. Dallis v. Aetna Life Ins. Co., 574 F.Supp. 547 (N.D. Ga. 1983). Insurers or subscribers who wish to alter this standard formulation are often frustrated by regulatory obstacles that are hostile to departures from the prevailing contractual model. See Hall and Anderson 1992.

74. Daniels 1988, at 97.

75. Hall 1985.

76. Tarasoff v. Regents of the University of California, 551 P.2d 334 (Cal. 1976).

77. Murray 1986. Murray observes that the same argument applies to the conflicted roles that physicians play when they work as sports team physicians and practice in military and company clinic settings. See Chapter 4 for further discussion.

78. For another analysis along these lines, see Schuck 1994, at 932 ("there are strong reasons to suspect that informed consent, at least the law in books, is often honored in the breach and almost impossible to enforce as a practical matter).

79. President's Commission 1982, at 108 (according to physician opinion survey (with a bias toward overreporting), written consent is obtained only in 1–2 percent of cases of blood tests or prescriptions, and informal, oral consent in only about half of these cases); Appelbaum, Lidz, and Meisel 1987, at 132; Shultz 1985, at 230, 259. See Novak v. Texada, Miller, Masterson and Davis Clinic, 514 So.2d 524 (La. Ct. App. 1987) (informed consent does "not extend to a routine flu injection. To hold otherwise would lead to results in the day-to-day practice of medicine never intended by the legislature"); Lidz, Meisel, Zerubavel et al. 1984, at 315 ("Informed consent in the pristine form envisioned by law and by ethicists was only rarely, if ever, to be found in [this empirical study of one] Hospital.").

80. Sinclair v. Block, 633 A.2d 1137 (Pa. 1993).

81. An outstanding, comprehensive survey and analysis of the multitude of research findings is contained in Meisel and Roth 1983, at 267–346. These authors observe that these empirical results are flawed by these studies' methods for measuring understanding (e.g., testing patient recall some time after the disclosure) and by their lack of sensitivity to the quality of disclosure (i.e., perhaps indicting more the manner in which informed consent is typically conducted than patients' ability to understand). Nevertheless, the evidence is fairly dismal. Even with explicit prompting, patients frequently are unable to answer even the simplest questions about the basic nature of the procedure, let alone its risks and alternatives. E.g., Leeb, Bowers, and Lynch 1976 (only 35 percent retained basic information seven days after surgery, even though they were told they were participants in a study, that the information was important, and that they would be questioned on it afterward); Hastings Center Rep. 1988, at 45 (reporting on British study that found, two to five days after operation, "[27 percent] did not known which organ had been operated on, and [44 percent] were unaware of how the surgery had been performed"); Muss et al. 1979 (finding that, during the course of treatment, about half of cancer patients were not aware of the purposes of chemotherapy and were unaware of potential lethal complications of infection and bleeding); Wallace 1986 (in various studies, patients forget 28–71 percent of information from their doctors within minutes of receiving it); see also Fellner and Marshall 1970; Ingelfinger 1972; Sprung and Winick 1989, at 1351; U.S. Congress, Office of Technology Assessment 1988, at 41.

82. Faden and Beauchamp 1986, at 276–77, 284–85 (discussing the two senses of informed consent: the subjective goal of patient comprehension versus the operative manifestation through objective standards for physician action); Weisbard 1986 (similar).

83. The caselaw is summarized in Annotation 1978.

84. See Katz 1984, at 76.

85. For instance, there is no accurate way to tell, ex ante, what a presently injured plaintiff would have decided prior to treatment, if fully informed, let's say, of a one-in-1000 risk of blindness. Only the rare injury results in suit; the other 999 patients are not heard from. Of course, once injured, the plaintiff regrets the decision, but what would he have actually decided if confronted only with the rare statistical possibility? Therefore, the law has no choice but to adopt an objective, reasonable-person test for risk aversion, despite the logical inconsistency with pure theory. See Twerski and Cohen 1988.

86. 858 P.2d 598, 606 (Cal. 1993).

87. The House of Lords was sharply critical of the U.S. patient-oriented standard when it adopted a professional custom standard of disclosure in Sidaway v. Bd of Governors, [1985] 2 W.L.R. 480.

88. Schwartz and Grubb 1985, at 19, 23. See also Miller 1987; Miller 1992.

89. E.g., Katz 1984, at 228 ("the radically different climate of physician-patient decision making that I envision cannot be implemented by judicial, legislative, or administrative orders"). See President's Commission 1982, at 30, 204, 252.

> ("The Commission recognizes that further evolution of legal standards toward a firmer protection of individual self-determination in medical decisions must be tempered by a recognition of the law's limits as an instrument of social control. . . . [T]he Commission is concerned that efforts to draw the law further into regulating the subtler aspects of relations between patients and health care professionals may prove ineffective, burdensome and ultimately counterproductive.

For further development of this theme, see Dworkin 1996.

90. In re Karen Ann Quinlan, 355 A.2d 647 (N.J. 1976); Canterbury v. Spence, 464 F.2d 772 (D.C. Cir. 1972).

91. For a history of insurers' reluctance to second-guess medical treatment decisions and the legal liabilities that result when they do, see Hall and Anderson 1992.

92. Haavi Morreim reasons that global disclosure suffices for cost-constraining incentives that operate on a global level, such as a year-end bonus for coming in under budget; she maintains that decision-specific disclosure is necessary only when incentives are so structured, such as rewarding physicians 15 cents on the dollar for every test they deny. Morreim 1991b, at 114. This neat dichotomy treats too simplistically the complexity of actual rationing mechanisms. First, it does not address the case where a nontreatment decision is rule-based. Second, there is no clean line between global and individual incentives. As discussed at length in Chapter 5, many other factors affect the significance of an incentive: its percentage size in relation to the doctor's income and in relation to the payments from that particular HMO, the number of patients covered, the nature of the treatment (whether primary care or specialist referral), the number of doctors in the pool, and the strength of offsetting incentives created by peer review, patient grievance, and malpractice mechanisms.

93. Menzel 1990.

94. E.g., Mechanic 1979, at 111; Mechanic 1986, at 214; Begley 1986, at 240; Morreim 1991b.

95. For further elaboration on this distinction, see Elhauge 1994, at 1537.

96. Therefore, Menzel himself is reluctant to ascribe full moral weight to merely presumed consent. He argues that treatment-specific disclosure is still required by informed consent doctrine even when presumed consent exists. Menzel 1993.

97. Or, as Menzel 1990 puts the point, where prior consent exists to the risk of an event occurring, no complaint can be made when the event transpires, even if there was no explicit consent to the event itself.

98. See text at notes 79–80 supra.

99. See Lidz and Meisel 1982, Vol. II, at 317, 333–34.

100. Epstein 1976, at 110 ("custom prevails because it is the best evidence on the terms of agreement"); Epstein 1986, at 201.

101. Mathis v. Morrisey, 13 Cal. Rptr. 2d 819 (Ct. App. 1992); Parris v. Sands, 25 Cal. Rptr. 2d 800 (Ct. App. 1993).

102. Siliciano 1991; Hall 1989.

103. Bovbjerg 1975.

104. Presumably, informed consent cannot ratify a negligent treatment recommendation, since this would constitute the waiver of malpractice liability, which is generally disallowed. Tunkl v. Regents of the Univ. of Cal., 383 P.2d 441 (Cal. 1963).

105. Text at note 30 above.

106. Handler 1986.

107. Brody 1992, at 115–18. In response to the objection that this standard makes it too easy for doctors to assert simple empty-mindedness as a defense, Brody responds that malpractice law serves as some check since at some point it would constitute malpractice to ignore too many factors. Nevertheless, Brody fails to explain how this approach to informed consent would keep it from collapsing completely into ordinary negligence law.

108. See Menzel 1990, at 145 ("[O]ne does not always need to give the information straight out. One might at first only suggest it, then wait for the patient to respond and ask. . . . [I]f the patient does not inquire further, a provider is not obligated to inform him or her more precisely.").

109. Canterbury v. Spence, 464 F.2d 772, n. 36 (D.C. Cir. 1972). The court continues: "The patient may be ignorant, confused, overawed by the physician or frightened by the

hospital, or even ashamed to inquire. . . . [A] rule which presumes a degree of sophistication which many members of society lack is likely to breed gross inequities."

110. Madsen v. Park Nicollet Medical Center, 431 N.W.2d 855, 859 (Minn. 1988) ("The informed consent/nondisclosure doctrine does not involve negligence in the administration of treatment, in failure to treat, or in failure to properly diagnose"); Atkins v. Strayhorn, 273 Cal. Rptr. 231 (Ct. App. 1990) (informed consent does not apply to failure to treat condition doctor did not believe patient had); Townsend v. Turk, 266 Cal. Rptr. 821 (Ct. App. 1990) ("'Dr. Turk did not believe further testing was necessary to assist . . . in making the correct decisions. . . . Dr. Turk could "hardly 'disclose what he did not believe.'"'"). See also the cases cited in note 54 above holding that informed refusal law applies only when patients reject treatment the physician recommends.

111. Special Project 1986.

112. Karlsons v. Guerinot, 394 N.Y.S.2d 933 (App. Div. 1977) (no informed consent violation for failing to recommend amniocentesis or to warn of risk of giving birth to deformed child); Atlanta Obstetrics and Gynecology Group v. Abelson, 392 S.E.2d 916 (Ga. Ct. App. 1990) (same as *Karlsons*); Munro v. Regents of the Univ. of Cal., 263 Cal. Rptr. 878, 885 (Ct. App. 1989) (no informed consent violation for failing to recommend genetic test for Tay-Sachs disease).

113. Elias and Annas 1994, at 1611–13.

114. See Brett and McCullough 1986. Likewise, I know of no successful suits against holistic healers charging that they failed to disclose the unconventional nature of their treatment practices.

Naturally, if the patient brings the issue up himself, the doctor is expected to speak truthfully about his decision, unless there is ethical and medical justification for employing a placebo.

115. See Chapter 4 for documentation and further discussion.

116. Gillick 1988, at 749 ("many of those who die in nursing homes are tacitly allowed to die without further attempt at salvation"; "doctors and nurses frequently decide quietly to approach nursing home residents with benign neglect of medical problems"); Lo et al. 1985 (documenting that doctors regularly withhold CPR, sometimes without consent or over the patient's and family's objection); Rosenthal 1990b, at A1, B20 (reporting that medical teams frequently simply go through the motions by performing half-hearted resuscitation efforts behind drawn curtains, charades known as "Hollywood codes"); Orentlicher 1992 (surveying the range of situations in which patient choice is suppressed by medical norms).

117. Gray, Capone, and Most 1991; Hackler and Hiller 1990; Marsh and Staver 1991; Murphy 1988; Schneiderman, Jecker, and Jonsen 1990. For opposing views, see Lo and Steinbrook 1983; Loewy 1991; Youngner 1990; Scofield 1991, at 28.

118. Meisel 1979, at 453 and n.133; Appelbaum, Lidz and Meisel 1987, at 69–70.

119. See generally 45 C.F.R. § 46 (1994).

120. Capron 1990, at 125, 155–56.

121. Appelbaum, Lidz, and Meisel 1987, at 251–52.

122. Ost 1984, at 301–312; Katz 1984, at 122–24; Jones 1990, at 421.

123. Hellman and Hellman 1991, at 1586.

124. It may be reasonable to assert inalienability in the context of refusing life-sustaining treatment or making other treatment decisions so monumental or innately personal that they cannot be delegated at all. Thus, it is one thing to waive disclosure of the risks of treatment or nontreatment and quite another to place in the doctor's hands the very deci-

sion of whether or not to die. However, this argument does not apply to informed consent to rationing of marginally beneficial care, where the life-and-death stakes are extremely attenuated. Moreover, even if the argument did reach this far, it is not as absolute as this account portrays. Delegation of the decision *is* allowed for incapacitated patients. This is further illustrated by the Ulysses paradigm developed in Chapter 4. Here, the insensitivity to costs that results from the very existence of insurance—what economists call "moral hazard"—is an analogous form of disability that warrants a delegation of rationing authority.

125. President's Commission 1982, at 44–45.

126. By far, the best development of this argument I have found is Shapiro 1988a.

127. The two authors who make this point particularly cogent are Childress 1982, at 147–48; Strasser 1986, at 268–69, 274–75.

128. E.g., Rodwin 1989, at 1405–06; Mehlman 1990, at n.37. These critics also observe that physicians manipulate the consent process to obtain the result they desire by the tone and sequence in which they convey the risk information, and some go so far as to suggest that true consent is never obtained simply because of the coerciveness of medical authority that is inherent in any doctor–patient relationship. See, e.g., Burt 1979, at 44–45 (all social relations have a "coercive attribute" which cannot be abolished, only reallocated); Flick 1991, at 1149–50 ("'People are idiots.' They need to be protected from themselves, and others, because people do not always know or choose the possibility they ought to prefer. The underlying theory is human fallibility and finitude.").

129. For general surveys and their dire assessments for the possibility of truly informed consent, see Thompson 1982 (this research "dispels the notion that physicians can adequately 'inform' patients simply by presenting the required information to them in a simple, jargon-free manner"); Merz and Fischhoff 1990, at 323 ("the notion of consent as informed is a legal fiction. The present law simply cannot ensure attainment of that goal"); Twerski and Cohen 1988, at 627–41. See generally Fischhoff 1985, at 170; McNeil, Pauker, Sox, and Tversky 1982; Redelmeier, Rozin, and Kahneman 1993; Schneider 1996.

130. Marquis 1983. See also Garnick, Hendricks, and Thorpe, et al. 1993, at 204 ("almost all privately insured people understand the basic elements of their insurance plans"). It is troubling, however, that understanding drops off markedly as the complexity of insurance coverage increases. Marquis 1983.

131. Davidson 1988.

132. Also, involving patients in medical decision making produces better compliance with the treatment regimen and enhances patient trust, which has a positive therapeutic effect of its own.

133. Havighurst 1992, at 1787.

134. Dworkin 1988, at 102 (quoting Harper and James 1959).

> The very foundation of the doctrine [of informed consent] is every man's right to forego treatment or even cure if it entails what for him are intolerable consequences or risks, however warped or perverted his sense of values may be in the eyes of the medical profession, or even of the community, so long as the distortion falls short of what the law regards as incompetency.

135. Indeed, to allow informed consent doctrine to default to the opposite of the recommended decision, where that decision is nontreatment, is *less* principled since the origins of informed consent lie in battery. Such a default rule would illogically invoke informed consent doctrine to *require* the patient to be cut where there is an *absence* of consent, in blatant contradiction of battery law.

136. Appelbaum 1993, at 669–76.

137. President's Commission 1982; Meisel and Roth 1983; Schneider 1994; Schneider 1996.

138. The one that comes closest asked 210 patients receiving blood pressure medication how much discussion they would like about their treatment alternatives. Barely half wanted "quite a lot" or "very extensive" discussion and one half preferred having no role in making the decision. Strull, Lo and Charles 1984.

139. Mehlman 1990.

140. Engelhardt 1986, at 279. Accord Green 1988, at 240 (providing sample of actual form with four models to choose from: physician decides; simple disclosure of risks; joint decision making; and patient controls); Schuck 1994, at 956 (advocating a contractual approach to setting variable disclosure standards).

141. Havighurst 1994, at 159–65.

142. Faden and Beauchamp 1986, at 240–41.

143. Compare Walker v. Pierce, 560 F.2d 609 (4th Cir. 1977) (holding that an obstetrician can refuse to accept low-income patients unless they agree to a sterilization following the delivery of their third child: "We perceive no reason why Dr. Pierce could not establish and pursue the policy which he publicly and freely announced").

144. Shultz 1985, at 223 n.16, 281–82, 282 n.278.

145. Ezekiel Emanuel uses collective choice among HMO plans as a paradigm for constructing a liberal communitarian theory of medical ethics. He reasons precisely as I do here that, when a subscriber chooses an insurance plan, he is bound by the internal code of ethics that the group has chosen to adopt. Emanuel 1991. See the next chapter for further elaboration of this point.

146. A contrasting body of law consists of the cases striking down exculpatory clauses that completely waive malpractice liability. The leading decisions are Tunkl v. Regents of the Univ. of Cal., 383 P.2d 441 (Cal. 1963); Emory University v. Porubiansky, 282 S.E.2d 903 (Ga. 1981); but see Schneider v. Revici, 817 F.2d 987 (2d Cir. 1987) (enforcing release of liability by breast cancer patient who chose dietary therapy over conventional treatment). Other decisions are collected and discussed in Mehlman 1990; Epstein 1988; Epstein 1986, at 201; Havighurst 1986, at 149; Robinson 1986, at 173; Ginsburg, Kahn, Thornhill and Gambardella 1986, at 253.

However, these decisions are easily distinguishable since, unlike the partial waiver of informed consent considered here, malpractice waiver is actively disfavored as a matter of public policy; therefore, the terms of the waiver are by definition unfair. Also, the bargaining circumstances in those cases are markedly one-sided, frequently involving a provider foisting the waiver agreement on an isolated patient at the time he seeks treatment. In contrast, the type of waiver contemplated here is one that the law recognizes as a permissible exercise of patient autonomy, it is negotiated by an employer on behalf of a large group of employees, and is agreed to at the time of insurance enrollment rather than in the midst of illness.

147. 552 P.2d 1178 (Cal. 1976).

148. 552 P.2d at 1186.

149. *Madden* was very narrowly construed by a lower-court decision in Wheeler v. St. Joseph Hospital, 133 Cal. Rptr. 775, 783 (Ct. App. 1976), which struck down an arbitration agreement in a hospital admission form, observing in part that the patient was given no choice if he wanted to be admitted to that hospital. As Mehlman observes, though, this half-hearted attempt to distinguish *Madden* should be read more as frustrated disagreement with the higher court decision. Mehlman 1990, at 407 n.147. *Madden* was decided

after *Wheeler* had already been briefed, and the lower court did not seriously examine whether Wheeler had the alternative of being admitted to another hospital on more favorable terms.

150. See, e.g., Broemmer v. Abortion Services of Phoenix, 840 P.2d 1013 (Ariz. 1992) (striking down a similar agreement to arbitrate with an abortion clinic, due to the adhesion nature of contract which offered no other option).

151. See Pear 1995. These seriously erode fiduciary responsibility, and are opposed by my argument, because of the following defects: (1) These clauses are not revealed to subscribers and therefore they do not receive patient consent; (2) they prohibit the disclosure of rationing rules, incentives, and mechanisms, which generic disclosure, I argue, is necessary in order to validate nondisclosure of treamtnet-specific decisions at the bedside; and (3) some would appear to prohibit truthful answers even when patients initiate questioning. The patient's right to complete candor in response to the patient's legitimate questioning cannot be waived under any circumstances.

152. For additional, more-or-less specific suggested disclosures, see Goold and Brody 1995, which is excerpted at note 23 above, and Havighurst 1995, at 187–90.

153. For reasons developed in Hall and Anderson 1992 and summarized in Chapter 3, the parties to a health insurance contract should be free to agree to be bound by rules that are developed after the contract is entered into, so long as the mechanism for adopting and changing rules is sufficiently specified in the contract.

154. Schuck 1994, at 954.

155. Requiring bedside disclosures in certain high-stakes situations may not be as difficult in practice as I imagine, however. Where the aggressive treatment option entails considerable medical risk or patient suffering, doctors may find it easy to use the required disclosure as an opportunity to discourage patients from choosing the option. Many commentators have observed that doctors can produce almost any patient choice they want by shading the competing benefits and costs to make any other choice appear unreasonable. See also Annas and Miller 1994, at 393–94 (arguing that thorough disclosure may be the best way to convince Americans to forgo expensive but largely futile life-sustaining treatment).

7

Conclusion: Deciding Who Decides

Who makes medical spending decisions is of vital but underrecognized importance. That is why I have analyzed the issue in such exhaustive detail. The danger is that we have wound our way through such a complex maze of arguments that even the most attentive readers will have lost their bearings. This chapter will attempt to map a path through this maze.

The best way to understand where we started and where we have ended is to recall the point made in Chapter 1: Health care rationing, like most social policy decisions, can be debated at three fundamentally different levels: (1) what should be done, (2) who decides what to do, and (3) how to choose the proper decision maker.[1] Most of this book has been addressed to the level (2) debate. I have not attempted to answer the level (1) question of which patients should receive which treatments or even what the more general substantive criteria should be for allocating medical resources. Instead, I have compared the merits and flaws of making these health care spending decisions by patients at the time of treatment, by doctors at the bedside, or through rules established by commercial or governmental institutions. This chapter summarizes the main points of this level (2) analysis, and makes a foray into the level (3) inquiry.

COMPARING DECISION MAKERS

The level (2) analysis of medical spending decisions has produced the inconclusive result that no single mechanism is uniformly to be favored or avoided. This failure to reach a clear resolution may be unsatisfying, but it should not be surprising. In his recent exposition on comparative institutional analysis, Neil Komesar warns that there are rarely any clear-cut winners. "In a world of institutional alternatives that are both complex and imperfect, institutional choice . . . by long lists of imperfections is deeply inadequate. . . . The same factors that cause one alternative institution to [appear ill suited to the task] often affect all the alternative institutions."[2] Sometimes, however, these factors apply with greater or lesser force to different institutions. By looking at all the positive and negative factors simultaneously for all three mechanisms and their various permutations, one hopes to find through comparative institutional analysis that some of the strengths of one institution offset weaknesses of others, and visa versa, in a fashion that yields a sensible combination among them.

To determine if this happy state of affairs is possible, I will summarize the major conclusions of this book in a manner that seeks to highlight where one type of institution is clearly superior or inferior to the others. The difficulty with any such summary, as Professor Komesar explains, is that it can only be done in the most general of terms. For each of several broad dimensions of medical care, we can only hope to identify for each of the major types of decision makers in which general direction the dimension cuts with some rough gauge of magnitude. As these multiple dimensions intersect, the resulting picture becomes quite chaotic. Nevertheless, some attempt must be made to tie together the various strands of thought developed in this book.

I will begin with the dual dimensions of cost and quality, broken into the simplest possible categories of low-cost versus high-cost and low-benefit versus high-benefit cases. We might ask: In which of the three major mechanisms do we have the most confidence for treatments that fall into each of these very general categories? Table 7-1 summarizes my tentative conclusions.

Patients are poorly suited to decide about high-cost treatments entirely on their own because this is the end of the cost spectrum for which insurance is most in demand. We might also have serious qualms about doctors exercing their own discretion when costs are high and they have a financial stake in the decision, since strong economic conflicts of interest might have a corrosive effect on patient trust. If doctors do not have an obvious stake in their cost-motivated decisions, then their role as rationers is more attractive because they are well situated to take a population-based view that makes marginal sacrifices for one patient only to provide more benefit to others. Similarly, for third parties, we have different reactions according to the exact situation. Insurers have an obvious economic bias, which is held in check to some extent by market forces, but which still makes us suspicious of their being too concerned about the costs of treatment. Democratic institutions are more likely than courts to take an appropriately balanced social view of costs. Otherwise, the cost dimension alone does not have a striking effect on our intuitions about appropriate decision mechanisms.

Table 7–1. Confidence in medical-spending decision makers for various categories of treatment

	Patients	Physician discretion		Third parties		
		No financial incentives	With financial incentives	Insurers	Courts	Citizens
High cost	No	?	No	No	?	Yes
Low cost	Yes	Yes	Yes	Yes	Yes	Yes
High benefit	Yes	Yes	Yes	Yes	Yes	Yes
Low benefit	Yes	Yes	?	Yes	?	Yes

The benefit spectrum produces few categorical insights. Both patients and doctors are well situated to recognize high versus low benefits as they may vary among individuals. Doctors are not especially accomplished at discerning patients' social values, but they have superior knowledge of the technical aspects of what works and what does not. Among third parties, insurers and regulators are able to draw on medical expertise and so suffer no absolute disability in assessing benefits, but they are only able to do so for aggregations of patients rather than individually. Courts can be trusted, but their views of benefits are more likely to be distorted by the extremes of the individualistic perspective and the adversarial tactics that are inherent in the litigation process.

We might gain somewhat more insight by combining these rough categories to form the following cost/benefit matrix. Simply aggregating the positions in the previous chart yields the tentative judgments shown in Table 7–2.

This purely mechanical process produces some conclusions that seem intuitively plausible. When benefits are high and costs are low, we trust just about any institution to get the obvious right answer. Childhood immunization is a case in point. However, when the stakes are raised and both costs and benefits are high, we place the most trust in unbiased mechanisms, especially democratic ones, because of the strong desire for social legitimacy. Expensive, life-saving transplants are a classic example.

Table 7–2. Confidence in medical-spending decision makers for cost/benefit categories of treatment

	Patients	Physician discretion		Third parties		
		No financial incentives	With financial incentives	Insurers	Courts	Citizens
High cost/High benefit	Mixed	Medium	Mixed	Mixed	Medium	Strong
High cost/Low benefit	Mixed	Medium	Low	Mixed	Uncertain	Strong
Low cost/High benefit	Strong	Strong	Strong	Strong	Medium	Strong
Low cost/Low benefit	Strong	Strong	Medium	Strong	Medium	Strong

Other conclusions seem less convincing. High-cost, low-benefit cases (such as redundant MRI scans) should produce clear answers, but our institutional confidences are mixed in a pattern that is not intuitively clear. The one point that stands out is, when more implicit, less overt rationing is called for, we again have more faith in unbiased physicians and third-party mechanisms. Where both costs and benefits are low and therefore the right answer is uncertain (e.g., antibiotics for probable viral infections), we appear to have equally strong confidence in most institutions, for reasons that are not apparent. It is also anomalous that democratic institutions receive consistently strong support in this rote summary despite the many flaws identified in Chapter 3, and it is strange that patients and insurers have precisely the same mixed set of ratings.

Naturally, this rough sketch is far too simplistic to provide much practical guidance. Among the factors it omits are the types of health benefits at stake and how they are measured. Health benefits might be classified broadly as concentrated (rare diseases) versus widespread (common diseases), certain versus uncertain, and subjective (value laden) versus objective (broad consensus). Benefits can be concentrated or widespread according to the numbers and demographics of the people affected by the condition. Compare the clotting factor for hemophiliacs with blood transfusions for ordinary patients. For some conditions and treatments, such as new, experimental treatments for cancer, a few patients receive clear benefits but most do not, yet we have very little information about which patients fall into which categories. For other treatments, the physiological benefits are clear, but the importance attached to those outcomes varies widely according to individual, subjective tastes. Consider, for instance, life-sustaining treatment for people with diminished capacity.

Third-party mechanisms are least able to account for variable or subjective benefits and best suited for situations where benefits are certain and uniform, for these are the ones most adaptable to rules. Patients and doctors are better situated to make case-specific judgment calls. Where third-party mechanisms are appropriate, there may be concern about using democratic institutions where the benefits are concentrated or localized for fear that the majority may be callous about conditions it believes will not affect it. Interest-group politics can also produce the opposite bias, namely, inattention to low-benefit conditions that are widely diffused, and excessive attention to concentrated high benefits because of their vocal advocates. Judicial safeguards are especially important where there is a risk of majoritarian tyranny.

A somewhat different political dynamic affects our intuitions according to whether health conditions and rationing dilemmas are highly visible or are obscured from public view. We have observed that visibility may call for heightened public legitimacy but that it may also handicap us from setting necessary resource constraints. This is illustrated by the paradox of identifiable versus statistical lives that arises when society is willing to "waste" huge sums of money in a futile attempt to save one person in severe distress but will spend very little on basic safety measures to prevent the crisis from occurring in the first place. This disparity occurs because in the latter event we have no psychological connection with the "statistical" lives that are being invisibly saved. Keeping some rationing decisions hidden, such as shortened hospital stays, may suppress this irrationality, but bringing some others such as aggressive life-support into the open may produce greater rationality. Some rationing decisions such as organ transplants are unavoidably visible and so require a mechanism that confers the greatest public legitimacy.

Competing mechanisms for resource allocation can also be evaluated with these "visibility" or "rationality" factors in mind. Individual patients tend to under-commit resources to preventive services or to illnesses that are hard to detect. These same biases are likely to affect democratic institutions. Physicians suffer from a reciprocal bias that causes them to overcommit to serious, visible illness. Their rescue and nonabandonment ethic leads them to favor those in the worst condition or those for whom they have already begun treatment, rather than those who might stand to receive the greatest benefit. Where conditions are perceived by the public as more threatening than they really are or treatments are perceived as more beneficial than is realistic, then less visible mechanisms such as physician bed-side rationing might be preferred. But third-party rules are called for where physicians' own biases are prominent, or where inherent visibility coupled with high stakes (for example, organ transplants) calls for heightened public legitimacy.

Many similar categorizations are also possible using equally general categories. We might attempt to assess resource allocation mechanisms according to whether they affect preventive, acute, or chronic care or the type of harm at risk (mental, physical, life, mobility, etc.). We might also attempt to devise new hybrid institutions and actors that combine the best and avoid the worst of the imperfect options that exist now. One especially appealing idea is Robert Veatch's suggestion, discussed at the end of chapter 3, for "medically-trained agents" to oversee treating physicians.

While these and other categorizations offer some useful insight, they are all ultimately unsatisfying because they offer no clear guide to action. These categorizations are too general to classify very many particular treatment decisions, and these multiple, intersecting dimensions produce too many conflicting vectors to offer a definitive resolution even of those cases whose characteristics are clear. As a consequence, at bottom we are not much further along in answering the level (2) question of who should make these decisions. We now understand much more about how resource allocation decisions present themselves, but the only definitive conclusion is that none of our major candidates should be ruled out.

CHOOSING DECISION MAKERS

Because this level (2) analysis has proven to be so indeterminant, we might try shifting our focus to the third-level question in order to obtain some greater sense of resolution. Just as the inability to settle on definitive first-order rationing criteria leads us to analyze who should decide, so the inability to conclusively choose a decision maker prompts us to examine ways of deciding who decides. The fundamental premise of a liberal democracy is that where consensus is lacking on questions of social policy, we look for some higher-level consensus on the best mechanism for putting the social policy question to individual or collective choice. At this third level, there are three basic options: the market, the legislature, and the courts.

I have suggested in the last three chapters that the market is a proper vehicle for selecting the best mix, or best range of mixes, among imperfect decision makers. This market mechanism can operate via the process of selecting a health insurance plan. If consumers are given an informed choice among different types of insurance that deliver care in different institutional settings, their decisions will, to a large extent, dictate a resolution of the dilemmas confronted at the second level. This motif of informed insurance selection has also been sounded by a number of other commentators as a solution to these and other vexing problems of medical ethics.[3] They observe that many of the most pressing and unresolved problems of health care public policy can be decided by individual choice through the mechanism of insurance selection.

For instance, our society continues to debate what intensity of life-support is appropriate for terminally ill and comatose patients and who should decide. Much of this debate might be mooted if those who insist on aggressive, spare-no-expense treatment at the end of life had to either pay for this treatment out of pocket or show that they elected insurance explicitly covering such treatment for a higher premium.[4] Likewise, health care resource allocation decisions more generally can be resolved by having subscribers elect at the time of insurance enrollment among particular treatments to be rationed, such as expensive organ transplants, or among generic standards of medical urgency to be applied in specific cases.[5]

In surveying the range of social and economic mechanisms for answering these crucial questions, I have consistently returned in this book to the notion that individuals should have a large voice in how best to allocate authority for making spending decisions, a voice that they can exercise when they select a particular insurance plan.[6] In Chapter 2, I argue that we should honor consumers' desire, expressed when they purchase comprehensive insurance, to remain partially or fully insulated from the costs of treatment due to the anxiety and stress of illness, whereas consumers who purchase catastrophic insurance signal their desire to make their own spending decisions. In Chapter 4, I argue that those who purchase one of the classic HMO models, if properly informed, signal their desire for some form of bedside rationing, and in Chapter 3 I concede that rule-based rationing is authorized by specific exclusions in insurance coverage. Chapter 5 demonstrates that informed insurance enrollment can validate an otherwise ethically suspect use of financial incentives that encourage physicians to trim marginally beneficial care. Even more controversially, I argue in Chapter 6 that informed insurance enrollment can validate physicians not fully disclosing to patients at the time of treatment some of the marginal cost/benefit trade-off decisions they make.

A market in insurance selection is different than the market mechanism rejected in the second chapter. There we discussed requiring consumers to make their own first-level spending decisions about particular items of treatment. That approach is deeply flawed because it requires consumers to know a great deal more than they do about the technical aspects of medicine, it requires them to go partially without the financial protection that they desire from insurance, and it ignores the vulnerable psychological state patients are in when they are sick. In contrast, consumers are much more able and willing to make the types of decisions expressed when they choose insurance. Insurance subscribers are essentially being asked what type of physician, what style of medicine, and what institutional structure they prefer. Subscribers may not have extensive experience with these matters, but they are at least capable of forming their own opinions about them. And through the convention of annual open enrollment, they have the opportunity to switch when they discover they have made a mistake.

The leading alternatives to this market mechanism are the political process and the courts. By advocating a market solution, I do not contend that it is uniquely and exclusively favored. Elected representatives also have a legitimate voice in the third-level debate, which they frequently express through laws such as those regulating utilization review activities, the content of health insurance, and physician payment incentives. A judicial process can also determine who possesses rationing authority by adjudicating disputes over insurance coverage and by reviewing the statutory and constitutional accuracy of government decisions. Space does not permit a full-scale comparative analysis of these competing approaches for selecting the best medical spending decision makers. At this point in the book, the most I can attempt to do is outline the basic justification for a primarily market approach to deciding who should decide.

The fullest embodiment of the market mechanism I favor is found in various proposals for health care reform using a managed competition structure. This structure was at the heart of President Clinton's rejected 1993 plan, and it is at the heart of the Medicare reforms recently crafted by Republican legislators. Managed competition is also taking hold in the private marketplace and at a smaller- scale governmental level. Some version of managed competition already exists for large private employers, federal employees, many state employees (for example, California), and several state Medicaid programs (for example, Arizona and Tennessee).

Ideally, consumers would be given a choice among a range of comprehensive health insurance options, from catastrophic coverage and medical savings accounts, to various forms of managed care, to unrestricted fee-for-service. The optimum range of choice will not be feasible in many nonmetropolitan locations that lack market depth, but it should be possible to offer at least one version of these three basic insurance types to most people. This insurance could be paid from a variety of governmental or private sources as long as individual subscribers are required to bear some of the differential costs for selecting one option over the other. Obviously, this would require a subsidy for those with low incomes. If such a subsidy is not feasible, then choices for low-income subscribers would have to be made in the political rather than the market arena.

Next, we must consider how best to structure insurance contracts so that options over decision-making authority are clear to subscribers who have to choose, and to the courts that enforce the contracts. At various points in this book, I have articulated language and concepts for telling consumers about the incentives, rules, and mechanisms for making cost/benefit trade-off decisions.[7] Elsewhere, I have developed additional ideas about how to structure decision making and dispute resolution under health insurance, ideas that are more complex and untested,[8] and there are other attractive contenders.[9] I have no doubt that these ideas can be refined and improved. Certainly, it is not possible to devise an optimal approach to contract structure and disclosure without extensive empirical testing of how best to present this large and complex body of information. Also, subscribers should be given the opportunity as frequently as is feasible to reconsider their decisions and switch plans based on their experiences.

As noted several times throughout the book, these assumptions of free and informed insurance selection are undermined by large and obvious defects in insurers' actual disclosure practices, subscribers' actual comprehension and attention spans, and the range of actual choice available in existing public and private insurance systems. Whether these inevitable real-world defects undermine the resulting medical spending decisions depends on which framework for moral and political analysis one adopts. The principle of promoting autonomy, by itself, is not capable of identifying what conditions are necessary for proper application of the principle.[10] Understanding when constraints in choice undermine the individual autonomy rationale requires that, in the remainder of this chapter, we approach the rationale from a somewhat broader theoretical perspective.

THE POLITICAL MORALITY OF INSURANCE SELECTION

In theory, it is an attractive solution to virtually any question of medical ethics that it be individually resolved through the informed choice of an insurance plan, since almost all questions of medical ethics entail the delivery or refusal of services potentially paid for by insurance. Because so much of the argument in this book rests at its core on the notion that people are bound to the decisions inherent in the insurance coverage they select, it is crucial to examine this position critically from a variety of moral and political perspectives.

I will employ the two systems of moral and political critique that are best suited to our political history and social culture: classic individual liberalism, and the emerging body of thought known as *communitarianism*. Neither liberalism nor communitarianism squarely answers how best to organize health insurance markets or write insurance contracts. Both systems of thought leave ample room for wide-ranging debate and creative solutions within a pluralistic society. But the contrasts in these two bodies of moral and political theory markedly affect the terms in which the debate is conducted, and therefore the likely end point of the debate.

The Limits of Medical Liberalism

Liberalism is a system of political, economic, and moral thought that attempts to reconcile the demands of maintaining a stable society with those of respecting individual value preferences.[11] It is broadly consistent with classic liberal principles to resolve medical/moral dilemmas by reference to the type of insurance individuals choose.[12] On the surface, this liberal solution to virtually any question of medical ethics fails only in specialized areas such as pregnancy, pediatrics, and contagious disease where one's enrollment and spending decisions directly and tangibly affect the rights and interests of others.

The obvious difficulty with this scheme is the practical limitations imposed by the insurance product and the insurance market. For insurance selection to operate in this idealized fashion, not only must the full array of individual preferences be available for each of the multitude of value dimensions in medical treatment, each of these value points on each of the value dimensions must exist in impossibly complex combinations with each of the other possible choices.

I, for instance, do not want to accept anything less than insurance that pays for the following, but I do not want to pay for anyone else's preference that is any more costly than: (1) coverage of medically necessary but not elective abortions; and (2) no payment for life-support if terminally ill and in pain but payment if permanently comatose; and (3) physician authority to trim marginally beneficial diagnostic tests but no direct financial incentive to do so; and (4) full disclosure of the risks of invasive treatment that is being proposed but only notice and simple explanation of other treatment being performed and only bare notice of important treatment alternatives being omitted; and (5) a very generous standard of medical appropriateness for cancer treatment but a moderate standard for heart treatment and a very stringent standard for both once I am 80 years old; and (6). . . . If even one of these items is absent in the options available in the marketplace, my election of insurance is morally compromised since each item has an important moral dimension about which I would not have a chance to express my individual preference.

I stress that this full product differentiation is necessary only for liberalism's vision to be perfectly implemented. But this is not necessary at all in order for liberalism to be only minimally satisfied. In our pluralistic society, freedom of choice and autonomous action are strongly held values that should be maximized when doing so is feasible. In health care reform debates, this might favor a voucher system for public programs so that beneficiaries can select their own insurance plan from many private sector alternatives rather than receiving a single, "socialized" uniform benefit package. There are a variety of other important ideas on how best to refine this maximalist version of the liberal vision, which seeks the most expansive range of choice that is feasible. But I do not intend to pursue these refinements here. Instead, it is more important first to set the lower limits of acceptable choice. The minimalist version of liberal ethics, which I will now explore, asks whether restrictions in the choice of insurance are ever so severe that the decision to enroll carries no legitimacy of consent whatsoever for the ethical compromises contained in the insurance package. In other words, acknowledging that any restriction in choice entails a moral compromise of the ethical ideal, is there a point at which choice is so constrained that liberalism attaches absolutely *no* moral force to a subscriber's enrollment decision?

Individual Choice in the Private Sector

In the private sector, "coercion" or "duress" is the legal and moral concept used to define minimally acceptable choice. It is only when pressures to act or decide . rise to a coercive level that we conclude the resulting action is robbed of all voluntariness and thus all moral significance. Coercion is required for moral negation, even though we might conclude that lesser forms of pressure are morally inferior. A contract signed with a gun to the head has no legal force whatsoever, whereas one signed under extreme financial distress or as the result of hard bargaining may still be partially or fully enforceable. A coerced confession to a crime is entirely inadmissible whereas the prosecution is free to use a confession obtained through blatant trickery or lies. Using these guideposts, when might we conclude that the limitations in choice among health insurance options similarly deny any moral relevance to the subscriber's accepting various controversial resource allocation decisions contained in the insurance package?

I will look first at private insurance, which is usually supplied by employers. Analytical philosophers have developed several insightful distinctions that clarify that private choices are not coerced by limited insurance options, however dire the individual's level of need, since employers and insurers have no moral or legal duty to provide health insurance of any sort. Alan Wertheimer provides the most comprehensive and cogent treatment of coercion to date.[13] He demonstrates that coercion is not simply a phenomenological test of psychic pressure; it entails a moral evaluation of the source of this pressure. The judgment of coercion turns on a two-pronged inquiry of (1) whether there was a deprivation of reasonable or meaningful choice and (2) whether a wrong was committed in creating this lack of choice. For instance, we would never say that a patient's election of heart surgery is coerced simply by virtue of the life-or-death urgency that compelled consent, since the doctor is not responsible for bringing about the patient's condition.

However, we might say that a psychiatrist coerces a patient into having sex with him if he incorrectly insists this is necessary for effective therapy.

In more difficult cases where the moral judgment is less clear, Wertheimer's analysis requires us to focus on whether an allegedly coerced party faces more of an opportunity than a threat, that is, whether the offer that is "too good to refuse" worsens rather than improves his baseline situation. Wertheimer applies this test at its extreme to Joel Feinberg's dastardly example of a "Lecherous Millionaire" who agrees to pay for the lifesaving operation on a woman's only child (not his own) if she agrees to be his mistress.[14] Such an offer may be illegal as soliciting prostitution and it is certainly immoral, unconscionable, exploitative, and therefore a far departure from the liberal ideal, but it is not coercive.[15] Because the Millionaire is not responsible for the woman's plight and is not obligated to pay for her child's treatment, he can only be viewed as increasing her preexisting range of options, however despicable his motives might be. This distasteful conclusion is fundamental to our very social fabric since, as Jeffrie Murphy has observed, if inequalities of fortune were to invalidate agreements, "then the law of contracts—in fact, the whole of capitalism—is in serious moral trouble indeed."[16]

These analytical insights reveal that, in the private sphere, so far as classic liberalism is concerned, a limited range of health insurance options does not absolutely defeat the moral force that arises from an individual's election of that insurance, even if only a single option is presented or the alternatives are so compromised as to threaten coverage for essential treatment. Coercion is absent for the simple reason that individual private employers and insurers have no preexisting moral or legal obligation to offer insurance of any particular sort and are not responsible for the compelling need that employees have to obtain insurance. Therefore, any form of private insurance improves the moral baseline condition of subscribers, however morally repugnant the resulting package of benefits and payment rules might be. This moral repugnance might create an intolerable departure from the liberal ideal and therefore give rise to public regulations that require more of insurers and employers, but it does not create grounds under classic liberalism for entirely invalidating the moral force of the choice the subscriber made in selecting this insurance package over another, or over nothing.

Flaws in the Private Insurance Market

The core problem with liberalism, then, is that it is both too demanding and too forgiving of the quality of the choice mechanism that is used to express individual preferences. Liberalism is too demanding in its idealized vision of autonomy, which seems never to be fully satisfied with the range of options and the inevitable costs and constraints that attach to choices within the range. My election of insurance is not fully autonomous unless I can have exactly the package of services I want and no more, and unless this choice is not hampered by any deficit in wealth or any imperfections in the market that burden my choice. On the other hand, at the extreme of realism where liberalism recognizes the practical limitations on available choice, it is satisfied far too easily under the coercion criterion by any limitation, however severe, and for virtually whatever reason.

Although the real-world conditions in which health insurance is actually sold fall in between these two extremes, they are much closer to the minimalist end than to the decent array of choice required for individualistic values to be well served. In the present market for private health insurance, looking only at those who presently can afford it, most people have no choice of insurance plans at all, and those that do have only a limited array of options. Over three-quarters of all private health insurance is sold through employer groups, and in most instances, employers make one choice for the entire work force.[17] Although many large employers allow employees to elect from a handful of options, those options usually vary only along one or two dimensions relating to the size of the deductible and the basic type of insurance (HMO, indemnity, or PPO). Very little differentiation exists in the particulars of coverage beyond how much the patient must pay out of pocket. The primary variables are the coverage for preventive and behavioral services. Virtually no variation exists on the core dimension of the standard of professional care for medical and surgical services.[18] Even where core variation exists, such as between HMOs and standard indemnity, insurance contracts are woefully deficient in explaining to subscribers some aspects of the actual terms of coverage and conditions of treatment they are electing. The most notable example is the failure, noted in Chapter 6, of HMOs to inform subscribers how physicians are compensated and the effects that payment incentives might have on treatment decisions.

More disturbing than these observations about the present state of the health insurance market is the realization that these conditions are largely impermeable aspects of even the most visionary types of market reform. Severe practical limitations on the feasible range of freedom are inevitable in any market of private insurance despite the most abiding hopes of reformers. Proponents of managed competition hope that all subscribers, and perhaps all people, will have the same range of options presently enjoyed by employees of large firms. At most, this suggests perhaps a dozen choices, mostly of the sort already in the market, with some enhancement in the types and amount of consumer information available for comparison shopping.[19]

This is a far cry from the hundreds or thousands of options necessary to achieve the perfect liberal resolution of the numerous complex value choices entailed in resource-constrained health care. Moreover, the limitations in consumers' attention spans and the complexities of reporting valid and understandable measures of basic comparative performance ensure that little time and energy will remain during the annual open enrollment to contemplate fundamental mysteries of the universe such as the meaning and value of life. Research shows that subscribers' ability to understand the basic content of their health insurance policies drops off sharply as the complexity of the plan increases.[20] It is for these very reasons that many of the most prominent managed competition advocates maintain that the content of insurance contracts should be largely uniform or be allowed to vary only by limited and carefully controlled categories so that consumers can focus their attention more directly on which insurers have the best doctors and the best systems for managing costs, rather than having to worry about exactly what services are covered.

Such uniformity may be good for economic efficiency, but it would greatly erode the liberal foundation for enforcing the restrictions contained in limited health insurance. On the other hand, consumer choice cannot be used to solve all moral problems given the incomprehensible confusion that results when every important aspect of health insurance varies from one policy to another. It is impossible to focus consumers' attention simultaneously on every single important feature of an insurance contract, yet liberal and market principles cannot tell us which features to hold constant and which to vary.

As discussed above, liberalism takes a polarized attitude toward this multitude of limitations. The idealized version, which often predominates in ethical discourse, declares that any accommodation of these limitations in choice denies a desirable level of individual autonomy, however unachievable that level may be in practical reality. In contrast, the minimalist version of liberal analysis, which sometimes predominates in political discourse, too willingly accepts all of these limitations because they are all unavoidable results of free markets. Even if some limits are imposed by government or industry fiat, this is done for legitimate, choice- and market-preserving reasons and thus does not constitute morally disabling coercion. Classic liberalism, therefore, does not provide the more nuanced analytical tools for determining what degree of freedom is acceptable or pragmatically optimal for validating ethically controversial choices. Additional insight can be gained, however, from a newer branch of liberalism developed by philosopher John Rawls.

Individual Choice in the Public Sector

Rawls takes us beyond this impasse in individual liberalism by developing principles of distributive (or social) justice that identify primary social goods to which everyone has a claim for equal distribution.[21] Although the content of Rawls's own package of primary social goods is notoriously abstract (containing items such as liberty, opportunity, and a sense of self-worth), other philosophers have used Rawls's analysis to build a case for a basic level of health care.[22] Because health more than any other tangible good is necessary to pursue the range of other social goods, there exists a fundamental social obligation to provide everyone with a decent minimum level of medical treatment.

No one has yet or is ever likely to develop this analysis to the level of concreteness necessary to prescribe an actual benefits package.[23] Still, it is useful to think abstractly about meeting or failing this "basic," "bare," or "decent" minimum. One can imagine a variety of heuristic devices with which to conceptualize what might go into an actual bare minimum level of support: It is the least amount of health care we can imagine ourselves tolerating in the worst of circumstances. It is whatever level of health care is necessary to keep us from cringing at the thought that others might be offered less. Or it is the level of health care coverage that could be purchased with the money that a high-minded, noncorrupt legislature would be willing to appropriate, given other competing social demands.[24]

However conceived, this bare minimum analysis allows us to rework the liberal solution with a new tool. This is accomplished by again speaking in terms of coercion. Where coercion is asserted in a private realm, it makes perfect sense to say that injustice in a person's social and economic baseline is no grounds for an individual rights-based claim to avoiding contractual obligations that exploit the situation. A grocer may require even a starving homeless person to pay for a loaf of bread, and doctors may charge even dying patients for their treatment. In contrast, in the public realm, social injustice provides strong grounds for claiming coercion against the government. The arrested criminal suspect who is denied minimally humane food and sleep has solid grounds for claiming that a resulting confession is coerced, and denying a prisoner minimally decent medical care is an unconstitutional imposition of "cruel and unusual punishment."

In the public health care sphere, we can say that the election of a morally compromised insurance package is socially coerced if it is made on pain of being denied a decent bare minimum level of health care. If the social minimum is not reasonably available to me,[25] my insurance selection cannot be used to validate the resulting moral compromises in my medical treatment. On the other hand, I can be forced to accept any degree of health care rationing, however severe the consequence, if I make a fully informed election of my rationed insurance over against a health care option that provides at least this basic social minimum.

This social coercion line of analysis is attractive because it extends liberal thinking from classic private markets to mixed private and public systems. It also holds some prospect for developing a meaningful moral standard other than conventional private coercion. Everyone has an elemental humanitarian claim to a decent minimum of health care; satisfying this claim is a moral obligation of society that falls on government if private markets or individual altruism fails. This support might be supplied through several different mechanisms. The government could supply it directly through state-owned-and-run clinics and hospitals; it could provide a safety-net insurance program similar to Medicaid; or it could distribute vouchers in an amount sufficient to purchase the bare minimum package in the private marketplace. However it is provided, if a subscriber to either a private or a public insurance plan has an option that meets the bare minimum, the moral compromises that exist in the insurance the subscriber actually selects are valid, even if the resulting insurance falls below the bare minimum in some respect. Conversely, it is a coercive denial of positive liberty to force a morally compromised form of insurance on pain of denying a basic minimum of health care.

This is as far as liberalism has been able to carry us, however. We are still stymied on two fronts in our search for a practical and concrete way to invoke insurance selection as a means to solve moral problems in health care resource allocation. First, without an actual, specified minimum benefits package, the vision of a normative standard becomes a chimera. Second, this normative analysis still does not resolve the tough moral compromises necessary to even implement an affordable basic package. For instance, we know from present experience that we cannot afford a basic package structured as unrestricted fee-for-service indemnity, yet medical ethics until recently treated as morally controversial any restriction in the choice of physician, and it still treats as controversial any incentives for physicians to consider the costs of treatment. Although it is unacceptable to propose as the bare minimum an exemplary level of service that even many middle-class citizens do not enjoy and cannot afford, it is still the case that some important items of coverage will have to be deleted and some controversial limitations on practice setting and practice style will have to be enforced in order to even set the moral baseline. The extension of liberalism into the public sphere cannot be used to determine through individual choice which compromises are allowable in creating this basic package. Without this moral baseline firmly in place, we cannot be certain that the value choices entailed in insurance selection against the baseline are morally grounded.

The Communitarian Vision

I now turn to communitarian theory to explore whether it is capable of taking us beyond these limitations in liberalism. I choose to apply communitarian theory because it offers an appealing alternative to classic liberalism, which has been subjected to increasing criticism for its excessive focus on individual rights.[26] On first inspection, communitarianism is quite promising for addressing mixed issues of ethics and economics.[27] It has established itself not as the utter rejection of liberalism but rather as a critique of the individualistic excesses of classic liberalism.[28] Communitarian thought is sensitive to the social contexts in which individuals act and therefore it potentially incorporates the interconnected complexities of the modern world, which does not neatly divide into the purely private and public realms imagined by classic liberalism. In particular, communitarianism is well suited to analyzing issues in the context of both public and private insurance selection, since the act of purchasing insurance can itself be viewed as the formation of a prototypical community. As discussed below, insurance by its nature is a community-forming vehicle in which individuals are required to set aside a portion of their individualism and share a common set of interests and expectations.

Various branches of communitarian thought emphasize different types of communities, from political, to social, to ideological, to familial. Elsewhere in society, communitarians bemoan the disintegration of traditional communities such as extended families and tight-knit neighborhoods.[29] Largely ignored but perfectly compatible with communitarianism are economic communities of interest. The only economic community to which communitarians have devoted substantial attention so far is the workplace. Health care has the good fortune of possessing another economic community-forming vehicle in the form of insurance.[30]

The central feature of a community—the reciprocal sharing of common interests and responsibilities—precisely describes an insurance pool.[31] Even though the collective aspect of insurance has become diluted through the corporatization of the enterprise and the individualization of the product, in its core design insurance is still very much a mutual enterprise. One who purchases insurance for a defined risk in a defined amount joins a fairly homogenous community of shared economic interest. What then does communitarian thought have to say about the resulting restrictions in freedom entailed by selection of a resource-constrained insurance plan? I will address this query at three levels: What restrictions on choice are permissible within a community? What is a community and how is one formed? And, interspersed throughout these two inquiries, what implications are there for health insurance and resource allocation?

Collective Choice

Within communities, communitarian theory is less concerned with the quality of choice than is liberalism. Communitarians do not view restrictions on individual choice as necessarily a compromise of the ethical ideal. Instead, where these restrictions are essential to the nature of the community, they *define* the ethical ideal. This is because communitarianism does not see individuals and their personal values as necessarily in opposition to their communities. Instead, communities are said to be constitutive of individual identities.[32] Therefore, it is a false polarization to say I am opposed to or suppressed by a community. Instead, I am defined in part by my community ties, both their liberalizing and their constraining aspects.[33]

Putting the point in a less metaphysical fashion, the claim is that people can express value preferences collectively as well as individually. We often rationally choose to suppress individual desires in order to achieve some end that is possible only through collective action.[34] A real threat of armed invasion by a foreign power may convince me to support a draft army that forces me and my neighbors to go to war, even though I personally do not want to volunteer my life individually to protect anyone but my own family. My desire for defense can only be realized by collective compulsion. Liberalism accommodates this example as the special case of a purely "public commodity"—one that is collectively produced and collectively consumed—but communitarianism generalizes this example to potentially any expression of collective will. For any number of individual preferences, individual initiative will not suffice because we are unable to achieve the full expression of these preferences without a collective rule of action or restraint.

Therefore, communitarians see limited options not as the negative suppression of individual choice but as the positive exercise of collective choice. Although individuals may still object, they are not being subjected to social compulsion; having participated in the community decision, they are more accurately viewed as exercising collective self-restraint or self-command. In the health arena, this vision of collective action fits most comfortably with public health regulation that results in chlorinating the water supply and immunization from contagious diseases.[35] But this collective view also has strong force in the realm of health insurance. An employer who selects a single health insurance plan with one or more ethically controversial features is exercising the collective preference of the entire work force. Likewise, a government that structures a public program expresses to some degree the will of the electorate.

The communitarian characterization of collective choice is especially persuasive for health insurance because of the attributes of insurance that require that group rather than individual decisions be made. If I were willing to pay for each item of my health care out-of-pocket, I legitimately could complain if treatment options were denied to me. When health care is covered by insurance, however, it necessarily must be subject to a uniform set of rules covering a group of subscribers. And the more that health insurance takes the form of managed care, the more we realize that these restrictions apply to the delivery of services as well as to the financing of services. This insight is captured in the newly popular slogan that, in the era of managed care, primary care physicians must begin to think in terms of *optimizing* the *health* of *populations* rather than *maximizing* the *treatment* of *individuals*. As David Eddy observes:

> When people decide to pool their resources to share the financial risks of health care, they must accept the fact that those resources will have to be shared in a way that maximizes the benefit to the entire group. Individuals cannot expect to draw without limit from the resource pool to maximize their personal care, regardless of the consequences to the other people who contributed to the pool. . . . When the size of the pool is fixed, health plans bear a deep responsibility for ensuring that the resources are allocated fairly—to maximize the health of the entire group, not just particular subsets.[36]

Preserving perfectly individualized treatment choice is not feasible in the realm of resource-constrained insurance, and communitarian thought helps us to realize that this is more of an advantage than a detriment. Even for those who can afford care out-of-pocket, Chapter 2 explains that health insurance might still be preferred simply because of the peace of mind (and possible therapeutic benefit) that comes from not having to worry about money at a time of personal crisis.

With this understood, collective constraints are legitimate when an insured group, following a sufficiently stringent decision rule, decides to exercise collective choice for the betterment of the whole. Money that is spent on the transaction costs of arranging for more choice takes away from the primary benefits to the entire group, so at some level the group rationally desires to restrict the coverage available to its members. Too often, we think of our health insurance as giving us individual entitlements to make limitless demands on anonymous resources. A communitarian vision helps us to see that insurance creates a collective interest in a shared resource that entails both individual rights to demand support and individual obligations of restraint.

Despite these rosy characterizations, the fact remains that individual subscribers are bound by the restrictions in insurance contracts no matter how severe or personally repugnant. The group may have decided not to pay for sex-change operations, but an individual member may vehemently object and may have had no choice in being made part of the group. Liberalism sees these as severe restraints on freedom whereas communitarianism tolerates or even celebrates them as acts of autonomous community self-determination. Majoritarian oppression of minority preferences is not a major concern in communitarian thought. As a result, it has been criticized for fostering totalitarian attitudes that marginalize individual preferences as not morally significant when they are in conflict with the community's fundamental values.[37]

Communitarianism attempts to avoid this charge of harsh intolerance by striking a middle road between the extremes of radical individualism and fascism. Whereas liberalism checks state power with individual rights, the communitarian approach is to stress the ways in which communities owe obligations of support to their members. Restrictions that deny basic social support are more easily and directly criticized under a communitarian framework than under liberalism because communitarian thought grounds the community's obligation in living, breathing societies and institutions. As a consequence, medical treatment cannot be denied (or forced) that infringes a basic obligation of support or a basic human right as defined by an insurance community.

This is so, however, only if and to the extent that the community in fact embraces a basic minimum. Communitarianism views a limitation in available treatment as not ethically problematic, no matter how much a particular individual's values may differ, if the limitation is fundamental to the community. Communitarianism has not developed a criterion of fundamentalness, but I will suppose it suffices that the value choice is one the community has made explicitly and therefore has incorporated into the insurance contract that defines an insurance community.

So far, this explanation is largely consistent with classic liberalism because it implicitly assumes freedom of choice among insurance communities. If people are completely free to leave one group and join another, any restriction within a group is truly voluntary. In other arenas of communitarian thought, restrictions in choice are a much greater problem than for health insurance because the nature of many communities is largely or entirely "ascriptive"—membership is imposed, not chosen.[38] We are born into a family with an established nationality and ethnicity. We have more choice over neighborhoods and jobs but still face significant obstacles in making changes.

Because health insurance is a commercial product sold in a competitive market, however, our membership in an insurance community is potentially much more freely chosen. Health insurance under managed competition reforms would enable subscribers who object to an insurance plan's limitations to opt into another plan once a year through the vehicle of annual open enrollment. Nevertheless, as discussed above, most insurance is not sold in a free-choice environment at present, and where it is, the range of choice even under open enrollment is severely constrained by the practical limitations needed to maintain a smooth-functioning market of competing insurers.

This is the critical juncture where communitarianism departs from liberalism. Even where the insurance at issue is public rather than private and therefore there may be no choice whatsoever, communitarianism sees nothing ethically deficient in any of the restrictions the insurance may impose, regardless of how severe. All that is required for moral and political legitimacy is a sufficiently explicit community decision, either by contract or, for public programs, by statute or regulation. In either event, at this first level of inquiry, communitarianism offers no principles to critique the legitimacy of insurance restrictions. Even the concept of the basic minimum carries little force. The community itself determines the acceptable minimum; moral compromises in health care delivery are legitimate if made consistently with whatever health insurance the community chooses to make available.

Moreover, unlike liberalism, communitarianism does not demand that the basic minimum exist as a fallback to a morally compromised insurance package. Moral compromises are permissible if necessary to create what that insurance group itself considers minimally acceptable health care. Communitarianism is consistent with a single-payer government insurance system that offers no options, regardless of how controversial or value-laden the contents of the single benefit package are. On the other hand, patients are entitled to the level of care that the community considers to be a decent minimum level of support, regardless of an individual's prior expression of preference. Therefore, communitarianism offers more protection against individual improvidence than does classic liberalism.

The Nesting of Communities and the Bounds of Ethical Debate

This tidy resolution of the problems of resource-constrained insurance is internally consistent and avoids the minimalist and maximalist extremes of liberalism. The communitarian middle ground appears to leave us, however, with an unsatisfyingly thin basis for ethical critique. Moral compromises contained in health insurance are valid under communitarian principles as long as they are explicit and the end result satisfies the community's own standard of a bare minimum.

Whether they are a good or bad idea is a matter for purely personal opinion, which may be largely irrelevant in any event given practical limitations in the range of choice. Once the contract is signed or the legislation is adopted, that concludes the matter, since the existence and extent of normative inquiry seems to rest exclusively within the community's own terms of existence. Communitarianism itself defines no particular level of support but looks to actual communities to determine what they deem sufficient. At most, communitarian theory might generate participation standards that require inclusiveness in the community's processes and a very general fairness criterion that requires roughly equal treatment within the community, but communitarian theory requires no absolute level of material support, nor does it prescribe the terms under which equality should be judged.[39]

Communitarianism broaches these issues by inquiring into how communities are formed and reformed. A community whose formation or membership is determined with excessive fiat, or one whose social policies are excessively harsh, might be declared an illegitimate community. Communitarianism has been much less explicit and successful in developing this higher normative perspective. Some communitarians seem content to accept actual communities however and wherever they find them. Others, however, have suggested that there are larger principles of community formation to be found within communitarian principles.

This enlargement of the sphere of communitarian critique occurs through the nesting of communities. Smaller communities exist within larger ones, and these boundaries are not only geographical but hierarchical in the sense that nested communities must adhere to the more general principles established by their host communities. Insurance communities must be formed under the rules of a private market, which rules themselves form a larger market community. And these market rules must be consistent with substantive social policies adopted by a political community, according to its own internal rules. This political community must adhere to constitutional principles, which are the foundational rules for generating communities. The validity of these constitutional principles can either be left to the unanswerable authority of actual historical "constitutional moments,"[40] or they can be further analyzed under the most general principles of justice derived from a particular tradition of rationality, such as a Rawlsian "original position" analysis.[41]

Fortunately, we need not carry things this far to produce some meaningful critique of health insurance, because it already exists within overarching communities that are well formed. We have an existing market system which we are in the process of reevaluating and reforming, following established legislative processes within our federation of constitutional sovereigns. The higher principles that form these host communities provide the terms by which to evaluate the ethical and public policy legitimacy of individual nested insurance communities.

Within the innermost circle—that of a particular insurance plan—we can debate the fairly mundane questions of how to interpret the terms of insurance coverage as they apply in specific cases. This is primarily the everyday work of lawyers, doctors, and utilization reviewers seeking to determine the meaning of "experimental" or "medically necessary." In a more dynamic mode, one can attempt at this first level to influence the substantive terms of coverage established by discrete insurance communities. This is a matter for negotiation between labor unions and employers, and for public insurance it is the subject of political debate within legislative bodies. The content of individual plans is influenced by individual subscribers' choice of plans, where they have such a choice. Here, the debate occurs via commercial marketing that seeks to change the decisions people make.

This debate need not be left solely to economic and political forces, however. Employers, insurers, and governments are open to more robust moral and public policy persuasion about the wisdom of their resource allocation decisions. As Michael Walzer demonstrates, these issues can be debated and resolved by reference to a criterion of internal coherence, which seeks to clarify the distributive principles actually held by particular social and economic communities.[42] Or, as Alasdair MacIntyre argues, this debate can be informed by broader-gauged historical traditions of moral, political, and even religious thought.[43]

Expanding outward, the next level of inquiry is whether different insurance communities are properly formed within the substantive and procedural rules of the prevailing market and government systems. This inquiry, conducted primarily by government regulators and the legal community, asks whether market and government administrative rules are being followed. Market rules might entail how much information consumers are given and how insurance policies are priced; government rules specify the proper process and level of public participation in making collective resource allocation decisions.

The third level of communitarian critique inquires into the broadest social rules for how market and political systems should function in the realm of health insurance. Through legislative processes, society as a whole considers the minimum content of private health insurance and how the selection process should be conducted, or through constitutional processes, society determines how the legislative process should function. It is at these highest levels that communitarian thought sets the allowable range of choice among insurance communities or adopts mandatory community standards that define the required bare minimum. These reconstitutive moments are rare and difficult to achieve, but hopefully we are still in the midst of one.

Regardless of whether society ultimately prefers market or government systems in general, it must decide in what circumstances patients, doctors, or various outsiders are best positioned to make medical spending decisions. Society certainly should not make this choice solely according to the analytical musings of an academic lawyer, nor could it very well do so, for I have failed to give any definite answer to these inquiries. My purpose is not to settle this debate, only to lay the groundwork for further thought by exposing the subtleties and complexities contained in these imperfect options. My objective will be met if the reader is convinced to avoid the attraction of absolutist taboos and simplistic-sounding solutions and instead is motivated to give this intractable problem hard thought that spawns creative ideas, if not permanent solutions.

Notes

1. I owe this insight to political theorist Frederick Schauer. See Schauer 1992.
2. Komesar 1995, at 6, 27.
3. See generally Menzel 1990; Morreim 1991b; Emanuel 1991; Veatch 1991a, at 183–85; Allen 1995.
4. See Morreim 1994b; Crandall 1995.
5. Havighurst 1992; Havighurst 1994.
6. This idea is receiving limited recognition in some states. One example comes from the debate over whether patients' free choice of physician should be preserved through state "any-willing-provider" laws or whether these laws are aimed at suppressing the burgeoning managed care sector. Maryland avoided this contentious debate by requiring that a "point-of-service" option be offered in every managed care contract, but at a price to be paid entirely by the subscriber. Md. Ann. Code art. 48a, Ch. 55, sec. 699. Likewise, several states avoid mandating controversial insurance benefits such as in vitro fertilization or acupuncture by requiring instead that they be offered as optional riders for an extra premium.
7. See primarily the end of Chapter 6.
8. See Ellman and Hall 1994; Hall and Anderson 1992.
9. Havighurst 1994 presents an especially thorough and cogent contract model that shares similarities with mine but also important differences.
10. Elhauge 1994, at 1530–34.
11. For recent comprehensive accounts of liberalism, see Holmes 1993; Nagel 1991.
12. This is the essential insight in Emanuel's lengthy work, *The Ends of Human Life*, which he attributes to communitarian theory, but as several commentators have observed, using private insurance selection to express and realize divergent value preferences is fully supported by classic liberalism as well. See Brody 1993; Daniels 1992; Hall et al. 1994. For additional development of the ethical relevance of insurance selection, see Veatch 1993.
13. Wertheimer 1987. Richard Epstein does the most convincing job of extending this framework to health care financing, although he speaks in terms of negative versus positive liberty, rather than coercion. Epstein 1996.
14. Ibid. at 229.
15. On the distinction between exploitation and coercion, see Wertheimer 1992, at 211; Feinberg 1988, at 176–275.
16. Murphy 1981, at 79, 82.
17. Institute of Medicine 1993; Medical Benefits 1994, vol. 11, no. 16, at 9 (84 percent of employers with health insurance offer only one plan).
18. Havighurst 1994.
19. Even then, the types of information that reformers desire to give consumers, and the types of information consumers usually want to receive, do not relate to the ethical dimensions of health care. Instead, this information is focused on the comparative quality and cost of care among competing groups of physicians and hospitals.

20. Marquis 1983.

21. Rawls 1971.

22. President's Commission 1985; Daniels 1985; Buchanan 1984.

23. For a thorough discussion of these difficulties and limitations, see Elhauge 1994. See also AMA 1994a.

24. For the most part, these are my formulations. Other formulations include the level of care enjoyed by the broad middle class, Elhauge 1994, and care required to restore normal species functioning or a normal opportunity range, Daniels 1981.

25. Note that "reasonably" encompasses difficult value judgments about how often I can choose and the differential costs of my options.

26. Leading sources in this growing literature include Etzioni 1993; Glendon 1991; Sandel 1984.

27. For a general overview of the relevance of communitarian thought to bioethics, see Callahan 1994. See also Dworkin 1993.

28. For a general introduction to communitarian thought, in addition to the sources in the surrounding text, see Bell 1993; Buchanan 1989; Philips 1993; Feinberg 1988, at 81–123.

29. Etzioni 1993.

30. It is this vehicle that Ezekiel Emanuel uses to form a complete communitarian system of health care ethics and resource allocation, in the form of competing insurance plans modeled on HMOs. Emanuel 1991. Emanuel's vision contains a stronger version of community than is necessary for his purposes since he sees an essential element of these insurance plans being a democratic, member-run system for setting spending priorities and ethical policies. The essential purpose of Emanuel's vision is achieved even without this level of participation, as long as members are free to leave insurance plans they disagree with and join those with which they are like-minded.

31. Jerry 1987, at 15–18.

32. Sandel 1982.

33. Jing-Bao Nie and Kirk Smith do a wonderful job of explaining this point by reference to the Chinese concept of yin and yang. Nie and Smith 1995.

34. Sunstein 1986.

35. Forster 1982.

36. Eddy 1994, at 821.

37. Kymlicka 1988; Nino 1989.

38. Sagoff 1994.

39. Walzer 1983.

40. Ackerman 1991.

41. This enlargement of communitarian thought is essentially what Rawls accomplishes in his most recent work, even though Rawls disavows the communitarian label for other reasons. Rawls envisions a "social union of social unions" which relegates most concrete substantive policy to an analysis of procedural justice, namely, whether the social policies have been adopted and enforced consistent with society's rules for how the relevant social decision-making institutions should operate. Rawls 1993.

42. Walzer 1983. This approach to ethical analysis is also similar to that developed by Tristram Engelhardt in *The Foundations of Bioethics*, even though he is not an avowed communitarian. Engelhardt argues that a secular pluralist society requires that we adopt a "procedural" or "geographical" medical ethics whose first task is to map out and clarify the moral communities in which disputes arise before advocating the substantive content of a particular moral community.

43. MacIntyre 1988.

Bibliography

Aaron, H.J. and Schwartz, W.B. (1990). "Rationing Health Care: The Choice Before Us," 247 *Science* 418.

Aaron, H.J. and Schwartz, W.B. (1984a). *The Painful Prescription: Rationing Hospital Care* (Washington, DC: Brookings Institution).

Aaron, H.J. and Schwartz, W.B. (1984b). "Rationing Hospital Care: Lessons from Britain," 310 *New Engl. J. Med.* 52.

Ackerman, B.A. (1991). *We the People* (Cambridge, MA: Belknap Press of Harvard University Press).

Allen, W.L. (1995). "Conscientious Objection in Health Care Financing and the Need for Pragmatic Toleration," in *Health Care Crisis: The Search for Answers*, eds. R.I. Misbin et al. (Frederick, MD: University Publishing Group).

AMA Council on Ethical and Judicial Affairs (1995a). "Ethical Considerations in the Allocation of Organs and Other Scarce Medical Resources Among Patients," 155 *Arch. Intern. Med.* 29.

AMA Council on Ethical and Judicial Affairs (1995b). "Ethical Issues in Managed Care," 273 *JAMA* 330–335.

AMA Council on Ethical and Judicial Affairs (1994a). "Ethical Issues in Health Care System Reform," 272 *JAMA* 1056–1062.

AMA Council on Ethical and Judicial Affairs (1994b). *Code of Medical Ethics: Current Opinions with Annotations* (Chicago, IL: American Medical Association).

AMA Council on Ethical and Judicial Affairs (1991). "Gender Disparities in Clinical Decision Making," 266 *JAMA* 559–562.

AMA Council on Ethical and Judicial Affairs (1990). "Black-White Disparities in Clinical Decision Making," 263 *JAMA* 2344.

American Society of Internal Medicine (1990). "The Hassle Factor: America's Health Care System Strangling in Red Tape," 31 *The Internist*, No. 8 (special suppl.) 1.

Anderson, A.G. (1978). "When Conflicts of Interest: Efficiency, Fairness and Corporate Structure," 25 *UCLA Law Rev.* 738.

Anderson, G.F. and Hall, M.A. (1996). "When Courts Review Practice Guidelines" (submitted for publication).

Anderson, G.F., Hall, M.A. and Steinberg, E.P. (1993). "Medical Technology Assessment and Practice Guidelines: Their Day in Court," 83 *Am. J. Public Health* 1635.

Anderson, R.M. and May, R.M. (1990). "Immunization and Herd Immunity," 335 *Lancet* 641.

Anderson, W.H. (1988). "HMO Financial Incentives and Informed Consent (Letter)," 260 *JAMA* 791.

Angell, M. (1993). "The Doctor as Double Agent," 3 *Kennedy Institute of Ethics J.* 279–286.

Angell, M. (1987). "Medicine: The Endangered Patient-Centered Ethic," 17 *Hastings Cent. Rep.* (February) 12 (Suppl.).

Angell, M. (1985). "Cost Containment and the Physician," 254 *JAMA* 1203.

Angell, M. (1984). "Patients' Preferences in Randomized Clinical Trials," 310 *New Engl. J. Med.* 1385.

Annas, G.J. and Miller, F.H. (1994). "The Empire of Death: How Culture and Economics Affect Informed Consent in the U.S., the U.K., and Japan," 20 *Am. J. Law Med.* 357.

Annas, G.J. (1985). "The Prostitute, The Playboy, and the Poet: Rationing Schemes for Organ Transplantation," 75 *Am. J. Public Health* 187.

Annotation (1985). "Liability for Failure of Physicians to Inform Patient of Alternative Modes of Diagnosis or Treatment," 38 *A.L.R.4th* 900.

Annotation (1978). "Modern Status of Views as to General Measure of Duty to Inform Patient of Risks of Proposed Treatment," 88 *A.L.R.3d* 1008.

Anspach, R. (1993). *Deciding Who Lives: Fateful Choices in the Intensive-Care Nursery* (Berkeley: University of California Press).

Appelbaum, P.S. (1993). "Must We Forgo Informed Consent to Control Health Care Costs?," 71 *Milbank Q.* 669.

Appelbaum, P.S., Lidz, C.W. and Meisel, A. (1987). *Informed Consent: Legal Theory and Clinical Practice* (New York: Oxford University Press).

Arrow, K.J. (1985). "The Economics of Agency," in *Principals and Agents: The Structure of Business*, eds. J.W. Pratt and R.J. Zeckhauser (Boston, MA: Harvard Business School Press).

Arrow, K.J. (1963). "Uncertainty and the Welfare Economics of Medical Care," 53 *Am. Econ. Rev.* 941.

Ashby, J.L. (1984). "The Impact of Hospital Regulatory Programs on Per Capita Costs, Utilization, and Capital Investment," 21 *Inquiry* 45.

Ayanian, J.Z. (1994). "Race, Class, and the Quality of Medical Care," 271 *JAMA* 1207.

Ayres, I., Dooley, L.G. and Gaston, R.S. (1993). "Unequal Racial Access to Kidney Transplantation," 46 *Vand. Law Rev.* 805–861.

Baier, A. (1986). "Trust and Antitrust," 96 *Ethics* 231.

Bailey, M.A. (1994). "The Democracy Problem," 24 *Hastings Cent. Rep.* (July) 39–42.

Bailey, M.A. (1986). "Rationing Medical Care: Processes for Defining Adequacy," in *The Price of Health: Cost-Benefit Analysis and Efficiency in Medicine*, eds. G. Agich and C. Begley (Boston: Kluwer Academic).

Barnett, R.E. (1986). "Contract Remedies and Inalienable Rights," 4 *Soc. Phil. Politics* 179.

Bates, E.W. and Connors, K.A. (1987). "Assessing Process of Care Under Capitated and Fee-for-Service Medicare," *Health Care Financing Rev.* (Ann. Suppl.).

Beauchamp, T.L. and Childress, J.F. (1994). *Principles of Biomedical Ethics* (4th ed., New York: Oxford University Press).

Beauchamp, T.L. and Childress, J.F. (1979). *Principles of Biomedical Ethics* (New York: Oxford University Press).

Beecher, H. (1961). "Surgery as Placebo," 176 *JAMA* 1102.

Begley, C.E (1986). "Physicians and Cost Control," in *The Price of Health*, eds. G.J. Agich and C.E. Begley (Dordrecht: D. Reidel).

Bell, D. (1993). *Communitarianism and its Critics* (New York: Oxford University Press).

Berk, M. and Monheit, A. (1992). "The Concentration of Health Care Expenditures: An Update," 11 *Health Aff.* (Winter 1992) 145–149.

Besharov, D. and Silver, J. (1987). "Rationing Access to Advanced Medical Technology," 8 *J. Leg. Med.* 507.

Blackhall, L.J., Murphy, S.T., Frank, G., et al. (1995). "Ethnicity and Attitudes Toward Patient Autonomy," 274 *JAMA* 820–825.

Blakeslee, S. (1990). "Health Care Choices: Letting the People Decide," *N.Y. Times*, June 14, at B7, col.4.

Blank, R.H. (1988). *Rationing Medicine* (New York: Columbia University Press).

Blomquist, A. (1991). "The Doctor as Double Agent: Information Asymmetry, Health Insurance and Medical Care," 10 *J. Health Econ.* 411.

Blumenthal, D. (1983). "Federal Policy Toward Health Care Technology: The Case of the National Center," 61 *Milbank Mem. Fund Q.* 584.

Blumstein, J. (1981). "Rationing Medical Resources: A Constitutional, Legal, and Policy Analysis," 59 *Tx. Law Rev.* 1345.

Bobinski, M.A. (1994). "Autonomy and Privacy: Protecting Patients from their Physicians," 55 *U. Pitt. Law Rev.* 291.

Bodenheimer, T. and Grumbach, K. (1994). "Paying for Health Care," 272 *JAMA* 634.

Boozang, K.M. (1993). "Death Wish: Resuscitating Self-Determination," 35 *Ariz. Law Rev.* 23.

Bovbjerg, R. (1978). "Problems and Prospects for Health Planning: The Importance of Incentives, Standards, and Procedures in Certificate of Need," 1978 *Utah Law Rev.* 83.

Bovbjerg, R. (1975). "The Medical Malpractice Standard of Care: HMOs and Customary Practice," 1975 *Duke Law J.* 1375.

Bovbjerg, R., Held, P. and Diamond, L. (1987). "Provider–Patient Relations and Treatment Choice in the Era of fiscal Incentives: The Case of the End-stage Renal Disease Program." 65 *Milbank Q.* 177–202.

Boyd, N.F., Sutherland, H.J., Heasman, K.Z., et al. (1990). "Whose Utilities for Decision Analysis?," 10 *Med. Decis. Making* 58.

Boyd, T.H. (1989). "Cost Containment and the Physician's Fiduciary Duty to the Patient," 39 *DePaul Law Rev.* 131.

Boyle, J.F. (1984). "Should We Learn to Say No?," 252 *JAMA* 782.

Brakel, S.J. (1985). "Voluntary Admission," in *The Mentally Disabled and the Law*, eds. S.J. Brackel, J. Brakel and J. Perry (Chicago: The Foundation).

Brennan, T.A. (1991). *Just Doctoring: Medical Ethics in the Liberal State* (Berkeley: University of California Press).

Brett, A.S. (1992). "The Case Against Persuasive Advertising by Health Maintenance Organizations," 326 *New Engl. J. Med.* 1353.

Brett, A.S. and McCullough, L.B. (1986). "When Patients Request Specific Interventions," 315 *New Engl. J. Med.* 1347.

Brock, D.W. and Wartman, S.A. (1990). "When Competent Patients Make Irrational Choices," 322 *New Engl. J. Med.* 1595.

Brody, B.A. (1993). "Liberalism, Communitarianism, and Medical Ethics," 18 *Law and Social Inquiry* 393.

Brody, H. (1992). *The Healer's Power* (New Haven, CT: Yale University Press).

Brody, H. (1987a). *Stories of Sickness* (New Haven, CT: Yale University Press).

Brody, H. (1987b). "Cost Containment as Professional Challenge," 8 *Theor. Med.* 5.

Brody, H. (1980). *Placebos and the Philosophy of Medicine: Clinical, Conceptual, and Ethical Issues* (Chicago: University of Chicago Press).

Brook, R.H. (1989). "Practice Guidelines and Practicing Medicine," 262 *JAMA* 3027.

Brown, L.D. (1991). "The National Politics of Oregon's Rationing Plan," 10 *Health Aff.* (Summer) 28.

Buchanan, A.E. (1989). "Assessing the Communitarian Critique of Liberalism," 99 *Ethics* 852–882.

Buchanan, A.E. (1988). "Principal/Agent Theory and Decisionmaking in Health Care," 2 *Bioethics* 317.

Buchanan, A.E. (1984). "The Right to a Decent Minimum of Health Care," 13 *Philos. Public Aff.* 55–78.

Buchanan, A.E. and Brock, D.W. (1989). *Deciding for Others: The Ethics of Surrogate Decision Making* (New York: Cambridge University Press).

Burt, R.A. (1979). *Taking Care of Strangers: The Rule of Law in Doctor-Patient Relations* (New York: The Free Press).

Butler, P.A. (1992). *Flesh or Bones? Early Experience of State Limited Benefit Health Insurance Laws* (Boulder, CO: National Academy for State Health Policy).

Calabresi, G. and Bobbitt, P. (1978). *Tragic Choices* (New York: W.W. Norton).

Calabresi, G. and Melamed, A.D. (1972). "Property Rules, Liability Rules, and Inalienability: One View of the Cathedral," 85 *Harv. Law Rev.* 1089.

Califano, Jr., J.A. (1992). "Rationing Health Care: The Unnecessary Solution," 140 *U. Pa. Law Rev.* 1525.

Califano, Jr., J.A. (1986). *America's Health Care Revolution: Who Lives? Who Dies? Who Pays?* (New York: Random House).

Callahan, D. (1994). "Bioethics: Private Choice and Common Good," 24 *Hastings Cent. Rep.* (May 1994) 28–31.

Callahan, D. (1990). *What Kind of Life? The Limits of Medical Progress* (New York: Simon and Schuster).

Callahan, D. (1989). "Rationing Health Care: Will it be Necessary? Can it be Done Without Age or Disability Discrimination?," 5 *Issues Law Med.* 353.

Callahan, D. (1988). "Meeting Needs and Rationing Care," 16 *Law Med. Health Care* 261.

Callahan, D. (1987). *Setting Limits: Medical Goals in an Aging Society* (New York: Simon and Schuster).

Cantor, N.L. (1992). "Prospective Autonomy: On the Limits of Shaping One's Post-competent Medical Fate," 8 *J. Contemp. Health Law Pol'y* 13.

Capilouto, E., et al. (1992). "How Restrictive are Medicaid's Categorical Eligibility Requirements? A Look at Nine southern States." 29 *Inquiry* 451–453.

Capron, A.M. (1992). "Where Is the Sure Interpreter?," 22 *Hastings Cent. Rep.* (July–August 1992) 26–27.

Capron, A.M. (1990). "Human Experimentation," in *Medical Ethics*, ed. R. Veatch (Boston: Jones and Bartlett).

Capron, A.M. (1974). "Informed Consent in Catastrophic Disease Research and Treatment," 123 *U. Pa. Law Rev.* 340.

Carrese, J.A. and Rhodes, L.A. (1995). "Western Bioethics on the Navajo Reservation: Benefit of Harm?," 274 *JAMA* 826–829.

Cassel, C.K. (1985). "Doctors and Allocation Decisions: A New Role in the New Medicine," 10 *J. Health Polit. Policy Law* 549.

Cassell, E.J. (1991). *The Nature of Suffering and the Goals of Medicine* (New York: Oxford University Press).

Cassell, E.J. (1985). *The Healer's Art* (Cambridge, MA: MIT Press).

Cassell, E.J. (1982). "The Nature of Suffering and the Goals of Medicine," 306 *New Engl. J. Med.* 639.

Champagne, A., et al. (1991). "An Empirical Examination of the Use of Expert Witnesses in American Courts," 31 *Jurimetrics J.* 375.

Chassin, M. (1988). "Standards of Care in Medicine," 25 *Inquiry* 437.

Chavkin, D.F. and Treseder, A. (1977). "California's Prepaid Health Plan Program: Can the Patient be Saved?," 28 *Hastings Law J.* 685.

Childress, J.F. (1983). "Triage in Neonatal Intensive Care: The Limitations of a Metaphor," 69 *Va. Law Rev.* 547.

Childress, J.F. (1982). *Who Should Decide? Paternalism in Health Care* (New York: Oxford University Press).

Christensen, S. (1992). "The Subsidy Provided Under Medicare to Current Enrollees," 17 *J. Health Polit. Policy Law* (Summer 1992) 255.

Christopher, M.J., Biblo, J., Johnson, L. and Potter, R.L. (1995). "Ethical Issues in Managed Care: Guidelines for Clinicians and Recommendations to Accrediting Organizations," in *Health Care Crisis: The Search for Answers*, eds. R.I. Misbin et al. (Frederick, MD: University Publishing Group).

Churchill, L.R. (1994). *Self-Interest and Universal Health Care: Why Well-Insured Americans Should Support Coverage for Everyone* (Cambridge, MA: Harvard University Press).

Churchill, L.R. (1987). *Rationing Health Care in America: Perceptions and Principles of Justice* (Notre Dame, IN: University of Notre Dame Press).

Clark, R.C. (1989). "Contracts, Elites, and Traditions in the Making of Corporate Law," 89 *Colum. Law Rev.* 1703.

Clark, R.C. (1985). "Agency Costs Versus Fiduciary Duties," in *Principals and Agents: The Structure of Business*, eds. J.W. Pratt and R.J. Zeckhauser (Boston, MA: Harvard Business School Press).

Clouser, K.D. and Gert, B. (1990). "A Critique of Principalism," 15 *J. Med. Philo.* 219.

Cohen, M.H. (1995). "A Fixed Star in Health Care Reform: The Emerging Paradigm of Holistic Healing," 27 *Ariz. St. Law J.* 79.

Comment (1981). "Informed Consent: From Disclosure to Patient Participation in Medical Decisionmaking," 76 *Nw. U. Law Rev.* 172.

Comment (1962). "The Action of Abandonment in Medical Malpractice Litigation," 36 *Tulane Law Rev.* 834.

Cooter, R. and Freedman, B. (1991). "The Fiduciary Relationship: Its Economic Character and Legal Consequences," 66 *N.Y.U. Law Rev.* 1045.

Costich, J.F. (1991). "Denial of Coverage for "Experimental" Procedures: The Problem of De Novo Review under ERISA," 79 *Ky Law J.* 801.

Cousins, N. (1979). *Anatomy of an Illness as Perceived by the Patient: Reflections on Healing and Regeneration* (New York: W.W. Norton).

Council for Affordable Health Insurance (1993). The Financial Impact of Medical Savings Accounts on Health Care Spending and the Federal Budget (Washington, DC).

Crandall, L.A. (1995). "Health Care Reform and Payment for 'Non-Beneficial' Medical Interventions at the End of Life: Is There a Policy Solution?," in *Health Care Crisis: The Search for Answers*, eds. R.I. Misbin et al. (Frederick, MD: University Publishing Group).

Crane, D. (1975). *The Sanctity of Social Life: Physicians' Treatment of Critically Ill Patients* (New York: Russell Sage Foundation).

Crossley, M.A. (1993). "Of Diagnoses and Discrimination: Discriminatory Nontreatment of Infants with HIV Infection," 93 *Colum. Law Rev.* 1581.

Cunningham, F.C. and Williamson, J.W. (1980). "How Does the Quality of Health Care in HMOs Compare to That in Other Settings? An Analytic Literature Review: 1958 to 1979," 1 *Group Health J.* 4.

Curran, W.J., Hall, M.A. and Kaye, D.H. (1990). *Health Care Law, Forensic Science, and Public Policy* (Toronto: Little, Brown).

Daniels, N. (1993). "Rationing Fairly: Programmatic Considerations," 7 *Bioethics* 224–233.

Daniels, N. (1992). "Liberalism and Medical Ethics," 22 *Hastings Cen. Rep.* (Dec. 1992) 41–43.

Daniels, N. (1991). "Is the Oregon Rationing Plan Fair?," 265 *JAMA* 2232.

Daniels, N. (1988). *Am I My Parents' Keeper? An Essay on Justice Between the Young and the Old* (New York: Oxford University Press).

Daniels, N. (1987). "The Ideal Advocate and Limited Resources," 8 *Theor. Med.* 69.

Daniels, N. (1986). "Why Saying No to Patients in the United States Is So Hard: Cost Containment, Justice, and Provider Autonomy," 314 *New Engl. J. Med.* 1380.

Daniels, N. (1985). *Just Health Care* (Cambridge, England: Cambridge University Press).

Daniels, N. (1981). "Health-Care Needs and Distributive Justice," 10 *Philo. Public Aff.* 146.

Danis, M., et al. (1994). "Stability of Choices About Life-sustaining Treatments," 120 *Ann. Intern. Med.* 568–573.

Davidson, B.N. (1988). "Designing Health Insurance Information for the Medicare Beneficiary: A Policy Synthesis," 23 *Health Serv. Res.* 685–720.

Davis, K.B. (1985). "Judicial Review of Fiduciary Decisionmaking—Some Theoretical Perspectives," 80 *Nw.U.L.Rev.* 1–99.

Developments (1995). "Confronting the New Challenges of Scientific Evidence," 108 *Harv. L. Rev.* 1481–1606.

Developments (1990). "Medical Technology and the Law," 103 *Harv. Law Rev.* 1519.

Developments (1985). "Privileged Communications," 98 *Harv. Law Rev.* 1451.

Developments (1981). "Conflicts of Interest in the Legal Profession," 94 *Harv. Law Rev.* 1244.

Deyoet, R.A., et al. (1987). "Reducing Roentgenography Use: Can Patient Expectations be Altered?," 147 *Arch. Intern. Med.* 141.

Diver, C.S. (1983). "The Optimal Precision of Administrative Rules," 93 *Yale Law J.* 65.

Doenges, J.L. (1959). "Third Party Medicine," *The Freeman* (August 1959).

Donabedian, A. (1983). "Quality, Cost, and Clinical Decisions," 468 *Ann. Am. Acad. Pol. Soc. Sci.* 196.

Donahue, P. (1994). "Federal Tax Treatment of Health Care Expenditures: Is it Part of the Health Care Problem,?" 46 *Wash. Univ. J. Urban Contemp. Law* 141.

Dougherty, C.J. (1990). "Health Care for Consenting Adults," 2 *Bioethics Books* 35.

Dranove, D. and White, W.D. (1987). "Agency and the Organization of Health Care Delivery," 24 *Inquiry* 405.

Dresser, R.S. (1982). "Ulysses and the Psychiatrists: A Legal and Policy Analysis of the Voluntary Commitment Contract," 16 *Harv. C.R.-C.L. Law Rev.* 777.

Dubois, R.W. and Brook, R.H. (1988). "Assessing Clinical Decision Making: Is the Ideal System Feasible?," 25 *Inquiry* 59.

Dubos, R.J. (1968). *Man, Medicine, and Environment* (New York: Praeger).

Dworkin, G. (1988). *The Theory and Practice of Autonomy* (Cambridge, England: Cambridge University Press).

Dworkin, R.B. (1996). *Limits: The Role of the Law in Bioethical Decision Making* (Bloomington, IN: University of Indiana Press).

Dworkin, R.B. (1993). "Medical Law and Ethics in the Post-Autonomy Age," 68 *Ind. Law J.* 727–742.

Dyer, A.R. (1986). "Patients, Not Costs, Come First," 16 *Hastings Cent. Rep.* (February) 5.

Easterbrook, F.H. and Fischel, D.R. (1991). *The Economic Structure of Corporate Law* (Cambridge, MA: Harvard University Press).

Easterbrook, F.H. and Fischel, D.R. (1986). "Close Corporations and Agency Costs," 38 *Stan. Law Rev.* 271.

Eddy, D.M. (1994). "Rationing Resources While Improving Quality," 272 *JAMA* 817.

Eddy, D.M. (1993). "Broadening the Responsibilities of Practitioner: The Team Approach," 269 *JAMA* 1849.

Eddy, D.M. (1991a). "Rationing by Patient Choice," 265 *JAMA* 105.

Eddy, D.M. (1991b). "What Care is 'Essential'? What Services are 'Basic'?," 265 *JAMA* 782.

Eddy, D.M. (1991c). "Oregon's Methods: Did Cost-effectiveness Analysis Fail?," 266 *JAMA* 2135.

Eddy, D.M. (1991d). "The Individual vs. Society: Is There a Conflict?," 265 *JAMA* 1446.

Eddy, D.M. (1991e). "Oregon's Plan: Should it be Approved?," 266 *JAMA* 2439.

Eddy, D.M. (1990). "Connecting Value and Costs: Whom Do We Ask, and What Do We Ask Them?," 264 *JAMA* 1737.

Eddy, D.M. (1984). "Variations in Physician Practice: The Role of Uncertainty," 3 *Health Aff.* (Summer) 75.

Editorial (1988). "The Last Word," 18 *Hastings Cent. Rep.* (June) 45.

Egan, T. (1990). "Oregon Lists Illnesses by Priority to See Who Gets Medicaid Care," *N.Y. Times*, May 3, at 1.

Eisenberg, J.M. (1986). *Doctors' Decisions and the Cost of Medical Care* (Ann Arbor, MI: Health Administration Press).

Eisenberg, J.M. and Williams, S.V. (1981). "Cost Containment and Changing Physicians' Practice Behavior," 246 *JAMA* 2195.

Elhauge, E. (1994). "Allocating Health Care Morally," 82 *Calif. Law Rev.* 1449.

Elhange, E. (1996). "The Limited Potential of Technology Assessment," *Va. Law Rev.* (in press).

Elias, S. and Annas, G.J. (1994). "Generic Consent for Genetic Screening," 330 *New Engl. J. Med.* 1611–1613.

Elixhauser, A. (1993). "Health Care Cost-Benefit and Cost-Effectiveness Analysis (CBA/CEA) From 1979 to 1990: A Bibliography," 31 *Med. Care* 7 (Suppl. July).

Elkowitz, A. (1986). "Physicians at the Bedside: Practitioners' Thoughts and Actions Regarding Bedside Allocation of Resources," 7 *J. Med. Hum. Bioethics* 122.

Ellis, R.P. (1985). "The Effect of Prior-Year Health Expenditures on Health Coverage Plan Choice," in 6 *Advances in Health Economics and Health Services Research*, eds. R. Scheffler and L. Rossiter (Greenwich, CT: JAI Press).

Ellman, E.J. (1989). "Monitor Mania: Physician Regulation Run Amok!," 1989 *Loy. U. Chi. Law J.* 721.

Ellman, I.M. and Hall, M.A. (1994). "Redefining the Terms of Health Insurance to Accommodate Varying Consumer Risk Preferences," 20 *Am. J. Law Med.* 187–201.

Ellsbury, K.E. (1989). "Can the Family Physician Avoid Conflict of Interest in the Gatekeeper Role?," 28 *J. Fam. Pract.* 698.

Elster, J. (1992). *Local Justice: How Institutions Allocate Scarce Goods and Necessary Burdens* (New York: Russell Sage Foundation).

Elster, J. (1982). "Sour Grapes—Utilitarianism and the Genesis of Wants," in *Utilitarianism and Beyond*, eds. A. Sen and B. Williams (New York: Cambridge University Press).

Elster, J. (1979). *Ulysses and the Sirens: Studies in Rationality and Irrationality* (New York: Cambridge University Press).

Emanuel, E.J. and Emanuel, L.L. (1994). "The Economics of Dying: The Illusion of Cost Savings at the End of Life," 330 *New Engl. J. Med.* 540.

Emanuel, E.J. and Emanuel, L.L. (1992). "Four Models of the Physician-Patient Relationship," 267 *JAMA* 2221.

Emanuel, E.J. (1991). *The Ends of Human Life: Medical Ethics in a Liberal Polity* (Cambridge, MA: Harvard University Press).

Emerson, R.W. (1940). "Self Reliance," in *Complete Essays and Other Writings of R. Emerson*, ed. B. Atkinson (New York: The Modern Library).

Emmet, D. (1994). *The Role of the Unrealisable: A Study in Regulative Ideals* (New York: St. Martin's Press).

Employee Benefit Research Institute (1992). *Public Attitudes on Setting Health Care Limits* (Washington, DC).

Ende, J., et al. (1980). "Measuring Patients' Desire for Autonomy: Decision Making and Information-Seeking Preferences Among Medical Patients," 4 *J. Personality Soc. Psychol.* 977.

Engelhardt, H.T. (1986). *The Foundations of Bioethics* (New York: Oxford University Press).

Enthoven, A.C. (1980). *Health Plan: The Only Practical Solutions to the Soaring Cost of Medical Care* (Reading, MA: Addison Wesley).

Epstein, A.M. (1990). "The Outcomes Movement—Will it Get Us Where We Want to Go?," 323 *New Engl. J. Med.* 266.

Epstein, R.A. (1996). *Mortal Peril: regulating Health Care in America* (draft manuscript).

Epstein, R.A. (1992). "Why is Health Care Special?," 40 *U. Kan. Law Rev.* 307.

Epstein, R.A. (1988). "Market and Regulatory Approaches to Medical Malpractice: The Virginia Obstetrical Non-Fault Status," 74 *Va. Law Rev.* 1451.

Epstein, R.A. (1986). "Medical Malpractice, Imperfect Information, and the Contractual Foundation for Medical Services," 49 *Law Contemp. Probs.* 201.

Epstein, R.A. (1976). "Medical Malpractice: The Case for Contract," 1976 *Am. Bar Found Res. J.* 87.

Erde, E.L. (1996). "Conflicts of Interest in Medicine: A Philosophical and Ethical Morphology," *in Conflicts of Interest in Clinical Practice and Research*, eds. R.G. Spece, D.S. Shimm, and A.E. Buchanan (New York: Oxford University Press).

Etzioni, A. (1993). *The Spirit of Community: Rights, Responsibilities, and the Communitarian Agenda* (New York: Crown).

Etzioni, A. (1991). "Health Care Rationing: A Critical Evaluation," 10 *Health Aff.* (Summer) 88.

Evans, R.W. (1983). "Health Care Technology and the Inevitability of Resource Alloca-
    tion and Rationing Decisions," 249 *JAMA* 2208.
Faden, R.R. and Beauchamp, T.L. (1986). *A History and Theory of Informed Consent* (New
    York: Oxford University Press).
Fajfar, M. (1992). "An Economic Analysis of Informed Consent to Medical Care," 80
    Georgetown Law Rev. 1941.
Families USA (1993). *No Sale: The Failure of Barebones Insurance* (Washington, DC).
Feinberg, J. (1988). *Harmless Wrongdoing* (New York: Oxford University Press).
Feinberg, J. (1983). "Autonomy, Sovereignty, and Privacy: Moral Ideals in the Constitu-
    tion?," 58 *Notre Dame Law Rev.* 445.
Feinberg, J. (1978). "Voluntary Euthanasia and the Inalienable Right to Life," 7 *Philo.
    Public Aff.* 93.
Fellner, C.H. and Marshall, J.R. (1970). "Kidney Donors—The Myth of Informed Con-
    sent," 126 *Am. J. Psychiatr.* 1245.
Figa, S.F. and Figa, H.M. (1990). "Redefining Full and Fair Disclosure of HMO Benefits
    and Limitations," 14 *Seton Hall Legislative J.* 151.
Finn, P.D. (1977). *Fiduciary Obligations* (Sydney: Law Book Co.).
Fischel, D.R. (1982). "The Corporate Governance Movement," 35 *Vand. Law Rev.* 1259.
Fischhoff, B. (1985). "Cognitive and Institutional Barriers to 'Informed Consent'" in *To
    Breathe Freely*, ed. M. Gibson (Totowa, NJ: Rowman & Allanheld).
Fleck, L.M. (1994). "Just Caring: Oregon, Health Care Rationing, and Informed Demo-
    cratic Deliberation," 19 *J. Med. Philo.* 367.
Fleck, L.M. (1992). "Just Health Care Rationing: A Democratic Decisionmaking Ap-
    proach," 140 *U. Penn. Law Rev.* 1579.
Fleck, L.M. (1990). "Justice, HMOs, and the Invisible Rationing of Health Care Resources,"
    4 *Bioethics* 97.
Fleck, L.M. (1987). "DRGs: Justice and the Invisible Rationing of Health Care Resources."
    12 *J. Med. Philo.* 165–196.
Flick, M.R. (1991). "The Due Process of Dying," 79 *Cal. Law Rev* 1121.
Fondacaro, M.R. (1995). "Toward a Synthesis of Law and Social Science: Due Process
    and Procedural Justice in the Context of National Health Care Reform," 72 *Den-
    ver Law Rev.* 303–358.
Ford, E.S. and Cooper, R.S. (1995). "Racial/Ethnic Differences in Health Care Utiliza-
    tion of Cardiovascular Procedures: A Review of the Evidence," 30 *Health Serv.
    Res.* 237.
Forster, J. (1982). "A Communitarian Ethical Model for Public Health Interventions: An
    Alternative to Individual Behavior Change Strategies," 3 *J. Public Health Policy*
    150–163.
Fox, D.M. (1979). "The Segregation of Medical Ethics: A Problem in Modern Intellec-
    tual History," 4 *J. Med. Philo.* 81.
Fox, R. and Swazey, J. (1984). "Medical Morality is Not Bioethics—Medical Ethics in
    China and the United States," 27 *Perspec. Bio. Med.* 336.
Fox, R. and Swazey, J. (1974). *The Courage to Fail: A Social View of Organ Transplants
    and Dialysis* (Chicago: University of Chicago Press).
Frank, J.D. (1973). *Persuasion and Healing: A Comparative Study of Psychotherapy*
    (Baltimore: Johns Hopkins University Press).
Frankel, T. (1983). "Fiduciary Law," 71 *Cal. Law Rev.* 795.
Frankford, D.M. (1994a). "Scientism and Economism in the Regulation of Health Care,"
    19 *J. Health Polit. Policy Law* 773.

Frankford, D.M. (1994b). "Managing Medical Clinicians' Work Through the Use of Financial Incentives," 29 *Wake Forest Law Rev.* 71–105.

Frankford, D.M. (1992). "Privatizing Health Care: Economic Magic to Cure Legal Medicine," 66 *South. Calif. Law Rev.* 98.

Frankfurt, H.G. (1971). "Freedom of the Will and the Concept of a Person," 68 *J. Philo.* 5.

Franks, P. and Clancy, C.M. (1992). "Gatekeeping Revisited—Protecting Patients from Overtreatment," 327 *New Engl. J. Med.* 424.

Freedman, B. (1987). "Equipoise and the Ethics of Clinical Research," 317 *New Engl. J. Med.* 141.

Freedmen, M. (1966). "Professional Responsibility of the Criminal Defense Lawyer: The Three Hardest Questions," 64 *Mich. Law Rev.* 1469.

Freidson, E. (1985). "The Reorganization of the Medical Profession," 42 *Med. Care Rev.* 11.

Freidson, E. (1970a). *Profession of Medicine: A Study of the Sociology of Applied Knowledge* (New York, NY: Dodd, Mead).

Freidson, E. (1970b). *Professional Dominance: The Social Structure of Medical Care* (New York: Atherton Press).

Fried, C. (1981). *Contract as Promise: a Theory of Contractual Obligation* (Cambridge, MA: Harvard University Press).

Fried, C. (1975). "Rights and Health Care—Beyond Equity and Efficiency," 293 *New Engl. J. Med.* 241.

Friedman, D. (1986). "Comments on 'Rationing and Publicity,'" in *The Price of Health*, eds. G.J. Agich and C.E. Begley (Boston: D. Reidel).

Friedman, E. (1986). "Doctors and Rationing: The End of the Honor System," 13 *Prim. Care* 349.

Friendly, H.J. (1975). "Some Kind of Hearing," 123 *U. Pa. Law Rev.* 1267.

Frohoch, F.M. (1992). *Healing Powers: Alternative Medicine, Spiritual Communities, and the State* (Chicago: University Chicago Press).

Fuchs, V.R. (1984). "The 'Rationing' of Medical Care," 311 *New Engl. J. Med.* 1572.

Fuller, L.L. (1978). "The Forms and Limits of Adjudication," 92 *Harv. Law Rev.* 353.

Furrow, B.R. (1988). "The Ethics of Cost-Containment: Bureaucratic Medicine and the Doctor as Patient-Advocate," 3 *Notre Dame J. Law Ethics Public Policy* 187.

Gabel, J.R. and Jensen, G.A. (1989). "The Price of State Mandated Benefits," 26 *Inquiry* 419.

Gardbaum, S.A. (1992). "Law, Politics, and the Claims of Community," 90 *Mich. Law Rev.* 685.

Garnick, D.W., Hendricks, A.M., Thorpe, K.E., et al. (1993). "How Well Do Americans Understand Their Health Coverage?," 12 *Health Aff.* 204.

Garvin, M. (1996). *Health Maintenance Organizations, in Health Care Corporate Law: Managed Care* (Boston: Little, Brown).

Gauthier, D. (1986). *Morals by Agreement* (New York: Oxford University Press).

Gaylin, W. (1993). "Faulty Diagnosis: Why Clinton's Health-Care Plan Won't Cure What Ails Us," *Harper's Mag.* (October 1993).

Geist, R.W. (1974). "Incentive Bonuses in Prepayment Plans," 291 *New Engl. J. Med.* 1306.

Gewirth, A. (1986). "Professional Ethics: The Separatist Thesis," 96 *Ethics* 282.

Gianelli, D.M. (1992). "Canadian Case Quandary: Should IQ Figure into Transplant Decisions?," *Am. Med. News,* July 27, at 1.

Gibbard, A. (1983). "The Prospective Pareto Principle and Equity of Access to Health Care," in *Securing Access To Health Care* 153, Vol. II (Washington, DC:

President's Commission for the Study of Ethical Problems in Medicine and Bio-medical and Behavioral Research).

Gifford, F. (1986). "The Conflict Between Randomized Clinical Trials and the Therapeutic Obligation," 11 *J. Med. Philo.* 347.

Gillick, M.R. (1988). "Limiting Medical Care: Physicians' Beliefs, Physicians' Behavior," 36 *J. Am. Geriatr. Soc.* 747.

Gillon, R. (1988). "Ethics, Economics and General Practice," in *Medical Ethics and Economics in Health Care*, eds. G. Mooney and A. McGuire (Oxford: Oxford University Press).

Gilmore, G. (1977). *The Ages of American Law* (New Haven: Yale University Press).

Ginsburg, W.H., Kahn, S.J., Thornhill, M.C. and Gambardella, S.C. (1986). "Contractual Revisions to Medical Malpractice Liability," 49 *Law Contemp. Probs.* 253.

Glantz, L. (1988). "Withholding and Withdrawing Treatment: The Role of the Criminal Law," 15 *Law Med. Health Care* 231.

Glendon, M.A. (1991). *Rights Talk: The Impoverishment of Political Discourse* (New York: The Free Press).

Glover, J.J. and Povar, G.J. (1991). "The Ethics of Cost-Conscious Physician Reimbursement," in *Paying the Doctor, Health Policy and Physician Reimbursement*, ed. J.D. Moreno (New York: Auburn House).

Goetz, C. and Scott, R. (1981). "Principles of Relational Contracts," 67 *Va. Law Rev.* 1089.

Gold, M., Hurley, R., Lake, T., et al. (1995). "A National survey of the Arrangements Managed-Care Plans Make with Physicians." 333 *New Engl. J. Med.* 1678–1693.

Gold, M., Nelson, L., Lake, T., et al. (1995). "Behind the Curve: A Critical Assessment of How Little Is Known About Arrangements Between Managed Care Plans and Physicians," 52 *Med. Care Res. Rev.* 307–341.

Goldberg, S.L. (1996). "A cure for What Ails? Why the Medical Advocate is Not the Answer to Problems in the Doctor-Patient Relationship," 1 *Widener Law Symposium J.* 324–363.

Good, D. (1988). "Individuals, Interpersonal Relations, and Trust," in *Trust: Making and Breaking Cooperative Relations,* ed. D. Gambetta (New York, NY: Basil Blackwell).

Goodman, J. and Musgrave, G. (1994). *Patient Power: The Free Enterprise Alternative to Clinton's Health Plan* (Washington, DC: The Cato Institute).

Goodman, J. and Musgrave, G. (1992). *Patient Power: Solving America's Health Care Crisis* (Washington, DC: The Cato Institute).

Goodwin, B. (1992). *Justice by Lottery* (Chicago: University of Chicago Press).

Goold, S.D. (1996). "Allocating Health Care," 21 *J. Health Polit. Policy Law* 69–98.

Goold, S.D. and Brody, H. (1995). "Rationing Decisions in Managed Care Settings: An Ethical Analysis," in *Health Care Crisis? The Search for Answers*, eds. R.I. Misbin et al. (Frederick, MD: University Publishing Group).

Gorvitz, S. (1986). "Baiting Bioethics," 96 *Ethics* 356.

Goss, M.E. (1961). "Influence and Authority Among Physicians in an Outpatient Clinic," 26 *Am. Soc. Rev.* 39.

Gramm, P. (1994). "Why We Need Medical Savings Accounts," 330 *New Engl. J. Med.* 1752.

Gray, B.H. (1991). *The Profit Motive and Patient Care: The Changing Accountability of Doctors and Hospitals* (Cambridge, MA: Harvard University Press).

Gray, W.A., Capone, R.J. and Most, A.S. (1991). "Unsuccessful Emergency Medical Resuscitation—Are Continued Efforts in the Emergency Department Justified?," 325 *New Engl. J. Med.* 1393.

Green, J.A. (1988). "Minimizing Malpractice Risks by Role Clarification," 109 *Ann. Intern Med.* 234.

Green, R. (1990). "Method in Bioethics: A Troubled Assessment," 15 *J. Med. Philo.* 179.

Griffin, A. and Thomasma, D.C. (1983). "Pediatric Critical Care," 143 *Arch. Intern. Med.* 325.

Grumet, G. (1989). "Health Care Rationing Through Inconvenience: The Third Party's Secret Weapon," 321 *New Engl. J. Med.* 607–611.

Gutman, A. (1985). "Communitarian Critics of Liberalism," 14 *Philo. Pub. Aff.* 308.

Hackler, J.C. and Hiller, F.C. (1990). "Family Consent to Orders not to Resuscitate: Reconsidering Hospital Policy," 264 *JAMA* 1281.

Hadley, J., Steinberg, E.P. and Feder, J. (1991). "Comparison of Uninsured and Privately Insured Hospital Patients: Condition on Admission, Resource Use and Outcome," 265 *JAMA* 374.

Hadorn, D.C. (1992a). "Emerging Parallels in the American Health Care and Legal-Judicial Systems," 18 *Am. J. Law Med.* 73.

Hadorn, D.C. (1992b). "The Problem of Discrimination in Health Care Priority Setting," 268 *JAMA* 1454.

Hadorn, D.C. (1992c). "Necessary Care Guidelines," in *Basic Benefits and Clinical Guidelines*, ed. D. Hadorn (Boulder, CO: Westview Press).

Hadorn, D.C. (1991a). "Setting Health Care Priorities in Oregon: Cost-Effectiveness Meets the Rule of Rescue," 265 *JAMA* 2218.

Hadorn, D.C. (1991b). "The Oregon Priority-Setting Exercise: Quality of Life and Public Policy," 21 *Hastings Cen. Rep.* (June 1991) 11.

Hadorn, D.C. and Brook, R.H. (1991). "The Health Care Resource Allocation Debate: Defining Our Terms," 266 *JAMA* 3328.

Hall, M.A. (1995). "Hospital and Physician Disclosure of Information Concerning a Patient's Crime," 63 *Det. Law Rev.* 145.

Hall, M.A. (1994a). *Is Community Rating Essential to Managed Competition?* (Washington, DC: The AEI Press).

Hall, M.A. (1994b). *Reforming Private Health Insurance* (Washington, DC: The AEI Press).

Hall, M.A. (1991). "The Defensive Effect of Medical Practice Policies," 54 *Law Contemp. Probs.* 119.

Hall, M.A. (1989). "The Medical Malpractice Standard Under Health Care Cost Containment," 17 *Law Med. Health Care* 347.

Hall, M.A. (1988). "Institutional Control of Physician Behavior: Legal Barriers to Health Care Cost Containment," 137 *U. Pa. Law Rev.* 431.

Hall, M.A. (1985). "Hospital and Physician Disclosure of Patient Crimes." 62 *Univ. Det. Law Rev.* 145–160.

Hall, M.A., et al. (1996). "Judicial Protection of Managed Care Consumers: An Empirical Study of Insurance Coverage Disputes," 24 *Seton Hall Law Rev.* 101.

Hall, M.A., et al. (1994). "Medical Liberalism's Past and Future," 34 *Jurimetrics J.* 234–244.

Hall, M.A. and Anderson, G.F. (1992). "Health Insurers' Assessment of Medical Necessity," 140 *U. Penn. Law Rev.* 1637.

Halper, T. (1985). "Life and Death in a Welfare State: End-Stage Renal Disease in the United Kingdom," 63 *Milbank Mem. Fund Q.* 52.

Handler, J.F. (1986). *The Conditions of Discretion: Autonomy, Community, Bureaucracy* (New York: Russell Sage Foundation).

Haney, D. (1992). "Splitting Ounces of Prevention, Pounds of Cure," *Los Angeles Times*, May 31, at A8 (Washington edition).

Hardin, G.J. (1980). *Promethean Ethics: Living with Death, Competition and Triage* (Seattle: University of Washington Press).

Hardwig, J. (1987). "Robin Hoods and Good Samaritans: The Role of Patients in Health Care Distribution," 8 *Theor. Med.* 47.

Harper, F. and James, F. (1959). *The Law of Torts* (Boston: Little, Brown).

Harris, J. (1985). *The Value of Life: An Introduction to Medical Ethics* (Boston: Routledge & Kegan Paul).

Havighurst, C.C. (1995). *Health Care Choices: Private Contracts as Instruments of Health Reform* (Washington, DC: The AEI Press).

Havighurst, C.C. (1992). "Prospective Self-Denial: Can Consumers Contract Today to Accept Health Care Rationing Tomorrow?," 140 *U. Pa. Law Rev.* 1755.

Havighurst, C.C. (1986). "Private Reform of Tort-Law Dogma: Market Opportunities and Legal Obstacles," 49 *Law Contemp. Probs.* 143–172.

Havighurst, C.C. (1978). "Health Maintenance Organizations and the Health Planners," 1978 *Utah Law Rev.* 123.

Havighurst, C.C. (1977). "Health Care Cost-Containment Regulation: Prospects and an Alternative," 3 *Am. J. Law Med.* 309.

Havighurst, C.C. and Hackbarth, G. (1979). "Private Cost Containment," 300 *New Engl. J. Med.* 1298.

Healey, Jr., J.M. and Dowling, K.L. (1991). "Controlling Conflicts of Interest in the Doctor-Patient Relationship: Lessons from *Moore v. Regents of University of California*," 42 *Mercer Law Rev.* 989.

Hellman, S. and Hellman, D.S. (1991). "Of Mice but Not Men: Problems of the Randomized Clinical Trial," 324 *New Engl. J. Med.* 1585.

Hemenway, D., Killen, A., Cashman, S., et al. (1990). "Physicians' Responses to Financial Incentives: Evidence from a For-Profit Ambulatory Care Center," 322 *New Engl. J. Med.* 1059–1063.

Hiatt, H.H. (1975). "Protecting the Medical Commons: Who Is Responsible?," 293 *New Engl. J. Med.* 235.

Hilfiker, D. (1985). *Healing the Wounds: A Physician Looks at His Work* (New York, NY: Pantheon Books).

Hill, Jr., T.E. (1989). "The Kantian Conception of Autonomy," in *The Inner Citadel: Essays on Individual Autonomy*, ed. J. Christman (New York: Oxford University Press).

Hillman, A.L. (1990). "Health Maintenance Organizations, Financial Incentives, and Physicians' Judgments," 112 *Ann. Intern. Med.* 891.

Hillman, A.L. (1987). "Financial Incentives for Physicians in HMOs: Is There a Conflict of Interest?," 317 *New Engl. J. Med.* 1743.

Hillman, A.L., et al. (1992). "Contractual Arrangements Between HMOs and Primary Care Physicians: Three-tiered HMOs and Risk Pools," 30 *Med. Care* 136.

Hillman, A.L., et al. (1991). "HMO Managers' Views on Financial Incentives and Quality," 10 *Health Aff.* (Winter) 207.

Hillman, A.L., et al. (1989). "How do Financial Incentives Affect Physicians' Clinical Decisions and the Financial Performance of Health Maintenance Organizations?," 321 *New Engl. J. Med.* 86.

Hillman, B.J., et al. (1990). "Frequency and Costs of Diagnostic Imaging in Office Practice—A Comparison of Self-Referring and Radiologist-Referring Physicians," 323 *New Engl. J. Med.* 1604.

Hirshfeld, E.B. (1992). "Should Ethical and Legal Standards for Physicians be Changed to Accommodate New Models for Rationing Health Care?," 140 *U. Penn. Law Rev.* 1809.

Hirshfeld, E.B. (1990). "Should Third Party Payors of Health Care Services Disclose Cost Control Mechanisms to Potential Beneficiaries?," 14 *Seton Hall Legislative J.* 115.

Holleman, W.L., Edwards, D.C. and Matson, C.C. (1994). "Obligations of Physicians to Patients and Third-Party Payors," 5 *J. Clin. Ethics* 113.

Holmes, S. (1993). *The Anatomy of Antiliberalism* (Cambridge, MA: Harvard University Press).

Homan, R.K. (1993). Medical Care Resource Allocation Decisions: The Response to Multiple Agency Roles (unpublished paper presented at the 1994 Association for Health Services Research Annual Meeting).

Houston, R. (1938). "The Doctor Himself as a Therapeutic Agent," 11 *Ann. Int. Med.* 1415.

Howe, E.G. (1986). "Ethical Issues Regarding Mixed Agency of Military Physicians," 23 *Soc. Sci. Med.* 803.

Hsiao, W.C. (1995). "Medical Savings Accounts: Lessons from Singapore," 14 *Health Aff.* (Summer) 260–266.

Huber, P.W. (1993). *Galileo's Revenge: Junk Science in the Courtroom* (New York: Basic Books).

Huber, P.W. (1988). *Liability: The Legal Revolution and Its Consequences* (New York: Basic Books).

Hume, D. (1953). "Of the Original Contract," in *Political Essays* (New York: Liberal Arts Press).

Hunter, K. (1991). *Doctors' Stories: The Narrative Structure of Medical Knowledge* (Princeton: Princeton University Press).

Iglehart, J. (1996). "Politics and Public Health." 334 *New Engl. J. Med.* 203–207.

Ingelfinger, F. (1980). "Arrogance," 303 *New Engl. J. Med.* 1507.

Ingelfinger, F. (1972). "Informed (But Uneducated) Consent," 287 *New Engl. J. Med.* 465.

Institute of Medicine, Committee for Evaluating Medical Technologies (1985). *Assessing Medical Technologies* (Washington, DC: National Academy Press).

Institute of Medicine (1993). *Employment and Health Benefits: A Connection at Risk*, eds. M.J. Field and H.T. Shapiro (Washington, DC: National Academy Press).

Institute of Medicine, Committee on Utilization Management by Third Parties (1989). *Controlling Costs and Changing Patient Care?: The Role of Utilization Management*, eds. B.H. Gray and M.J. Field (Washington, DC: National Academy Press).

Jacobson, P.D. and Rosenquist, C.J. (1988). "The Introduction of Low-Osmolar Contrast Agents in Radiology: Medical, Economic, Legal and Public Policy Issues," 260 *JAMA* 1586.

James, W. (1988). *Immunization: The Reality Behind the Myth* (South Hadley, MA: Bergin & Garvey).

Jecker, N.S. (1990). "Integrating Medical Ethics with Normative Theory: Patient Advocacy and Social Responsibility," 11 *Theor. Med.* 125.

Jecker, N.S. and Berg, A.O. (1992). "Allocating Medical Resources in Rural America: Alternative Perceptions of Justice," 34 *Soc. Sci. Med.* 467.

Jensen, G.A. (1993). "Regulating the Content of Health Plans," in *American Health Policy: Critical Issues for Reform*, ed. R.B. Helms (Washington, DC: The AEI Press).

Jensen, G.A. and Morlock, R.J. (1994). "Why Medical Savings Accounts Deserve a Closer Look," 4 *J. Am. Health Policy* 14.

Jerry, R.H. (1987). *Understanding Insurance Law* (New York: Matthew-Bender).

Jesilow, P., Geis, G. and Pontell, H. (1991). "Fraud by Physicians Against Medicaid," 266 *JAMA* 3318.

Jones, C.J. (1990). "Autonomy and Informed Consent in Medical Decisionmaking: Toward a New Self-Fulfilling Prophecy," 47 *Wash. Lee Law Rev.* 379.

Jonsen, A.R., Siegler, M. and Winslade, W.J. (1986). *Clinical Ethics: A Practical Approach to Ethical Decisions in Clinical Medicine* (2nd ed., New York, NY: Macmillan).

Kalb, P. (1989). "Controlling Health Care Costs By Controlling Technology: A Private Contractual Approach," 99 *Yale Law J.* 1109.

Kalb, P. and Miller, D. (1989). "Utilization Strategies for Intensive Care Units," 261 *JAMA* 2389.

Kamm, F. (1993). *Morality and Mortality* (Oxford: Oxford University Press).

Kahneman, D., Slovic, P. and Tversky, A., eds. (1982). *Judgment Under Uncertainty: Heuristics and Biases* (New York: Cambridge University Press).

Kapp, M.B. (1984). "Legal and Ethical Implications of Health Care Reimbursement by Diagnosis Related Groups," 12 *Law Med. Health Care* 245.

Kasper, J.F., et al. (1992). "Developing Shared Decision-Making Programs to Improve the Quality of Health Care," 4 *Quality Rev. Bull.* 183.

Katz, J. (1984). *The Silent World of Doctor and Patient* (New York: The Free Press).

Katz, J. (1977). "Informed Consent—A Fairy Tale? Law's Vision," 39 *U. Pitt. Law Rev.* 137.

Katz, P. (1985). "How Surgeons Make Decisions," in *Physicians of Western Medicine,* eds. R.A. Hahn and A.D. Gaines (Hingham, MA: D. Reidel Pub. Co.).

Keeler, E. B., et al. (1996). "Can Medical Savings Accounts for the Nonelderly Reduce Health Care Costs?" 275 *JAMA* 1666.

Keeler, E.B. and Rolph, J.E. (1983). "How Cost Sharing Reduced Medical Spending of Participants in the Health Insurance Experiment," 249 *JAMA* 2220.

Kennedy, D. (1976). "Form and Substance in Private Law Adjudication," 89 *Harv. Law Rev.* 1685.

Kidd, A.M. (1953). "Limits of the Right of a Person to Consent to Experimentation on Himself," 117 *Science* 211.

Kilner, J.F. (1990). *Who Lives? Who Dies?: Ethical Criteria in Patient Selection* (New Haven: Yale University Press).

Klein, R. (1993a). "Rationality and Rationing: Diffused or Concentrated Decision Making?," in *Rationing of Health Care in Medicine*, ed. M. Tunbridge (London: Royal College of Physicians).

Klein, R. (1993b). "Dimensions of Rationing: Who Should do What?," 307 *Br. Med. J.* 309–311.

Kleinman, A. (1988). *The Illness Narratives: Suffering, Healing, and the Human Condition* (New York: Basic Books).

Komesar, N.K. (1995). *Imperfect Alternatives: Choosing Institutions in Law, Economics, and Public Policy* (Chicago: University of Chicago Press).

Komrad, M.S. (1983). "A Defence of Medical Paternalism: Maximising Patients' Autonomy," 9 *J. Med. Ethics* 38.

Ku, L. and Fisher, D. (1990). "The Attitudes of Physicians Toward Health Care Cost-Containment Policies," 25 *Health Serv. Res.* 25.

Kuflik, A. (1986). "The Utilitarian Logic of Inalienable Rights," 97 *Ethics* 75.

Kuflik, A. (1984). "The Inalienability of Autonomy," 13 *Philo. Public Aff.* 271.

Kymlicka, W. (1988). "Liberalism and Communitarianism," 18 *Can. J. Philo.* 181–204.

La Puma, J. and Lawlor, E.F. (1990). "Quality-Adjusted Life-Years: Ethical Implications for Physicians and Policymakers," 263 *JAMA* 2917.

Lamm, R.D. (1994). "Rationing and the Clinton Health Plan," 19 *J. Med. Philo.* 445.

Lamm, R.D. (1992). "Rationing of Health Care: Inevitable and Desirable," 140 *U. Pa. Law Rev.* 1511.

Lantos, J.D., Singer, P.A., Walker, R.M., et al. (1987). "The Illusion of Futility in Clinical Practice," 87 *Am. J. Med.* 81.

Lasker, R.D., Shapiro, D.W. and Tucker, A.M. (1992). "Realizing the Potential of Practice Pattern Profiling," 29 *Inquiry* 287–297.

Laudicina, S. (1992). *Impact of State Basic Benefit Laws on the Uninsured* (Washington, DC: Blue Cross and Blue Shield Association).

Lave, J. and Lave, L. (1970). "Medical Care and its Delivery: An Economic Appraisal," 35 *Law Contemp. Prob.* 252.

Leape, L.L. (1995). "Translating Medical Science into Medical Practice: Do We Need a National Medical Standards Board?" 273 *JAMA* 1534–1537.

Leeb, D., Bowers, D.G. and Lynch, J.B. (1976). "Observations on the Myth of 'Informed Consent,'" 58 *Plast. Reconstr. Surg.* 280 (1976)

Leichter, H.M. (1992). "Political Accountability in Health Care Rationing: In Search of a New Jerusalem," 140 *U. Penn. Law Rev.* 1939.

Leonard, S.D. (1992). "Letter to the Editor," *N.Y. Times*, April 28, at A16.

Levine, R.J. (1991). "Informed Consent: Some Challenges to the Universal Validity of the Western Model," 19 *Law, Med. Health Care* 207.

Levinsky, N.G. (1990). "Age as a Criterion for Rationing Health Care," 322 *New Engl. J. Med.* 1813.

Levinsky, N.G. (1984). "The Doctor's Master," 311 *New Engl. J. Med.* 1573.

Levinson, D.F. (1987). "Toward Full Disclosure of Referral Restrictions and Financial Incentives by Prepaid Health Plans," 317 *New Engl. J. Med.* 1729.

Levmore, S. (1993). "Commissions and Conflicts in Agency arrangements: Lawyers, Real Estate Brokers, Underwriters, and Other Agents' Rewards," 36 *J. Law Econ.* 503–539.

Lidz, C.W., Meisel, A. and Zerubavel, E., et. al. (1984). *Informed Consent: A Study of Decisionmaking in Psychiatry* (New York, NY: Guilford Press).

Lidz, C.W., et al. (1983). "Barriers to Informed Consent," 99 *Ann. Intern. Med.* 539.

Lidz, C.W. and Meisel, A. (1982). "Informed Consent and the Structure of Medical Care," in *Making Health Care Decisions, Vol. II* (Washington, DC: President's Commission for the Study of Ethical Problems in Medicine and Biomedical and Behavioral Research).

Lipsky, M. (1980). *Street-Level Bureaucracy: Dilemmas of the Individual in Public Services* (New York: Russell Sage Foundation).

Llewellyn-Thomas, H., Sutherland, H. and Thiel, E. (1993). "Do Patients' Evaluations of a Future Health State Change When They Actually Enter that State?," 31 *Med. Care* 1002.

Lo, B., et al. (1985). "'Do Not Resuscitate' Decisions: A Prospective Study at Three Teaching Hospitals," 145 *Arch. Intern. Med.* 1115.

Lo, B. and Steinbrook, R. (1983). "Deciding Whether to Resuscitate," 143 *Arch. Intern. Med.* 1561.

Loewy, E. (1991). "Involving Patients in Do Not Resuscitate (DNR) Decisions: An Old Issue Raising its Ugly Head," 17 *J. Med. Ethics* 156.

Lohr, K.N., Brook, R.H., Kamberg, C.J., et al. (1986). "Effect of Cost Sharing on Use of Medically Effective and Less Effective Care," 24 *Med. Care* S31 (Suppl.).

Louisell, D.W. and Williams, H. (1960). *Medical Malpractice* (Albany: Matthew-Bender).

Lowey, E.H. (1980). "Cost Should Not Be a Factor in Medical Care," 302 *New Engl. J. Med.* 697.

Lu, E. (1993). "The Potential Effect of Managed Competition in Health Care on Provider Liability and Patient Autonomy," 30 *Harv. J. Legislation* 499.

Luban, D. (1988). *Lawyers and Justice: An Ethical Study* (Princeton, NJ: Princeton University Press).

Luft, H.S. (1982). "Health Maintenance Organizations and the Rationing of Medical Care," 60 *Milbank Mem. Fund Q.* 319.

Luft, H.S., et al. (1985). "Adverse Selection in a Large Multiple-Option Health Benefits Program," in 6 *Advances in Health Economics and Health Services Research,* eds. R. Scheffler and L. Rossiter, Vol. VI (Greenwich, CT: JAI Press).

Luhmann, N. (1973). *Trust and Power* (Chichester: John Wiley & Sons).

Lustig, B.A. (1992). "The Method of 'Principalism': A Critique of the Critique," 17 *J. Med. Philo.* 487.

MacIntyre, A. (1988). *Whose Justice? Which Rationality?* (Notre Dame, IN: University of Notre Dame Press).

MacIntyre, A. (1981). *After Virtue: A Study in Moral Theory* (Notre Dame, IN: University of Notre Dame Press).

Mackie, J.L. (1977). *Ethics: Inventing Right and Wrong* (New York: Penguin).

Macklin, R. (1993). *Enemies of Patients* (New York: Oxford University Press).

Macneil, I.R. (1978). "Contracts: Adjustment of Long-Term Economic Relations Under Classical, Neoclassical, and Relational Contract Law," 72 *Nw. U. Law Rev.* 854.

Mansfield, G. (1991). "Vaccinations May Cause New Problems," *Seattle Times*, April 8, at A11.

Marmor, T.R. and Blustein, J. (1992). "Cutting Waste by Making Rules: Promises, Pitfalls, and Realistic Prospects," 140 *U. Penn. Law Rev.* 1543.

Marquis, M.S. (1992). "Adverse Selection With a Multiple Choice Among Health Insurance Plans: A Simulation Analysis," 11 *J. Health Econ.* 129.

Marquis, M.S. (1983). "Consumers' Knowledge About Their Health Insurance Coverage," 5 *Health Care Fin. Rev.* 65–80.

Marquis, M.S. and Buchanan, J.L. (1994). "How Will Changes in Health Insurance Tax Policy and Employer Health Plan Contributions Affect Access to Health Care and Health Care Costs,?" 271 *JAMA* 939.

Marsh, F.H. and Staver, A. (1991). "Physician Authority for Unilateral DNR Orders," 12 *J. Leg. Med.* 115.

Marsh, F.H. and Yarborough, M. (1990). *Medicine and Money: A Study of the Role of Beneficence in Health Care Cost Containment* (Westport, CT: Greenwold Press).

Marylander, S. J. (1980). "Management Professionals vs. Medical Professionals," in *Hospital Administrator-Physician Relationships*, ed. J.O. Hepner (St. Louis: Mosby).

Mashaw, J.L. (1983). *Bureaucratic Justice: Managing Social Security Disability Claims* (New Haven: Yale University Press).

May, W.F. (1983). *The Physician's Covenant: Images of the Healer in Medical Ethics* (Philadelphia: Westminster Press).

McCaughey, E. (1994). "No Exit," *The New Republic*, February 7.

McConnell, T. (1984). "The Nature and Basis of Inalienable Rights," 3 *Law Philo.* 25.

McGraw, D. (1995). "Financial Incentives to Limit Services: Should Physicians be Required to Disclose these to Patients?" 83 *Gerogetown Law Rev.* 1821.

McNeil, B.J., Pauker, S.G., Sox, H.C. and Tversky, A. (1982). "On the Elicitation of Preferences for Alternative Therapies," 306 *New Engl. J. Med.* 1259.

Mechanic, D. (1992). "Professional Judgment and the Rationing of Medical Care," 140 *Penn. Law Rev.* 1713.

Mechanic, D. (1986). *From Advocacy to Allocation: The Evolving American Health Care System* (New York: The Free Press).

Mechanic, D. (1980). "Rationing of Medical Care and the Preservation of Clinical Judgment," 11 *J. Fam. Pract.* 431.

Mechanic, D. (1979). *Future Issues in Health Care: Social Policy and the Rationing of Medical Services* (New York, NY: Free Press).

Mechanic, D., Ettel, T., Davis, D. (1990). "Choosing Among Health Insurance Options: A Study of New Employees," 27 *Inquiry* 14.

Mechanic, D. and Schlesinger, M. (1996). "The Impact of Managed Care on Patients' Trust in Medical Care and their Physicians," 275 *JAMA* 1693–97.

Medica Foundation (1994). *The 17 Minute Report* (Minneapolis: Medica Foundation).

Mehlman, M.J. (1996). "Medical Advocates: A Call for a New Profession," 1 *Widener Law Symposium J.* 299–323.

Mehlman, M.J. (1993). "The Patient-Physician Relationship in an Era of Scarce Resources: Is there a Duty to Treat?," 25 *Conn. Law Rev.* 349.

Mehlman, M.J. (1990). "Fiduciary Contracting: Limitations on Bargaining Between Patients and Health Care Providers," 51 *U. Pitts. Law Rev.* 365.

Mehlman, M.J. (1986). "Health Care Cost Containment and Medical Technology: A Critique of Waste Theory," 36 *Case W. Res. Law Rev.* 778.

Mehlman, M.J. (1985). "Rationing Expensive Lifesaving Medical Treatments," 1985 *Wis. Law Rev.* 239.

Meisel, A. (1988). "A 'Dignitary Tort' as a Bridge Between the Idea of Informed Consent and the Law of Informed Consent," 16 *Law Med. Health Care* 210.

Meisel, A. (1979). "The 'Exceptions' to the Informed Consent Doctrine: Striking a Balance Between Competing Values in Medical Decisionmaking," 1979 *Wis. Law Rev.* 413.

Meisel, A. and Roth, L.H. (1983). "Toward an Informed Discussion of Informed Consent: A Review and Critique of the Empirical Studies," 25 *Az. Law Rev.* 267–346.

Menzel, P.T. (1993). "Double Agency and the Ethics of Rationing Health Care: A Response to Marcia Angell," 3 *Kennedy Institute of Ethics J.* 287–292.

Menzel, P.T. (1990). *Strong Medicine: The Ethical Rationing of Health Care* (New York: Oxford University Press).

Merz, J.F. and Fischhoff, B. (1990). "Informed Consent Does not Mean Rational Consent: Cognitive Limitations on Decision-Making," 11 *J. Leg. Med.* 321.

Meyer, H. (1994). "Support Grows for MSAs But Studies Question Actual Savings," *Am. Med. News*, November 7, at 3, 10.

Meyer, H. (1989). "Suit: HMO Failed to Disclose MD Cost Incentives," *Am. Med. News*, January 20, at 4.

Miles, S.H. (1991). "Informed Demand for 'Non-Beneficial' Medical Treatment," 325 *New Engl. J. Med.* 512.

Milgram, S. (1969). *Obedience to Authority: An Experimental View* (New York, NY: Harper & Row).

Mill, J.S. (1975). "On Liberty," in *Three Essays* (Oxford: Oxford University Press).

Mill, J.S. (1929). *Principles of Political Economy*, ed. W.J. Ashley (London: Longmans, Green).

Miller, F.H. (1992). "Denial of Health Care and Informed Consent in English and American Law," 18 *Am. J. Law Med.* 37.

Miller, F.H. (1987). "Informed Consent for the Man on the Clapham Omnibus: An English Cure for 'The American Disease'?," 9 *W. New Engl. Law Rev.* 169.

Miller, F.H. (1983). "Secondary Income From Recommended Treatment: Should Fiduciary Principles Constrain Physician Behavior?," in *The New Health Care for Profit:*

Doctors and Hospitals in a Competitive Environment, ed. B.H. Gray (Washington, DC: National Academy Press).

Miller, R.H. and Luft, H.S. (1994). "Managed Care Plan Performance Since 1980: A Literature Analysis," 271 *JAMA* 1512.

Minnesota Department of Health (1994). Medical Savings Accounts: A Feasibility Study for the Minnesota Legislature. (Unpublished government report)

Mitka, M. (1993). "High School Grads Say What's 'Medically Necessary,'" *Am. Med. News*, September 20.

Moerman, D.E. (1983). "Physiology and Symbols: The Anthropological Implications of the Placebo Effect," in *The Anthropology of Medicine*, eds. L. Romanucci-Ross, D.E. Moerman and L.R. Tancredi (New York: Praeger).

Moffit, R.E. (1994). "Personal Freedom and Responsibility: The Ethical Foundations of a Market-Based Health Care Reform," 19 *J. Med. Philo.* 471.

Monheit, A.C. and Harvey, P.H. (1993). "Source of Health Insurance for the Self Employed: Does Differential Taxation Make a Difference,?" 30 *Inquiry* 293.

Mooney, G. and Ryan, M. (1993). "Agency in Health Care: Getting Beyond First Principles," 12 *J. Health Econ.* 125–135.

Moore, S.H. and Martin, D.P. (1983). "Does the Primary-Care Gatekeeper Control the Costs of Health Care? Lessons from the SAFECO Experience," 309 *New Engl. J. Med.* 1400.

Moreno, J. (1995). *Deciding Together: Bioethics and Moral Consensus* (New York: Oxford University Press).

Morone, J.A. (1992). "The Bias of American Politics: Rationing Health Care in a Weak State," 140 *U. Penn. Law Rev.* 1923.

Morone, J.A. (1993). "The Health Care Bureaucracy: Small Changes, Big Consequences," 18 *J. Health Polit. Policy Law* 723.

Morreim, E.H. (1994a). "Redefining Quality by Reassigning Responsibility," 20 *Am. J. Public Health* 79.

Morreim, E.H. (1994b). "Profoundly Diminished Life: The Casualties of Coercion," 24 *Hastings Cen. Rep.* (January–Febuary 1994) 33.

Morreim, E.H. (1994c). "Of Rescue and Responsibility: Learning to Live with Limits," 19 *J. Med. Philo.* 455.

Morreim, E.H. (1991a). "Economic Disclosure and Economic Advocacy: New Duties in the Medical Standard of Care," 12 *J. Legal Med.* 275.

Morreim, E.H. (1991b). *Balancing Act: The New Medical Ethics of Medicine's New Economics* (Dordrecht: Kluwer Academic).

Morreim, E.H. (1991c). "Gaming the System: Dodging the Rules, Ruling the Dodgers." 151 *Arch. Intern. Med.* 443–447.

Morreim, E.H. (1989). "Fiscal Scarcity and the Inevitability of Bedside Budget Balancing," 149 *Arch. Intern. Med.* 1012.

Morreim, E.H. (1987). "Clinicians or Committees—Who Should Cut Costs?," 17 *Hastings Cent. Rep.* 34.

Morreim, E.H. (1985). "The M.D. and the DRG," 15 *Hastings Cent. Rep.* (June 1985) 30.

Morrisey, M. (1992). *Price Sensitivity in Health Care: Implications for Health Care Policy* (Washington, DC: National Federation of Independent Businesses).

Moyers, B. (1993). *Healing and the Mind* (New York: Doubleday).

Murphy, D.J. (1988). "Do-Not-Resuscitate Orders: Time for Reappraisal in Long-Term-Care Institutions," 260 *JAMA* 2098.

Murphy, D.J. and Finucane, T.E. (1993). "New Do-Not-Resuscitate Policies: A First Step in Cost Control," 153 *Arch. Intern. Med.* 1641.

Murphy, J.G. (1981). "Consent, Coercion, and Hard Choices," 67 *Va. Law Rev.* 79.

Murphy, J.G. (1970). *Kant: The Philosophy of Right* (New York: St. Martin's Press).

Murray, T.H. (1986). "Divided Loyalties for Physicians: Social Context and Moral Problems," 23 *Soc. Sci. Med.* 827.

Murray, T.H. (1984). "Divided Loyalties in Sports Medicine," 12 *Physician Sports* 134.

Muss, H.B., et al. (1979). "Written Informed Consent in Patient with Breast Cancer," 43 *Cancer* 1549.

Myerson, A.R. (1995). "Helping Health Insurers Say No," *N.Y. Times*, March 20, at D1.

Nagel, J.H. (1992). "Combining Deliberation and Fair Representation in Community Health Decisions," 140 *U. Penn. Law Rev.* 1965.

Nagel, J.H. (1991). *Equality and Partiality* (New York: Oxford University Press).

Nease, R.F., Kneeland, T., O'Connor, G.T., et al. (1995). "Variation in Patient Utilities for Outcomes of the Management of Chronic Stable Angina: Implications for Practice Guidelines," 273 *JAMA* 1185–1190.

Nelson, J.L. (1994). "Publicity and Pricelessness: Grassroots Decisionmaking and Justice in Rationing," 19 *J. Med. Philo.* 333.

Newdick, C. (1995). *Who Should we Treat/ Law, Patients and Resources in the NHS* (Oxford: Clarendon Press).

Newhouse, J.P. and The Insurance Experiment Group (1993). *Free For All? Lessons from the RAND Health Insurance Experiment* (Cambridge, MA: Harvard University Press).

Nichols, L.M. (1995). "MSAs and Risk Segmentation," 14 *Health Aff.* (Summer) 275–276.

Nie, J. and Smith, K. (1995). "Individualism and Communitarianism in the Ethics of Health Promotion: The Search for a Yin-Yang/Dialectic Model," in *Health Care Crisis? The Search for Answers*, eds. Misbin et al. (Frederick, MD: University Publishing Group).

Nino, C. (1989). "The Communitarian Challenge to Liberal Rights," 8 *Law Philo.* 37–52.

Northwestern National Life Insurance Company (1990). *Americans Speak Out on Health Care Rationing*.

Note (1969). "Scarce Medical Resources," 69 *Colum. Law Rev.* 620.

Novack, D.H. (1987). "Therapeutic Aspects of the Clinical Encounter," 2 *J. Gen. Intern. Med.* 346–355.

Novack, D.H., et al. (1989). "Physicians' Attitudes Toward Using Deception to Resolve Difficult Ethical problems," 261 *JAMA* 2980.

Nozick, R. (1974). *Anarchy, State, and Utopia* (New York: Basic Books).

Oberman, L. (1994). "Reform's Cost-Benefit Balancing Act," *Am. Med. News*, May 9, at 3, 35.

O'Connor, B.B. (1995). *Health Traditions: Alternative Medicine and the Health Professions* (Philadelphia: University of Pennsylvania Press).

Ohsfeldt, R. (1993). "Contractual Arrangements, Financial Incentives, and Physician-Patient Relationships," in *Sociomedical Perspectives on Patient Care Relationships*, eds. J.M. Clair and R.M. Allman (Lexington, KY: University Press of Kentucky).

Orentlicher, D. (1996). "Paying Physicians More to do Less: Financial Incentives to Limit Care." 30 *Univ. Richmond Law Rev.* 155–197.

Orentlicher, D. (1995). "Health Care Reform and the Patient-Physician Relationship," 5 *Health Matrix* 141.

Orentlicher, D. (1994). "Rationing and the Americans with Disabilities Act," 271 *JAMA* 308.

Orentlicher, D. (1992). "The Illusion of Patient Choice in End-of-Life Decisions," 267 *JAMA* 2101.

Ost, D.E. (1984). "The 'Right' Not to Know," 9 *J. Med. Philo.* 301–312.

Otten, A. (1989). "Intensive-Care Units Are Rejecting Patients Because of Crowding," *Wall St. J.*, May 23, at 1.

Ozar, D.T. (1987). "Cost Containment and Physicians' Decisions: Rethinking the Philosophy of Medicine," 8 *Theor. Med.* 81.

Ozminkowski, R.J., Friedman, B. and Taylor, Z. (1993). "Access to Heart and Liver Transplantation in the 1980s," 31 *Med. Care* 1027.

Paris, J.J., et al. (1993). "Beyond Autonomy—Physicians' Refusal to Use Life-Prolonging Extracorporeal Membrane Oxygenation," 329 *New. Engl. J. Med.* 354.

Paris, J.J., Crone, R.K. and Reardon, F. (1990). "Physicians' Refusal of Requested Treatment: The Case of Baby L," 322 *New Engl. J. Med.* 1012.

Parmley, W. (1994). "Clinical Practice Guidelines: Does the Cookbook have Enough Recipes?," 272 *JAMA* 1374.

Parsons, T. (1951). "Magic Science and Religion," in *The Social System* (Glencoe, IL: Free Press).

Paul-Shaheen, P., Clark, J.D. and Williams, D. (1987). "Small Area Analysis: A Review and Analysis of the North American Literature," 12 *J. Health Polit. Policy Law* 741.

Pauly, M.V. (1994). *An Analysis of Medical Savings Accounts: Do Two Wrongs Make a Right?* (Washington, DC: The AEI Press).

Pauly, M.V. (1990). "The Rational Nonpurchase of Long-Term-Care Insurance," 98 *J. Polit. Econ.* 153.

Pauly, M.V. (1980). "Overinsurance: The Conceptual Issues," in *National Health Insurance: What Now, What Later, What Never?*, ed. M.V. Pauly (Washington, DC: The AEI Press).

Pauly, M.V., Danzon, P., Feldstein, P.J. and Hoff, J. (1992). *Responsible National Health Insurance* (Washington DC: The AEI Press).

Pauly, M.V., Eisenberg, J., Radany, M., et al. (1992). *Paying Physicians: Options for Controlling Cost, Volume and Intensity of Services* (Ann Arbor, MI: Health Administration Press).

Pauly, M. and Goodman, J. (1995). "Tax Credits for Health Insurance and Medical Savings Accounts," 14 *Health Aff.* 126–139.

Pear, R. (1995). "Doctors Say H.M.O.'s Limit What They Can Tell Patients." *N.Y. Times*, December 21, at A1.

Pear, R. (1994). "Medicare Denials Vary Greatly State by State," *N.Y. Times*, March 29, at D23.

Pearlman, R.A., et al. (1982). "Variability in Physician Bioethical Decision-Making," 97 *Ann. Intern. Med.* 420.

Pellegrino, E.D. (1991). "Trust and Distrust in Professional Ethics," in *Ethics, Trust, and the Professions: Philosophical and Cultural Aspects*, eds. E.D. Pellegrino, R.M. Veatch and J.P. Langan (Washington, DC: Georgetown University Press).

Pellegrino, E.D. (1982). "Being Ill and Being Healed," in *The Humanity of the Ill*, ed. V. Kestenbaum (Knoxville: University Tennessee Press).

Pellegrino, E.D. (1979). "Toward a Reconstruction of Medical Morality: The Primacy of the Act of Profession and the Fact of Illness," 4 *J. Med. Philo.* 32.

Pellegrino, E.D. and Thomasma, D.C. (1993). *The Virtues in Medical Practice* (New York: Oxford University Press).

Pellegrino, E.D. and Thomasma, D.C. (1988). *For the Patient's Good: The Restoration of Beneficence in Health Care* (New York: Oxford University Press).

Pellegrino, E.D. and Thomasma, D.C. (1981). *A Philosophical Basis of Medical Practice* (New York: Oxford University Press).

Perry, C.B. (1994). "Conflicts of Interest and the Physician's Duty to Inform," 96 *Am. J. Med.* 375–380.

Peters, Jr., P.G. (1995). "Health Care Rationing and Disability Rights," 70 *Ind. Law J.* 491.

Peters, W. and Rogers, M. (1994). "Variation in Approval by Insurance Companies of Coverage for Autologous Bone Marrow Transplantation for Breast Cancer," 330 *New Engl. J. Med.* 473.

Peterson, D.T. (1985). "Letter to the Editor," 312 *New Engl. J. Med.* 1330.

Philips, D.L. (1993). *Looking Backward: A Critical Appraisal of Communitarian Thought* (Princeton, NJ: Princeton University Press).

Physician Payment Review Commission (1995). Annual Report to Congress (Washington, DC).

Physician Payment Review Commission (1989). "Risk-Sharing Arrangements in Prepaid Health Plans," in *Annual Report to Congress* (Washington, DC).

Pildes, R.H. (1991). "The Unintended Cultural Consequences of Public Policy," 89 *Mich. Law Rev.* 936.

Pollock, E.J. (1993). "HMO Held Liable for Refusing Coverage," *Wall St. J.*, December 28, at B5.

Pratt, J.W. and Zeckhauser, R.J. (1985). "Principals and Agents: An Overview," in *Principals and Agents: The Structure of Business*, eds. J.W. Pratt and R.J. Zeckhauser (Boston: Harvard Business School Press).

President's Commission for the Study of Ethical Problems in Medicine and Biomedical and Behavioral Research (1985). *Securing Access to Health Care* (Washington, DC: U.S. Government Printing Office).

President's Commission for the Study of Ethical Problems in Medicine and Biomedical and Behavioral Research (1982). *Making Health Care Decisions: The Ethical and Legal Implications of Informed Consent in the Patient-Practitioner Relationship* (Washington, DC: U.S. Government Printing Office).

Prillaman, H.L. (1990). "A Physician's Duty to Inform of Newly Developed Therapy," 6 *J. Contemp. Health Law Policy* 43.

Puma, J.L., et al. (1988). "Ethics, Economics, and Endocarditis: The Physician's Role in Resource Allocation," 148 *Arch. Intern. Med.* 1809.

Quill, T.E. and Cassel, C.K. (1995). "Nonabandonment: A Central Obligation for Physicians," 122 *Ann. Intern. Med.* 368–378.

Radin, M.J. (1987). "Market-Inalienability," 100 *Harv. Law Rev.* 1849.

Rakowski, E. (1993). "Taking and Saving Lives," 93 *Colum. Law Rev.* 1063.

Randall, V. (1993). "Racist Health Care: Reforming an Unjust Health Care System to Meet the Needs of African-Americans," 3 *Health Matrix* 127.

Rasell, M.E. (1995). "Cost Sharing in Health Insurance—A Reexamination," 332 *New Engl. J. Med.* 1164–1168.

Rawls, J. (1993). *Political Liberalism* (New York: Columbia University Press).

Rawls, J. (1971). *A Theory of Justice* (Cambridge, MA: Harvard University of Press).

Reagan, M.D. (1988). "Health Care Rationing: What Does it Mean?," 319 *New Engl. J. Med.* 1149.

Redelmeier, D.A., Rozin P. and Kahneman D. (1993). "Understanding Patients' Decisions: Cognitive and Emotional Perspectives," 270 *JAMA* 72 (1993).

Redelmeier, D. and Tversky, A. (1990). "Discrepancy Between Medical Decision for Individual Patients and for Groups," 322 *New Engl. J. Med.* 1162.

Reitemeier, P.J. and Brody, H. (1988). "Treatment Refusal for Economic Reasons," in *Medical Ethics: A Guide for Health Professionals*, eds. J.F. Monagle and D.C. Thomasma (Rockville, MD: Aspen).

Relman, A.S. (1990a). "The Trouble With Rationing," 323 *New Engl. J. Med.* 911.

Relman, A.S. (1990b). "Is Rationing Inevitable?," 322 *New Engl. J. Med.* 1809.

Relman, A.S. (1985a). "Dealing with Conflicts of Interest," 313 *New Engl. J. Med.* 749.

Relman, A.S. (1985b). "Cost Control, Doctors' Ethics, and Patient Care," 1 *Issues Sci. Tech.* 103.

Rhoden, N.K. (1988). "Litigating Life and Death," 102 *Harv. Law Rev.* 375.

Rhodes, R.P. (1992). *Health Care Politics, Policy, and Distributive Justice: The Ironic Triumph* (Albany: State University of New York Press).

Rice, T. and Morrison, K. (1994). "Patient Cost Sharing for Medical Services: A Review of the Literature and Implications for Health Care Reform," 51 *Med. Care Rev.* 235.

Rice, T. and Thorpe, K.E. (1993). "Income-Related Cost Sharing in Health Insurance," 12(2) *Health Affairs* 21–39.

Roberts, A.H., Kewman, D.G., Mercier, L. and Hovell, M. (1993). "The Power of Non-specific Effects in Healing: Implications of Psychosocial and Biological Treatments," 12 *Clin. Psychol. Rev.* 375–391.

Roberts, A.H. (1995). "The Powerful Placebo Revisited: Magnitude of Nonspecific Effects," 1 *Mind/Body Med.* 35–43.

Robertson, J.A. (1990). "Prior Agreements for Disposition of Frozen Embryos," 51 *Ohio St. Law J.* 407.

Robinson, G. (1986). "Rethinking the Allocation of Medical Malpractice Risks Between Patients and Providers," 49 *Law Contemp. Probs.* 173.

Robinson, J.C. (1993). "Payment Mechanisms, Nonprice Incentives, and Organizational Innovation in Health Care," 30 *Inquiry* 328–333.

Rodwin, M.A. (1995a). "Conflicts in Managed Care," 322 *New Engl. J. Med.* 604.

Rodwin, M.A. (1995b). "Strains in the Fiduciary Metaphor: Divided Physician Loyalties and Obligations in a Changing Health Care System," 21 *Am. J. Law Med.* 241–257.

Rodwin, M.A. (1993). *Medicine, Money and Morals: Physicians' Conflicts of Interest* (New York: Oxford University Press).

Rodwin, M.A. (1989). "Physicians' Conflicts of Interest: The Limitations of Disclosure," 321 *New Engl. J. Med.* 1405.

Rooney, J.P. (1992). "Give Employees Medial IRAs and Watch Costs Fall," *Wall St. J.*, September 28.

Rose-Ackerman, S. (1985). "Inalienability and the Theory of Property Rights," 85 *Colum. Law Rev.* 931.

Rosenblatt, R.E. (1981). "Rationing 'Normal" Health Care: The Hidden Legal Issues," 59 *Tex. Law Rev.* 1401–1420.

Rosenfeld, S.C. (1994). "So You Want to Join an H.M.O.? Good Luck," *N.Y. Times*, Aug. 9, at A23, col.2.

Rosenthal, E. (1990a). "Health Insurers Say Rising Fraud is Costing Them Tens of Billions," *N.Y. Times*, July 5, at A1, B7.

Rosenthal, E. (1990b). "Rules on Reviving the Dying Bring Undue Suffering, Doctors Contend," *N.Y. Times*, October 4, at A1, B20.

Rosoff, A.J. (1981). *Informed Consent: A Guide for Health Care Providers* (Rockville, MD: Aspen Systems Corp.).

Rothman, D.J. (1991). *Strangers at the Bedside: A History of How Law and Bioethics Transformed Medical Decision Making* (New York, NY: Basic Books).

Rozovsky, F.A. (1990). *Consent to Treatment: A Practical Guide* (2nd ed., Boston: Little, Brown).

Rubin, E.L. (1996). "The New Legal Process, The Synthesis of Discourse, and the Microanalysis of Institutions." 109 *Harv. Law Rev.* 1393–1438.

Rubin, H.R., et al. (1993). "Patients' Rating of Outpatient Visits in Different Practice Settings," 270 *JAMA* 835.

Rundle, R.L. (1989). "How Doctors Boost Bills by Misrepresenting the Work They Do," *Wall St. J.*, December 6, at A1, A8.

Russell, C. (1994). "How Much Do People Know About Health,?" *Washington Post*, March 1, at Health 6.

Sagoff, M. (1994). "Two Cheers for Community," (May 1994) *Hastings Cent. Rep.* 33–34.

Salkever, D.S. and Bice, T.W. (1979). *Hospital Certificate-of-Need Controls: Impact on Investment, Costs, and Use* (Washington, DC: The AEI Press).

Sandel, M.J. (1984). *Liberalism and its Critics* (New York: New York University Press).

Sandel, M.J. (1982). *Liberalism and the Limits of Justice* (Cambridge, England: Cambridge University Press).

Sanders, S.J. (1991). "Regulating Managed Care Plans Under Current Law: A Radical Reversion to Established Doctrine," 20 *Hofstra Law Rev.* 73.

Schafer, A. (1982). "The Ethics of the Randomized Clinical Trial," 307 *New Engl. J. Med.* 719.

Schauer, F. (1992). "The Right to Die as a Case Study in Third-Order Decisionmaking," 17 *J. Med. Philo.* 573–587.

Schauer, F. (1991). *Playing by the Rules: A Philosophical Examination of Rule-Based Decision-Making in Law and in Life* (Oxford: Clarendon Press).

Schelling, T.C. (1984). *Choice and Consequence* (Cambridge, MA: Harvard University Press).

Schieber, G.J., Poullier, J.P. and Greenwald, L.M. (1994). "Health System Performance in OECD Countries, 1980–1992," 13 *Health Aff.* (Fall) 101.

Schneider, C.E. (1996). The Practice of Autonomy: Patients, Doctors, and Medical Decisions (unpublished manuscript).

Schneider, C.E. (1994). "Bioethics with a Human Face," 69 *Ind. Law J.* 1075–1104.

Schneider, C.E. (1992). "Discretion and Rules: A Lawyers View," in *The Uses of Discretion*, ed. K. Hawkins (Oxford: Clarendon Press).

Schneiderman, L.J., Jecker, N.S. and Jonsen, A.R. (1990). "Medical Futility: Its Meaning and Ethical Implications," 112 *Ann. Intern. Med.* 949.

Schon, D. (1983). *The Reflective Practitioner: How Professionals Think in Action* (New York: Basic Books).

Schroeder, S.A. (1987). "Strategies for Reducing Medical Costs by Changing Physicians' Behavior," 3 *Int. J. Technol. Assess. Health Care* 39.

Schuck, P.H. (1994). "Rethinking Informed Consent," 103 *Yale Law J.* 899.

Schwartz, B. (1991). *Administrative Law* (3d ed., Boston: Little, Brown).

Schwartz, M.L. (1978). "The Professionalism and Accountability of Lawyers," 66 *Calif. Law Rev.* 669.

Schwartz, R. and Grubb, A. (1985). "Why Britain Can't Afford Informed Consent," 15 *Hastings Cent. Rep.* 19.

Schwartz, W.B. (1989). "We're Already Rationing Medical Care," *N.Y. Times*, October 16, at 21.

Schwartz, W.B. (1987). "The Inevitable Failure of Current Cost-Containment Strategies: Why They Can Provide Only Temporary Relief," 257 *JAMA* 220.

Schwartz, W.B. and Aaron, H. (1990). "The Achilles Heel of Health Care Rationing," *N.Y. Times*, July 9, at A15.

Scofield, G. (1991). "Is Consent Useful When Resuscitation Isn't," *Hastings Cent. Rep.* (November–December 1991) 28.

Scott, A.W. (1949). "The Fiduciary Principle," 37 *Cal. Law Rev.* 539.

Sealy, L.S. (1963). "Some Principles of Fiduciary Obligation," 1963 *Cambridge Law J.* 119.

Sealy, L.S. (1962). "Fiduciary Relationships," 1962 *Cambridge Law J.* 69.

Sehgal, A., Galbraith, A., Chesney, M., et al. (1992). "How Strictly Do Dialysis Patients Want Their Advance Directives Followed?," 267 *JAMA* 59.

Selby, J., Fireman, B., and Swain, B. (1996). "Effect of a Copayment on use of the Emergency Room in a Health Maintenance Organization." 334 *New Engl. J. Med.* 635–641.

Selker, H., Griffith, J., Dorey, F. and D'Agostino, R. (1987). "How Do Physicians Adapt When the Coronary Care Unit is Full?," 257 *JAMA* 1181.

Shapiro, M.H. (1994). "Regulation as Language: Communicating Values by Altering the Contingencies of Choice," 55 *U. Pitts. Law Rev.* 681.

Shapiro, M.H. (1988a). "Is Autonomy Broke?," 12 *Law Hum. Behav.* 353.

Shapiro, M.H. (1988b). "Introduction: Judicial Selection and the Design of Clumsy Institutions," 61 *S. Cal. Law Rev.* 1555.

Shapiro, M.H. (1987). "On Not Watering all the Flowers: Regulatory Theory and the Funding of Heart Transplantation," 28 *Jurimetrics* 21.

Shepherd, J.C. (1981). *The Law of Fiduciaries* (Toronto: Carswell).

Shultz, M. (1985). "From Informed Consent to Patient Choice: A New Protected Interest," 95 *Yale Law J.* 219.

Siegel, B.S. (1990). *Peace, Love & Healing* (New York: Harper Perennial).

Siegel, B.S. (1986). *Love, Medicine & Miracles* (New York: Harper & Row).

Silberman, C. (1991). "From the Patient's Bed," 13 *Health Management Q.* 12.

Siliciano, J. (1991). "Wealth Equity, and the Unitary Medical Malpractice Standard," 77 *Va. Law Rev.* 439.

Simon, W.H. (1982). "Legality, Bureaucracy, and Class in the Welfare System," 92 *Yale Law J.* 1198.

Singer, D., Carr, P., Mulley, A. and Thibault, G. (1983). "Rationing Intensive Care— Physician Responses to a Resource Shortage," 309 *New Engl. J. Med.* 1155.

Sislowitz, M. (1988). "Doctors' Faustian Deal," *N.Y. Times*, January 7, at 23.

Somers, H.M. and Somers, A.R. (1961). *Doctors, Patients and Health Insurance: The Organization and Financing of Medical Care* (Washington, DC: Brookings Institution).

Sorlie, P., Johnson, N., Backlund, E. and Bradham, D. (1994). "Mortality in the Uninsured Compared with the in Persons with Public and Private Health Insurance," 154 *Arch. Intern. Med.* 2408.

Special Project (1986). "Legal Rights and Issues Surrounding Conception, Pregnancy, and Birth," 39 *Vand. Law Rev.* 597.

Special Report (1987). "Guidelines for Coronary Angiography," 10 *J. Am. Coll. Cardio.* 935.

Spiro, H.M. (1986). *Doctors, Patients, and Placebos* (New Haven: Yale University Press).

Sprung, C.L. and Winick, B.J. (1989). "Informed Consent in Theory and Practice: Legal and Medical Perspectives on the Informed Consent Doctrine and a Proposed Reconceptualization," 17 *Crit. Care Med.* 1346.

Stacy, T. (1994). "Letter to the Editor," 331 *New Engl. J. Med.* 1158.

Stade, N.K. (1993). "Note, The Use of Quality-of-Life Measures to Ration Health Care: Reviving a Rejected Proposal," 93 *Colum. Law Rev.* 1985.

Starr, P. (1993). "The Framework of Health Care Reform," 329 *New Engl. J. Med.* 1666.

Steel, K., et al. (1981). "Iatrogenic Illness on a General Medical Service at a University Hospital," 304 *New Engl. J. Med.* 638.

Steinwald, O. and Sloan, F. (1981). "Regulatory Approaches to Hospital Cost Containment: A Synthesis of Empirical Research," in *A New Approach to the Economics of Health Care*, ed. M. Olsen (Washington, DC: American Enterprise Institute for Public Policy Research).

Stephens, G.G. (1989). "An Opposing View," 28 *J. Fam. Pract.* 698.

Stiglitz, J.E. (1987). "Principal and Agent," in *The New Palgrave: A Dictionary of Economics*, eds. J. Eatwell et al. (New York: Stockton Press).

Stone, A.A. (1985). "Law's Influence on Medicine and Medical Ethics," 312 *New Engl. J. Med.* 310.

Stone, D.A. (1979). "Physicians as Gatekeepers: Illness Certification as a Rationing Device," 27 *Public Policy* 227.

Strasser, M. (1988). "The New Paternalism," 2 *Bioethics* 103.

Strasser, M. (1986). "Mill and the Right to Remain Uniformed," 11 *J. Med. Philo.* 265.

Strauss, M., LoGerfo, J. and Yeltatzie, J., et. al. (1986). "Rationing Intensive Care Unit Services," 255 *JAMA* 1143.

Strull, W., Lo, B. and Charles, G. (1984). "Do Patients Want to Participate in Medical Decision Making?," 252 *JAMA* 2990.

Suchman, A.L. and Matthews, D.A. (1988). "What Makes the Doctor-Patient Relationship Therapeutic? Exploring the Connexional Dimension of Medical Care," 108 *Ann. Intern. Med.* 125–130.

Sullivan, R.J. (1989). *Immanuel Kant's Moral Theory* (Cambridge, England: Cambridge University Press).

Sulmasy, D.P. (1992). "Physicians, Cost Control, and Ethics," 116 *Ann. Intern. Med.* 920.

Summers, R. (1974). "Evaluating and Improving Legal Processes—A Plea for Process Values," 60 *Cornell Law Rev.* 1.

Sun, M. (1983). "Fishing for a Forum on Health Policy," 219 *Science* 37.

Sunstein, C.R. (1996). *Legal Reasoning and Political Conflict* (New York: Oxford University Press).

Sunstein, C.R. (1995a). "Incompletely Theorized Agreements," 108 *Harv. L. Rev.* 1732–1772.

Sunstein, C.R. (1995b). "Problems with Rules," 83 *Cal. L. Rev.* 953–1026.

Sunstein, C.R. (1986). "Legal Interference with Private Preferences," 53 *University Chi. Law Rev.* 1129.

The SUPPORT Principal Investigators (1995). "A Controlled Trial to Improve Care for Seriously Ill Hospitalized Patients: The Study to Understand Prognoses and Preferences for Outcomes and Risks of Treatment (SUPPORT)," 274 *JAMA* 1591–1598.

Symposium (1995a). "Moral and Conceptual Disputes About When Treatments are Medically Futile," 20 *J. Med. Philo.* 109–224.

Symposium (1995b). "Medical Futility," 25 *Seton Hall Law Rev.* 873.

Symposium (1990). "Grassroots Bioethics Revisited: Health Care Priorities and Community Values," 20 *Hastings Cent. Rep.* (September–October1990) 16–23.

Symposium (1989). "Contractual Freedom in Corporate Law," 89 *Colum. Law Rev.* 1395.

Symposium (1978). "In the Service of the State: The Psychiatrist as Double Agent," 8 *Hastings Cent. Rep.* (Special Suppl., April).

Tanenbaum, S. (1994). "Knowing and Acting in Medical Practice: The Epistemological Politics of Outcomes Research," 19 *J. Health Polit. Policy Law* 27.

Tanenbaum, S. (1993). "What Physicians Know," 329 *New Engl. J. Med.* 1268.

Taurek, J.M. (1977). "Should the Numbers Count?," 6 *Philo. Public Aff.* 293–316.

Terrion, H. (1993). "Informed Choice: Physicians' Duty to Disclose Nonreadily Available Alternatives," 43 *Case Western Reserve Law Rev.* 491–523.

Thomas, W.J. (1993). "The Oregon Medicaid Proposal: Ethical Paralysis, Tragic Democracy, and the Fate of a Utilitarian Health Care Program," 72 *Or. Law Rev.* 47.

Thompson, W.C. (1982). "Psychological Issues and Informed Consent," in *Making Health Care Decisions*, Vol. III (Washington, DC: President's Commission for the Study of Ethical Problems in Medicine and Biomedical and Behavioral Research).

Thurow, L. (1984). "Learning to Say 'No'," 311 *New Engl. J. Med.* 1569.

Tomlinson, T. and Brody, H. (1990). "Futility and the Ethics of Resuscitation," 264 *JAMA* 1276.

Toombs, S.K. (1992). *The Meaning of Illness, A Phenomenological Account of the Different Perspectives of Physician and Patient* (Boston: Kluwer Academic).

Toon, P.D. (1994). "Justice for Gatekeepers," 343 *Lancet* 585.

Toulmin, S. (1986). "Divided Loyalties and Ambiguous Relationships," 23 *Soc. Sci. Med.* 783.

Truog, R.D., Brett, A.S. and Frader, J. (1992). "The Problem With Futility," 326 *New Engl. J. Med.* 1560.

Turner, J.A., Deyo, R.A. and Loeser, J.D., et al. (1994). "The Importance of Placebo Effects in Pain Treatment and Research," 271 *JAMA* 1609–1614.

Turner, J.F., Mason, T., Anderson, D., et al. (1995). "Physicians' Ethical Responsibilities Under Co-Pay Insurance: Should Potential Fiscal Liability Become Part of Informed Consent?," 6 *J. Clin. Ethics* 68–72.

Tweed, V. (1994). "Medical Savings Accounts: Are They are Viable Option?," *Business Health*, October, at 40.

Twerski, A.D. and Cohen, N.B. (1992). "Comparing Medical Providers: A First Look at the New Era of Medical Statistics," 58 *Brooklyn Law Rev.* 5 (Symposium).

Twerski, A.D. and Cohen, N.B. (1988). "Informed Decision Making and the Law of Torts: The Myth of Justiciable Causation," 1988 *U. Ill. Law Rev.* 607.

Ubel, P. and Arnold, R (1995). "The Unbearable Rightness of Bedside Rationing." 155 *Arch. Intern. Med.* 1837–1842.

U.S. Congress, Office of Technology Assessment (1994). *Identifying Health Technologies That Work: Searching for Evidence* (Washington, DC).

U.S. Congress, Office of Technology Assessment (1993). *Benefit Design in Health Care Reform: Background Paper—Patient Cost Sharing* (Washington, DC).

U.S. Congress, Office of Technology Assessment (1992a). *Evaluation of the Oregon Medicaid Proposal* (Washington, DC).

U.S. Congress, Office of Technology Assessment (1992b). *Does Health Insurance Make a Difference?* (Washington, DC).

U.S. Congress, Office of Technology Assessment (1988). *The Quality of Medical Care Information for Consumers* (Washington, DC).

U.S. Dep't of Health and Human Servs. (1990). *Report to Congress: Incentive Arrangements Offered by Health Maintenance Organizations and Competitive Medical Plans to Physicians* (Washington, DC).

U.S. General Accounting Office (1993). *Medicaid: States Turn to Managed Care to Im-*

prove Access and Control Costs (Washington, DC: GAO/HRD), reprinted in *1993 Medicare & Medicaid Guide (CCH)* ¶ 41,392.

U.S. Government Accounting Office (1992). *Access to Health Insurance: State Efforts to Assist Small Businesses* (Washington, DC: GAO/HRD).

Veatch, R.M. (1993). "Why Justice Requires Multiple Insurance Plans," *Phi Kappa Phi J.* 22–31.

Veatch, R.M. (1991a). *The Patient-Physician Relation: The Patient as Partner*, Vol. II (Bloomington: Indiana University Press).

Veatch, R.M. (1991b). "Allocating Health Resources Ethically: New Roles for Administrators and Clinicians," 8 *Front. Health Serv. Mgt.* 3.

Veatch, R.M. (1990). "Physicians and Cost Containment: The Ethical Conflict," 30 *Jurimetrics J.* 461.

Veatch, R.M. (1986). "DRGs and the Ethical Reallocation of Resources," 16 *Hastings Cent. Rep.* (June 1986) 32–40.

Veatch, R.M. (1981). *A Theory of Medical Ethics* (New York, NY: Basic Books).

Veatch, R.M. and Spicer, C.M. (1992). "Medically Futile Care: The Role of the Physician in Setting Limits," 18 *Am. J. Law Med.* 15.

Ventres. W., Nichter, M., et al. (1993). "Limitation of Medical Care: An Ethnographic Analysis," 4 *J. Clin. Ethics* 134.

Vertinsky, I.B., et al. (1974). "Measuring Consumer Desire for Participation in Clinical Decision Making," 9 *Health Serv. Res.* 121.

Vladeck, B. (1981). "The Market vs. Regulation: The Case for Regulation," 59 *Milbank Q.* 209.

Waldo, D.R., et al. (1991). "Health Spending Through 2030: Three Scenarios," 10 *Health Aff.* (Winter) 231.

Wallace, L.M. (1986). "Informed Consent to Elective Surgery: The 'Therapeutic' Value?," 22 *Soc. Sci. Med.* 29.

Walsh, D.C. (1986). "Divided Loyalties in Medicine: The Ambivalence of Occupational Medical Practice," 23 *Soc. Sci. Med.* 789.

Walzer, M. (1983). *Spheres of Justice: A Defense of Pluralism and Equality* (New York, NY: Basic Books).

Weiner, J.P. (1986). "Assuring the Quality of Care in HMOs: Past Lessons, Present Challenges and Future Directions," 7 *Group Health Ass'n Am. J.* 10.

Weinstein, J.B. (1986). "Improving Expert Testimony," 20 *U. Rich. Law Rev.* 473.

Weisbard, A.J. (1986). "Informed Consent: The Law's Uneasy Compromise With Ethical Theory," 65 *Neb. Law Rev.* 749.

Welch, H.G. (1991). "Should the Health Care Forest be Selectively Thinned by Physicians or Clear Cut by Payers?," 115 *Ann. Int. Med.* 223.

Welch, H.G. (1984). "Antibiotic Resistance: A New Kind of Epidemic," 76 *Postgrad. Med.* No. 6, at 63.

Welch, W.P., et al. (1990). "Toward New Typologies for HMOs," 68 *Milbank Q.* 221.

Wennberg, J. and Gittelsohn, A. (1982). "Variations in Medical Care Among Small Areas," 246 *Sci. Am.* 120.

Wennberg, J. and Gittelsohn, A. (1973). "Small Area Variations in Health Care Delivery," 182 *Science* 1102.

Wertheimer, A. (1992). "Two Questions About Surrogacy and Exploitation," 21 *Philo. Public Aff.* 211.

Wertheimer, A. (1987). *Coercion* (Princeton: Princeton University Press).

Wessel, M.R. (1988). "Adversary Science and the Adversary Scientist: Threats to Responsible Dispute Resolution," 28 *Jurimetrics J.* 379.

Wessel, M.R. (1980). *Science and ConScience* (New York: Columbia University Press).

Wexler, D.B. and Winnick, B.J. (1991). *Essays in Therapeutic Jurisprudence* (Durham, NC: Carolina Academic Press).

Wikler, D. (1991). "What Has Bioethics to Offer Health Policy?," 69 *Milbank Q.* 233.

Wikler, D. (1988). "Ought the Young Make Health Care Decisions for Their Aged Selves?," 13 *J. Med. Philo.* 57.

Williams, A. (1992). "Cost-Effectiveness Analysis: Is it Ethical?," 18 *J. Med. Ethics* 7.

Williams, A. (1988). "Health Economics: The End of Clinical Freedom?," 297 *Br. Med. J.* 1183.

Williams, A. (1985). *Medical Ethics: Health Service Efficiency and Clinical Freedom* (Portfolio 2) (York, England: University of York, Center for Health Economics).

Williams, A. (1974). "'Need' as a Demand Concept (with Special Reference to Health)," in *Economic Policies and Social Goals*, ed. A.J. Culyer (New York: St. Martin's Press).

Wilson, J.Q. (1993). *The Moral Sense* (New York, NY: The Free Press).

Winslow, G.R. (1982). *Triage and Justice* (Berkeley: University of California Press).

Wolf, S.M. (1994). "Health Care Reform and the Future of Physician Ethics," 24 *Hastings Cent. Rep.* (March–April) 28.

Wolf, S.M. (1988). "Conflict Between Doctor and Patient," 16 *Law, Med. Health Care* 197.

Woolhandler, S. and Himmelstein, D.U. (1995). "Extreme Risk—The New Corporate Proposition for Physicians." 333 *New Engl. J. Med.* 1678–1683.

Wright, R.F. (1992). "Complexity and Distrust in Sentencing Guidelines," 25 *U.C. Davis Law Rev.* 617.

Wright, R.F. (1991). "Sentencers, Bureaucrats, and the Administrative Law Perspective on the Federal Sentencing Guidelines," 79 *Cal. Law Rev.* 1.

Yarborough, M.A. and Kramer, A.M. (1986). "The Physician and Resource Allocation," 2 *Clin. Geriatr. Med.* 465.

Youngner, S.J. (1990). "Futility in Context," 264 *JAMA* 1295.

Youngner, S.J. (1988). "Who Defines Futility?," 260 *JAMA* 2094.

Zaner, R.M. (1991). "The Phenomenon of Trust and the Patient-Physician Relationship," in *Ethics, Trust, and the Professions: Philosophical and Cultural Aspects*, eds. E.D. Pellegrino, R.M. Veatch and J.P. Langan (Washington, DC: Georgetown University Press).

Zawacki, B. (1985). "ICU Physician's Ethical Role in Distributing Scarce Resources," 13 *Crit. Care Med.* 57–60.

Index

Aaron, Henry, 85, 120
adversarialism. *See* physician-patient
  relationship
After Virtue, 130
agency. *See* physician agency
Agency for Health Care Policy and
  Research, 74, 86
AHCPR. *See* Agency for Health Care
  Policy and Research
alternative medicine, 24, 41–42, 67, 213
AMA. *See* American Medical Association
American Arbitration Association, 184
American Association of Retired People, 66
American Medical Association, 22, 74, 85
  code of medical ethics, 127
  and guidelines on physician discretion, 91
Anderson, Gerard, 74
Annas, George, 215
Appelbaum, Paul, 221
Arato v. Avedon, 208
Association of American Physicians and
  Surgeons, 132
autopaternalism, 151

Bailey, Mary Ann, 10
bare bones laws. *See* state law

Beauchamp, Tom, 223
bioethics, 127–129, 211. *See also*
  medical ethics; physician, ethics
  history of 128
  and physician training, 129
Blue Cross/Blue Shield, 65
Bluestein, Jan, 86
Bobbit, Philip, 95
Bodenheimer, Thomas, 45
British National Health Service, 141, 208
Brody, Howard, 103, 198, 206, 215
Brook, Robert, 85–86
Brougham, Lord, 133
Brown, Larry, 66
Bush Administration, 116

Calabresi, Guido, 95
California Public Employees Retirement
  System, 54
Callahan, Daniel, 92
Canterbury v. Spence, 209
cardiopulmonary resuscitation, 125–6, 216
case management, 102. *See also* managed
  care
catastrophic coverage. *See* insurance,
  catastrophic coverage

295